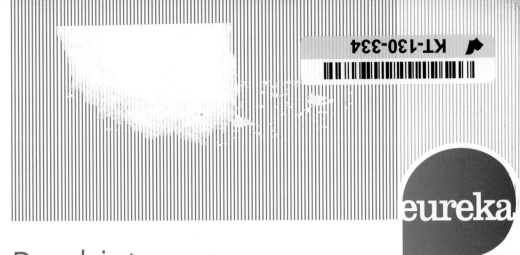

eureka

Psychiatry

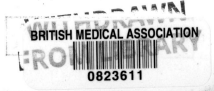

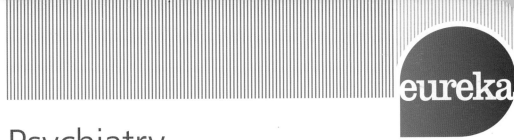

Psychiatry

Clare Fenton MBChB BSc MSc
MRCPsych
Specialty Registrar in Child and
Adolescent Psychiatry
Tees, Esk and Wear Valleys NHS
Foundation Trust
Northallerton, UK

Keri-Michèle Lodge MBChB BSc
MA MSc MRCPsych
Specialty Trainee in Psychiatry of
Intellectual Disability
Tees, Esk and Wear Valleys NHS
Foundation Trust
York, UK

Janine Henderson MRCPsych
MClinEd
MB BS Programme Director
Hull York Medical School
York, UK

Series Editors

Janine Henderson MRCPsych
MClinEd
MB BS Programme Director
Hull York Medical School
York, UK

David Oliveira PhD FRCP
Professor of Renal Medicine
St George's, University of London
London, UK

Stephen Parker BSc MS DipMedEd
FRCS
Consultant Breast and General
Paediatric Surgeon
St Mary's Hospital
Newport, UK

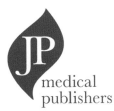

JP
medical
publishers

London • Philadelphia • New Delhi • Panama City

© 2016 JP Medical Ltd.

Published by JP Medical Ltd, 83 Victoria Street, London, SW1H 0HW, UK

Tel: +44 (0)20 3170 8910   Fax: +44 (0)20 3008 6180

Email: info@jpmedpub.com   Web: www.jpmedpub.com, www.eurekamedicine.com

ISBN: 978-1-909836-31-0

British Library Cataloguing in Publication Data
A catalogue record for this book is available from the British Library

Library of Congress Cataloging in Publication Data
A catalog record for this book is available from the Library of Congress

Publisher:	Richard Furn
Development Editors:	Thomas Fletcher, Paul Mayhew, Alison Whitehouse
Editorial Assistants:	Sophie Woolven, Katie Pattullo
Copy Editor:	Carrie Walker
Graphic narratives:	James Pollitt
Cover design:	Forbes Design
Page design:	Designers Collective

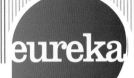

Series Editors' Foreword

Today's medical students need to know a great deal to be effective as tomorrow's doctors. This knowledge includes core science and clinical skills, from understanding biochemical pathways to communicating with patients. Modern medical school curricula integrate this teaching, thereby emphasising how learning in one area can support and reinforce another. At the same time students must acquire sound clinical reasoning skills, working with complex information to understand each individual's unique medical problems.

The *Eureka* series is designed to cover all aspects of today's medical curricula and reinforce this integrated approach. Each book can be used from first year through to qualification. Core biomedical principles are introduced but given relevant clinical context: the authors have always asked themselves, 'why does the aspiring clinician need to know this'?

Each clinical title in the series is grounded in the relevant core science, which is introduced at the start of each book. Each core science title integrates and emphasises clinical relevance throughout. Medical and surgical approaches are included to provide a complete and integrated view of the patient management options available to the clinician. Clinical insights highlight key facts and principles drawn from medical practice. Cases featuring unique graphic narratives are presented with clear explanations that show how experienced clinicians think, enabling students to develop their own clinical reasoning and decision making. Clinical SBAs help with exam revision while Starter questions are a unique learning tool designed to stimulate interest in the subject.

Having biomedical principles and clinical applications together in one book will make their connections more explicit and easier to remember. Alongside repeated exposure to patients and practice of clinical and communication skills, we hope *Eureka* will equip medical students for a lifetime of successful clinical practice.

Janine Henderson, David Oliveira, Stephen Parker

About the Series Editors

Janine Henderson is the MB BS undergraduate Programme Director at Hull York Medical School (HYMS). After medical school at the University of Oxford and clinical training in psychiatry, she combined her work as a Consultant Psychiatrist with postgraduate teaching roles, moving to the new Hull York Medical School in 2004. She has a particular interest in modern educational methods, curriculum design and clinical reasoning.

David Oliveira is Professor of Renal Medicine at St George's, University of London (SGUL), where he served as the MBBS Course Director between 2007 and 2013. Having trained at Cambridge University and the Westminster Hospital he obtained a PhD in cellular immunology and worked as a renal physician before being appointed as Foundation Chair of Renal Medicine at SGUL.

Stephen Parker is a Consultant Breast and General Paediatric Surgeon at St Mary's Hospital, Isle of Wight. He trained at St George's, University of London, and after service in the Royal Navy was appointed as Consultant Surgeon at University Hospital Coventry. He has a particular interest in e-learning and the use of multimedia platforms in medical education.

About the Authors

Clare Fenton is a Specialty Registrar in Child and Adolescent Psychiatry. She has been involved in clinical teaching throughout her career and recently published an interactive training module with the Royal College of Psychiatry. She recently completed a masters degree focusing on risk assessment in suicide.

Keri-Michèle Lodge is a Specialty Trainee in the Psychiatry of Intellectual Disability. She has been involved in designing and delivering teaching to medical students throughout her career and has written for the *Student BMJ*. She pursued her interest in education by completing an Academic Clinical Fellowship. Her recent research has focused on autism spectrum disorder.

Preface

All doctors, regardless of specialty, encounter patients with mental illness. Yet to the uninitiated, psychiatry can seem daunting. There are new terms to learn to describe symptoms which are difficult to understand. There are often no clear diagnostic tests and it is challenging to be faced with patients who may not think they are unwell, who may not trust you and may even be frightened of you; all this while you are asking them questions about personal and distressing issues.

Eureka Psychiatry demystifies the subject by providing clear, evidence-based explanations of mental disorders, their investigation and management. The first two chapters are dedicated to the anatomy and physiology underlying psychiatric pathology, and the clinical principles and skills required to diagnose and manage psychiatric patients. The following chapters describe the important psychiatric disorders and include clinical cases which provide insight into how psychiatrists diagnose patients. Later chapters cover psychiatric emergencies and the integration of psychiatric care. Finally, a chapter of exam-style SBAs helps you revise effectively.

Throughout the book, innovative graphic narratives help you develop personal observation skills to use when handling difficult clinical scenarios. Boxes give guidance on communication skills while artworks help to clarify key concepts.

Eureka Psychiatry has everything you need to become capable and confident in managing psychiatric patients and to succeed in your exams. We very much hope you will enjoy reading it.

Clare Fenton, Keri-Michèle Lodge, Janine Henderson
January 2016

Contents

Series Editors' Foreword	v
About the Series Editors	vi
About the Authors	vi
Preface	vii
Glossary	xi
Acknowledgements	xii

Chapter 1 First principles

Introduction	1
Overview of psychiatry	2
Theoretical basis of psychiatry	8
Ethical and legal issues in psychiatry	28
Classification of psychiatric disease	33
Global mental health	36

Chapter 2 Clinical essentials

Introduction	43
How to take a history	44
Psychiatric examination	53
Investigations	72
Management options	74

Chapter 3 Affective (mood) disorders

Introduction	97
Case 1 Low mood	98
Case 2 Overactivity	102
Depressive disorders	105
Bipolar affective disorder	115
Persistent mood disorders	121

Chapter 4 Schizophrenia and psychotic illness

Introduction	123
Case 3 Auditory hallucinations	124
Case 4 Self-neglect	127
Schizophrenia	128
Other psychotic disorders	138

Chapter 5 Anxiety disorders

Introduction	143
Case 5 Persistent pervasive symptoms of anxiety	144
Generalised anxiety disorder	147
Panic disorder	150
Phobias	151
Obsessive compulsive disorder	154
Acute stress reaction and post-traumatic stress disorder	157

Chapter 6 Suicide and self-harm

Introduction	161
Case 6 A serious overdose	162
Case 7 Repeated self-harm	164
Self-harm	166
Suicide	172

Chapter 7 Personality disorders

Introduction	177
Case 8 Emotional instability and relationship difficulties	178
Personality disorders	180

Chapter 8 Substance misuse and addictions

Introduction	185
Case 9 Excessive alcohol consumption	186
Case 10 Heroin use	189
Alcohol dependence	192
Drugs and psychoactive substances	197
Drug-induced psychiatric disorders	201

Chapter 9 Eating disorders

Introduction	203
Case 11 Rapid weight loss	204
Anorexia nervosa	206
Bulimia nervosa	210

Chapter 10 Perinatal psychiatry

Introduction	213
Case 12 Low mood 6 weeks after delivery	214
Postnatal blues	217
Postnatal depression	218
Postnatal psychosis	220

Chapter 11 Physical and psychological co-morbidity

Introduction	223
Case 13 Chronic neck pain	224
Somatisation and medically unexplained symptoms	226
Conversion disorders	228
Delirium	229
Psychiatric illness secondary to physical illness	231
Organic personality change	233
Sleep disorders	235
Psychosexual disorders	238

Chapter 12 Dementia and old-age psychiatry

Introduction	243
Case 14 Increasing forgetfulness	244
Dementia	247
Alzheimer's disease	248
Vascular dementia	250
Other dementias	251
Mental illness in the elderly	255

Chapter 13 Child and adolescent psychiatry

Introduction	259
Case 15 Disruptive behaviour in a 5-year-old	260
Developmental disorders	262
Behavioural disorders	265
Emotional disorders	269

Chapter 14 Psychiatry of intellectual disability

Introduction	271
Case 16 Angry outbursts at work	272
Intellectual disability	275
Mental illness in the context of intellectual disability	278

Chapter 15 Psychiatric emergencies

Introduction	281
Case 17 Refusal to be admitted to hospital	281
Case 18 Acute psychotic symptoms	284
Case 19 Acute confusion	286
Case 20 Suicidal behaviour	287
Case 21 Agitated and violent patient	289
Case 22 Acute alcohol withdrawal	290
Case 23 Fever, muscle stiffness and tremor	293

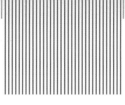

Chapter 16 Integrated care

Introduction   297
Case 24 Chronic psychosis and weight
    gain   300
Management of mild and moderate
    depression   302
Physical health problems in the chronically
    mentally unwell   304
Depression in the chronically physically
    unwell   305

Screening for postnatal depression   307
Alcohol dependence   308
Community care of dementia   309

Chapter 17 Self-assessment

SBA questions   313
SBA answers   325

Index   **333**

Glossary

5-HT	5- hydroxytryptamine (serotonin)	MAOI	monoamine oxidase inhibitor
AA	Alcoholics Anonymous	MMR	measles, mumps and rubella
ADHD	attention deficit hyperactivity disorder	MMSE	Mini Mental State Examination
ASD	autism spectrum disorder	MRI	magnetic resonance imaging
BMI	body mass index	MSE	mental state examination
BPS	biopsychosocial	NaSSA	noradrenergic and specific serotonergic antidepressant
CBT	cognitive behavioural therapy	OCD	obsessive compulsive disorder
CJD	Creutzfeld–Jakob disease	PHQ-9	Patient Health Questionnaire-9
CNS	central nervous system	REM	rapid eye movement
CT	computed tomography	SNRI	serotonin and noradrenaline reuptake inhibitor
DSM	Diagnostic and Statistical Manual of Mental Disorders	SPECT	single photon emission computed tomography
ECG	electrocardiography	SSRI	selective serotonin reuptake inhibitor
ECT	electroconvulsive therapy	TCA	tricyclic antidepressant
GABA	γ-aminobutyric acid	WHO	World Health Organization
GAD	generalised anxiety disorder		
GP	general practitioner		
ICD	International Classification of Diseases		

Acknowledgements

Thanks to the following medical students for their help reviewing chapters: Jessica Dunlop, Aliza Imam, Roxanne McVittie, Daniel Roberts and Joseph Suich.

Figures 8.4, 12.3, and 12.4a, b are reproduced from Collins D et al, *Eureka Neurology & Neurosurgery*. London: JP Medical, 2016.

We would like to thank John Gossa for his work preparing graphic narratives for this book.

CF, KL, JH

I would like to thank Ella and Nathaniel for their entertaining distractions and Elise for occasionally allowing me a full night's sleep while writing. Thanks to my husband for his invaluable support and motivation.

CF

I am grateful to my family for their patience and encouragement during the writing of *Eureka Psychiatry*. I thank Peter, Juliet, Chris and especially David for providing the inspiration and, most of all, I thank Lorna and Neve for their motivation.

KL

Chapter 1
First principles

Introduction. 1
Overview of psychiatry 2
Theoretical basis of psychiatry 8
Ethical and legal issues
in psychiatry. 28
Classification of psychiatric
disease 33
Global mental health. 36

Introduction

Psychiatry focuses on the prevention, diagnosis and treatment of mental health disorders.

Mental health disorders are common, often chronic conditions. To treat them to best effect, a thorough understanding of the patient's psychological and social experiences is required, with additional attention to the patient's physical condition. Despite mental health disorders being distinguished from physical conditions, they often appear as part of or in conjunction with them. Conditions that first appear to be psychiatric disorders are occasionally found to have a physical cause and vice versa.

Historically, mentally ill people were cared for by lay people and the clergy because their problems were considered to be spiritual rather than medical in origin. Psychiatry as a discipline increasingly established its medical identity from the early 1800s. Subsequent progress in neurosciences, genetics, social sciences and psychoanalytic theory in the 20th century established psychiatry as a medical specialty in its own right.

Over the centuries, there have been huge changes in the public perception of mentally ill individuals and in the treatment approaches used. However, negative views regarding the origins of mental illness persist in many societies. The stigma – sense of disgrace – attached to mental disorders further undermines a patient's well-being and increases their social isolation.

Overview of psychiatry

Starter questions

Answers to the following questions are on page 40.

1. Why is stigma more of a problem for psychiatric patients?
2. Why is psychiatry often considered unscientific and subjective?
3. Why do psychiatric patients have a shorter life expectancy?

Mental health

The World Health Organization (WHO) defines health as 'A state of complete physical, mental and social well-being, and not merely the absence of disease.' However, mental health is a state of mental well-being that is not defined simply by the absence of disease. It is a state in which each individual is able to work productively, achieve their own potential and cope effectively with the usual stresses of life. Mental health underpins the ability to experience emotions, engage effectively with others and enjoy life.

Each individual experiences a wide range of emotions in everyday life in response to ordinary events. In addition, many social, physical and psychological factors impact upon feelings and emotions:

- Social factors include life events, poor education, stressful working environments, discrimination, domestic violence and poverty
- Physical factors include physical ill-health, genetic factors, drugs and medications
- Psychological factors include a person's personality, cognitive style and response to traumatic events

The boundary between mental health and mental ill-health is hard to define as it is based on the observation of complex emotions and responses.

Prevention of mental health disorders

The prevention of mental health disorders and the promotion of mental well-being are the focus of a considerable number of research projects and public health campaigns. Mental health promotion focuses on improving living conditions and encouraging the adoption of healthy lifestyles. Strategies include:

- Early childhood interventions, e.g. preschool psychosocial activities for disadvantaged populations, child and youth development programmes and mental health promotion in schools
- Increasing access to education for women in disadvantaged circumstances
- Social support for elderly people
- Reducing poverty
- Violence prevention programmes

Psychiatry as a specialty

Psychiatry as a medical specialty 'feels' different from other branches of medicine. Students often feel unskilled and unprepared for working with mental health patients. Despite the advances that have been made, public perceptions and the stigma relating to mental health disorders still impact upon the practice of this specialty.

Students and psychiatry

Psychiatry can seem daunting because of the specific vocabulary that is used, the very detailed approach to patient assessment and the apparently complicated decision-making processes involved. A fear of psychiatric patients and mental health settings is compounded by misleading media portrayals. Inexperienced students are fearful of upsetting patients by saying the wrong thing.

You can take a number of approaches to overcome barriers to learning:

- Engage with the terminology used in psychiatry at an early stage (see Chapter 2).
- Become familiar with the signs and symptoms elicited in the mental state examination. This is just the psychiatrist's version of a physical examination. A careful observation and description of the patient's presentation is the first step in making a diagnosis
- Liaise closely with the nursing staff in mental health teams. They can help identify patients who will be able to work well with you. See as many patients as you can
- Ask questions. Decisions made by

psychiatrists and mental health teams depend not only on a sound knowledge of psychiatry, but also on a detailed knowledge of each individual patient and their circumstances. This can make decisions look subjective as they differ between patients, but the mental health teams will be able to explain the reasoning behind their decisions

- Be curious and interested. Patients have stories to tell and many will appreciate the opportunity to discuss these with you

Stigma and psychiatry

Stigma is a significant problem for individuals with mental illness. The stigma and discrimination that affect those with mental health conditions are experienced in many ways (**Table 1.1**).

Isolation

Historically, the stigma associated with mental health disorders has been exacerbated by the confinement of patients behind closed walls in asylums. Patients were set aside from

Stigma in mental health	
Area of impact	**Examples**
Expression of prejudicial attitudes	Wide range of attitudes including lack of understanding, blaming individuals for their mental illness and hostile, aggressive attitudes
Social activity	Exclusion from wide range of social activity, both deliberate and unintentional. Can result in severe social isolation
Violations of human rights	Lack of equality in access to care Inhumane treatment Degrading living circumstances Physical, psychological and sexual abuse as a consequence of vulnerability
Media portrayal	Negative projection of those with mental health in films and the media Inappropriate reporting of cases in the news relating to mental illness
Poor access to housing and employment	Discrimination in job applications Poor employment support
Poor funding for treatment	Funding not allocated to mental health services with the degree priority as for other specialties

Table 1.1 The impact of stigma in mental health

both ordinary life and other forms of health-care provision in general hospitals.

Internalising stigma

People with mental health problems internalise society's views, leading to shame, low self-esteem, withdrawal from others and poor social functioning. Modern psychiatric practice aims, wherever possible, to deliver care to patients in their own environment. This diminishes the boundary between physical and mental health problems, at the same time as reducing the stigma associated with the service as a whole.

Psychiatrists and stigma

Psychiatrists and other mental health workers experience stigma as a consequence of their profession. Psychiatrists have always occupied a slightly different role from other doctors due to their presence in legal proceedings and their role in the compulsory confinement of the severely mentally ill. As a result, psychiatrists may be feared and mistrusted in a way that other doctors are not.

Culture and psychiatry

Most psychiatric disorders present in all cultures, but the features displayed within them vary in different cultural settings. To understand the presentation of any illness you must be sensitive to the culture of the patient in which it arises.

Cultural beliefs

Different beliefs influence the nature of patient's symptoms, such as delusions, or their behaviour when distressed. What may appear to be a delusion in one culture may be a culturally accepted belief in another. This raises questions about the nature of psychiatry and psychiatric illness: one society may accept something as being within the bounds of normal behaviour, when in another culture it would be considered mental illness requiring treatment.

Ishaar is a 42-year-old Somali refugee. He fled his country during the civil war after his village was invaded by militia who raped and tortured his female relatives and killed his brother. He is visiting his general practitioner (GP) with persistent headaches.

Through the Somali interpreter, Ishaar describes terrible headaches, difficulty sleeping and poor appetite. He is preoccupied by guilty thoughts about the family members who are still in Somalia and blames himself for not having been able to prevent the violence that he witnessed. He believes the headaches are a punishment for this, caused by the curse of an evil spirit that is taking away his energy. He weeps while he is explaining this.

The Somali interpreter explains that many Somalis do not recognise mental illness and seeking help for a mental health disorder is often seen as shameful. In Somali society, it is common to interpret physical symptoms as a consequence of spiritual interference. He explains that Ishaar wants treatment for his headaches and is working with religious elders to help him cope with his distress.

The GP recognises that Ishaar is depressed and that his beliefs are part of his cultural background rather than delusions or psychotic symptoms. He works closely with the interpreter to explain how he is going to help Ishaar with his symptoms using medication and counselling.

Migrant populations

Specific groups, for example refugees and asylum seekers, often have a higher prevalence of disorders such as post-traumatic stress disorder as a consequence of experiencing or witnessing acts of war and violence. Their assessment requires a specific consideration of:

- Language and communication, using skilled interpreters

- Cultural differences, considering beliefs that affect the patient's presentation, e.g. in some cultures it is normal to believe that spiritual forces can impact upon bodily function
- How culture affects the patient's understanding of mental illness and willingness to accept treatment and access care
- The impact of the illness on the patient's social environment, employment and integration into the community

History of psychiatry

Evidence of primitive attempts to treat mental disorders date back to at least 5000 BC. Attitudes have ranged from supportive approaches offering sanctuary and support in asylums to physically abusive treatments aimed at casting out demons (**Figure 1.1**).

In the Roman era, mentally ill people were treated with physical treatments such as cold baths and purges, and medications such as opiates to induce sleep. By Saxon times, beating to exorcise the devils responsible for the illness was the standard approach.

Early hospitals for the mentally ill appeared in medieval times. However, many of these hospitals were associated with the mistreatment of their mentally ill patients and appalling standards of care. Many mentally ill individuals were taken under the care of the clergy, who tried to rid them of their 'religious madness' – any extreme belief in the existence of supernatural intervention in human affairs.

The asylum era

By the 17th century, abnormal beliefs that had previously been considered to be evidence of possession by the devil became a matter of illness. Doctors began to replace the clergy in caring for the 'insane', giving rise to the medical model of mental illness.

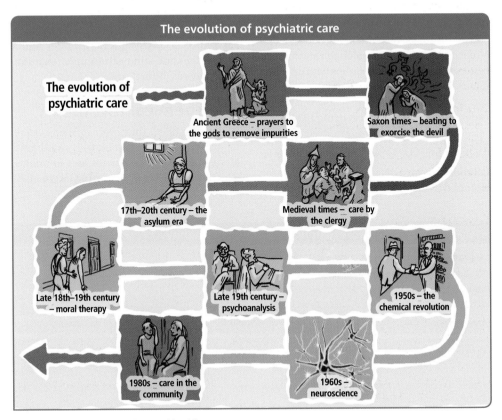

The evolution of psychiatric care

The evolution of psychiatric care

Ancient Greece – prayers to the gods to remove impurities

Saxon times – beating to exorcise the devil

17th–20th century – the asylum era

Medieval times – care by the clergy

Late 18th–19th century – moral therapy

Late 19th century – psychoanalysis

1950s – the chemical revolution

1980s – care in the community

1960s – neuroscience

Figure 1.1 The evolution of mental health care.

Asylums took over medical care, and many sufferers lived in them for many years. The asylums varied enormously from tiny, caring homely institutions to those where cruelty and corruption were rife. One notorious asylum was the Bethlam Hospital in London (known as Bedlam), where members of the public paid to view the mentally ill patients who were restrained in chains in their cells.

Little effective treatment was available, although numerous physical approaches to treatment arose in this era, many of which were dangerous (**Table 1.2**).

Moral therapy

A new movement of humane asylums, started by the Quaker religious movement, appeared in the UK in the late 18th century. These provided 'moral therapy' and rehabilitation of the patient into everyday life, avoiding all forms of punishment and restraint.

Madness became seen as a disorder of mind and body that required medical attention and treatment. Psychiatrists began to classify disorders, discriminating between different presentations, considering contributory factors and identifying disorders with different outcomes. This paved the way for the use of psychoanalysis and new psychoactive medications for specific disorders in the 1950s.

The rise of psychoanalysis

Psychoanalysis arose from the work of Sigmund Freud. A group of psychological theories and associated treatment techniques gained popularity in the early 20th century. Central to the original psychoanalytical approach were the following beliefs:

■ Behaviour, emotions and psychiatric disorder have their roots in underlying psychological processes
■ An individual's development is determined by events in childhood that have often been forgotten but continue to influence their attitudes and behaviour
■ Defence mechanisms, which protect the mind from difficult thoughts and ideas, are employed in situations that arouse anxiety
■ Human behaviour is affected by irrational but unconscious ideas and drives
■ Conflicts between conscious thoughts and unconscious thoughts give rise to psychological disturbance and emotional disturbances such as anxiety or depression

Although some of Freud's theories have been rejected, psychoanalytic thinking continues to have a significant impact on modern psychiatry. Most psychiatrists apply a biological approach to psychiatric disorder and a psychodynamic approach to understanding their patients' difficulties.

The chemical revolution

Prior to the 1950s, there were no medications to target specific psychiatric conditions. Medications such as opiates and bromides, which were generally sedating, were used

Historical treatment of insanity		
Application	Method	Aim
Water immersion therapy (17th century)	Patient fully immersed in freezing water until unconscious and could drown	'Kill the mad idea' by near-death immersion
Indoor water cures (18th century)	Cold shower rooms, bath boxes, dunking devices and chairs in which patients were restrained for hours	Keep the patient upright and immersed, so that less blood could travel to the brain in order to sedate the patient and reduce psychosis
Gyrating chair	Patient strapped into a chair and rotated at speed	Shake up the blood and tissues to restore equilibrium
Physical restraint, bloodletting, purging and induced vomiting	Varied, e.g. annual bloodletting	Tame the 'wild beast' that madness represented

Table 1.2 Historical approaches to the treatment of insanity

for everything. In the 1950s the introduction of lithium, followed by antidepressant and antipsychotic medications, brought about a major change in the treatment of inpatient populations. For some patients, successful treatment meant they were able to leave institutional care for the first time in many years and continue their treatment in the community (**Figure 1.2**).

The many medications now available to treat mental health conditions are known as psychotropic drugs. Their use has grown so much that they are now the leading class of medication sold in the USA, with antidepressants being the most frequently prescribed. There is a risk that the increased availability of these medications can result in overprescription and an overreliance on medication instead of counselling and psychotherapies for milder mental illness.

Neuroscience and psychiatry

Modern neuroscience began to develop more rapidly in the 1960s. Information about neurotransmitters and neurobiological changes has offered explanations for disorders such as Alzheimer's disease and has lead to advances in treatments for depression and psychotic disorders. As a result, there is no longer a clear discrimination between neurological and psychiatric ('functional') disorders (see page 8).

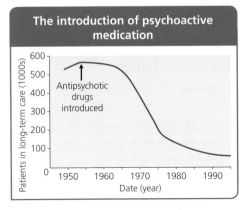

The introduction of psychoactive medication

Figure 1.2 The number of patients in long-term care before and after the introduction of psychoactive medication.

Community care

In the 1980s and 1990s, the delivery of psychiatric care changed from being based in large hospitals to being provided predominantly through community mental health services. Many psychiatric hospitals were closed, and most patients who had lived for years in long-stay hospitals were rehabilitated into the community.

Although some hospital beds remain for patients who are too unwell to be treated in the community, most services have been reconfigured to deliver care in the patient's home. New services include:

- **Crisis intervention services**, which provide rapid-response care for patients with acute illness
- **Early intervention services**, providing psychiatric input for patients with newly diagnosed psychotic illness
- **Home treatment teams**, to provide ongoing input for patients with mental disorders
- **Rehabilitation teams**, which focus on re-integrating patients into their social setting after significant illness
- **Assertive outreach teams**, providing care for patients who are limited in their engagement with mental health services

Collaboration with primary care

The physical health of patients with psychiatric disorder is often poor, with much higher rates of cardiovascular disease than in the general population. Smoking, a poor diet and a lack of exercise contribute to the latter. On average, patients with severe chronic mental health disorders die more than 15 years earlier than those without. In addition, more individuals with mental illness die by suicide.

Physical health must be regularly assessed in this population. A close collaboration between the mental health and primary care teams ensures that physical health conditions are monitored and treated.

Theoretical basis of psychiatry

Starter questions

Answers to the following questions are on page 40.

4. Why has the distinction between mind and body become less clear?
5. How do we know which neurotransmitters are implicated in different psychiatric disorders?

Modern psychiatry is founded on principles derived from the biological, psychological and social sciences.

Early classification systems which separated mental disorders into those caused by physical or anatomical changes in the nervous system and 'functional' disorders lacking a physical basis no longer hold. Twentieth century research demonstrated the genetic, biochemical and endocrinological dysfunctions underlying many 'functional' disorders. Accordingly the boundary between neurology and psychiatry is eroding. However, there are significant obstacles to elucidating the processes that underpin both healthy mental functioning and dysfunction:

■ The complexity of the human brain, which contains many different cell types (neurones) and relies on the healthy functioning of a vast array of chemicals responsible for the transmission of information between cells (neurotransmitters)
■ The disparities between humans and other species in brain functioning, which makes it difficult to develop animal models for research
■ The near impossibility of carrying out investigations in the live human brain
■ The lack of biochemical markers to confirm the diagnosis of particular conditions
■ The neuroplasticity of brain cells (see page 21). The connections between the cells are continually changing in response to environmental stimuli, developmental processes and experiences, medications, drugs and diseases

Neuroanatomy

The nervous system is made up of two main cell types: neurones and glial cells:

■ Neurones are the main functional cells in the brain. They process information and communicate with other cells via axons. These are projections from the cell body via which neurones communicate electrically and chemically (**Figure 1.3**)
■ Glial cells (glia) support the neurones by maintaining the cellular environment of the nervous system (**Table 1.3**). They make up about 80% of the cells in the nervous system

Anatomical divisions: the central and peripheral nervous systems

Anatomically, the nervous system has two main functional divisions (**Figures 1.4** and **1.5**):

■ The central nervous system (CNS), which comprises all the cells within the brain, brainstem and spinal cord
■ The peripheral nervous system, which comprises all the cells and nerves outside

A neurone

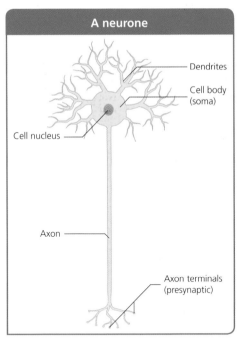

Dendrites

Cell body (soma)

Cell nucleus

Axon

Axon terminals (presynaptic)

Figure 1.3 The structure of a typical neurone.

the brain, brainstem and spinal cord. It includes the spinal and cranial nerves, sympathetic and parasympathetic nerves and nerves that supply the gut (enteric nervous system)

Functional divisions: somatic and autonomic

Functionally, the nervous system is divided into two types: somatic and autonomic. These link all the central and peripheral neuronal activity to allow continual adaptive responses to internal and environmental changes:

- The somatic system is involved in controlling conscious and unconscious sensation and voluntary movement. It conveys information to the brain (the afferent or sensory input) and from the brain to the muscles (the efferent or motor output)

- The autonomic nervous system (**Figure 1.5**) is the part of the efferent system that is responsible for controlling the internal organs. It also regulates homeostasis – the maintenance of stable internal bodily conditions. The autonomic nervous system has two divisions:
  - The sympathetic nervous system, best known for the fight or flight response
  - The parasympathetic nervous system, which maintains internal bodily conditions in a steady state

Cells in the nervous system		
Cell	**Type**	**Function**
Neurones		Excitation and nerve impulse conduction communicating with each other via synapses
Neuroglial cells	Astrocytes	Supporting framework for neurones Maintain the blood–brain barrier Store and release some neurotransmitters Guide neurones in embryo Immunological roles (antigen presenting cells, secretion of cytokines mediating immune response in the CNS)
	Oligodendrocytes	Myelination of CNS neurons
	Ependymal cells	Facilitate CSF movement Form a barrier with astrocytes between ventricles and CSF, and the brain Line central canal of spinal cord
	Microglial cells	Macrophages in brain
	Schwann cells	Myelination of peripheral nerves

Table 1.3 Types of cells in the nervous system. CSF, cerebrospinal fluid; CNS, central nervous system

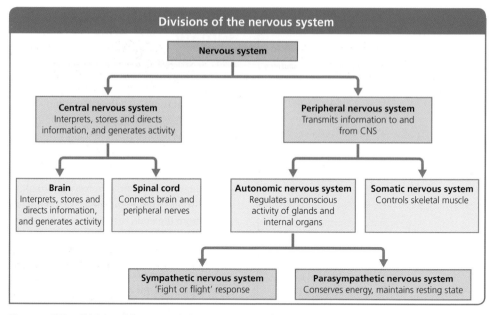

Figure 1.4 The divisions of the nervous system. CNS, central nervous system.

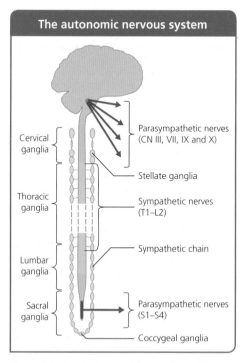

Figure 1.5 The divisions and innervations of the autonomic nervous system. CN, cranial nerve.

The emotion of fear arises in response to a real or perceived threat. It is accompanied by physical sensations including rapid breathing, an increased heart rate, increased muscle tone, sweating, 'butterflies in the stomach' and increased alertness. This is the fight or flight response, mediated by the sympathetic nervous system. It prepares the body to run away or stay and fight.

The central nervous system

The CNS is made up of the brain, brainstem and spinal cord (**Figures 1.6** and **1.7**).

The brain

The brain is composed of two cerebral hemispheres, each of which is made up of four major lobes. The cerebral hemispheres are responsible for the reception, processing and integration of information so that decisions and responses can be made.

The four main lobes have different functions (**Figure 1.8** and **Table 1.4**):

Divisions of the nervous system

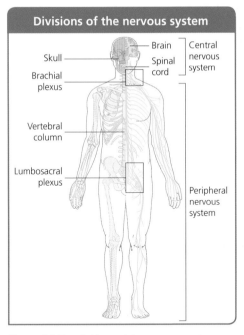

Figure 1.6 The divisions of the nervous system.

The central nervous system

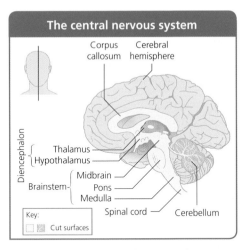

Figure 1.7 Gross anatomy of the central nervous system.

- Occipital lobe – interpretation of visual information
- Parietal lobe – sensory functioning
- Temporal lobe – language, learning, memory, interpretation of emotion, hearing, smell and taste
- Frontal lobe – motor function and thought processing

Lobes of the brain

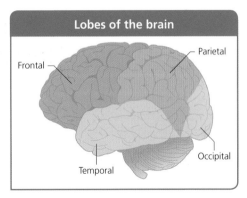

Figure 1.8 The lobes of the brain.

The frontal lobe controls many activities associated with personality. These include the ability to predict the consequences of current actions, the choice between good and bad actions and the suppression of socially unacceptable behaviours.

Pick's disease is a type of dementia that predominantly affects the frontal and temporal lobes. Patients initially exhibit marked personality and behavioural changes. As a result, it is often misdiagnosed in the early stages as other psychiatric disorders, for example depression.

Structural organisation of the cerebral hemispheres

The cerebral hemispheres are made up of grey matter and white matter.

The cortex, or grey matter, is the outer layer of the cerebral hemispheres consisting mainly of the cell bodies of neurones. These interconnect to form pathways from the cerebral cortex to the brainstem, spinal cord and nuclei (compact clusters of neurones) that lie deeper in the cerebral cortex. The cortex is the thinking, processing part of the brain.

The subcortical layer, or white matter, lies beneath the cortex. It contains the neuronal axons which have protein coatings called myelin sheaths. These form subcortical pathways connecting different areas of cortex and

Functional areas of the cortex and consequences of damage		
Area	Functions	Consequences of damage
Frontal lobe	Judgement Emotional responses Expressive language Word association Memory for habits Initiating activity	Disinhibition Poor judgement Lack of planning Impulsiveness Tactlessness Apathy Poor problem solving Socially inappropriate behaviour Emotional lability
Temporal lobe	Hearing Memory acquisition Some visual perception Categorisation of objects	Prosopagnosia (inability to recognise familiar faces) Selective attention deficit Identification of objects decreased Short-term memory loss Altered sexual interest Increase aggression
Parietal lobe	Visual attention Touch perception Goal-orientated voluntary movement Object manipulation Integrates senses to make sense of the world	Inability to name objects Agraphia (problems writing) Alexia (problems reading) Difficulty drawing objects Right/left confusion Dyscalculia (problems with maths) Apraxias (lack of awareness of own body parts and loss of skill such as dressing) Poor hand–eye coordination
Occipital lobe	Visual perception	Visual defects Colour agnosia Illusions/hallucinations Inability to recognise words Difficulty recognising drawn objects Difficulty reading and writing
Cerebellum	Coordination and control of movement and balance	Loss of fine movement Gait abnormalities Inability to reach and grasp Tremor Vertigo Slurred speech
Brain stem	Breathing Heart rate Sweating Blood pressure Digestion Thermoregulation Alertness Sleep Balance	Decreased vital capacity Dysphagia Dizziness Nausea Insomnia Poor balance

Table 1.4 Areas of the cerebral cortex, their function and consequences of damage to that area

linking the cortex to the rest of the CNS. The deep cortical nuclei lie within these subcortical pathways. These are three clusters of functionally related cells: the basal ganglia, the limbic system and the thalamus and hypothalamus.

Functional organisation of the cerebral hemispheres

The cortex is functionally organised into motor, sensory and association areas. It has key roles in memory, attention, cognition, perception, language and consciousness (**Table 1.4**).

The two hemispheres are connected via the corpus callosum, which is composed of neuronal axons.

> **In children who start to learn a musical instrument before the age of 6 years the corpus callosum is increased in volume.** This reflects the increased connectivity between the two sides of the brain supporting the improved coordination of the two hands involved in playing an instrument. This in turn further improves their future musical ability.

Lateralisation of function

The right and left hemispheres have different functions. Some activities such as motor control are bilateral but others are localised. For example, the left hemisphere is involved in the analysis of information and in speech. The right side of the brain is related to information synthesis, creativity and musicality.

Normal brain functioning requires all areas of the brain to be working in balance with each other. Particular changes in behaviour and functioning have been mapped to different areas of the brain (**Table 1.4**).

> **Frontal leucotomy (commonly known as lobotomy) involves severing fibres in the corpus callosum between the frontal lobes.** In the 1940s and 1950s, this was performed on severely disturbed patients with schizophrenia, anxiety and mania. Although it reduced the distressing symptoms, many patients experienced devastating changes including apathy, loss of initiative, decreased concentration and disinhibition.

The limbic system

The limbic system is a group of functionally linked areas that lie on the medial aspect of the temporal lobe (**Figures 1.9** and **1.10**). It has a number of roles of relevance to psychiatry including:

- Spatial memory and the acquisition of information
- Emotional reactions to external stimuli
- The interpretation of emotional reactions in others

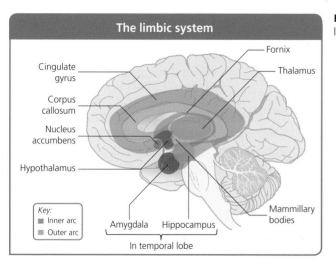

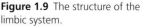

The limbic system

- Fornix
- Cingulate gyrus
- Thalamus
- Corpus callosum
- Nucleus accumbens
- Hypothalamus
- Mammillary bodies
- Amygdala   Hippocampus
- In temporal lobe

Key:
- Inner arc
- Outer arc

Figure 1.9 The structure of the limbic system.

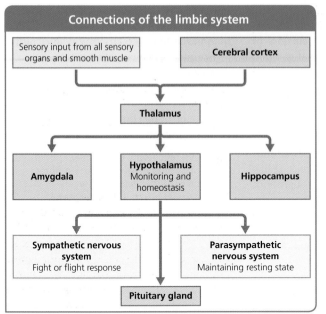

Figure 1.10 The functional connections of the limbic system.

- Complex motor control
- Pain perception
- Social interaction

The thalamus and hypothalamus

The thalamus and hypothalamus lie beneath the cortex. They integrate information from the cortex and maintain the body's internal homeostasis. The thalamus plays a role in consciousness by moderating the overall activity level in the brain. The hypothalamus controls automatic, unconscious behaviours.

The thalamus

The thalamus is made up of 12 nuclei, nine of which are organised into three groups (**Table 1.5**). The thalamus connects the cerebral cortex with the brainstem. It integrates and transmits information relating to sensation and movement in the control of:

- Memory formation
- Arousal
- Consciousness

Functions of the thalamic nuclei		
Group of nuclei	Function	Connection to
Anterior	Learning, memory and alertness	Limbic system
Medial nuclei	Emotion, cognition	Limbic system, frontal lobes
Lateral nuclei	Sensorimotor control	Sensorimotor cortex

Table 1.5 Functions of the thalamic nuclei

The hypothalamus

The hypothalamus lies on either side of the third ventricle. It is made up of 13 nuclei and receives input from the limbic system. It is connected to the pituitary gland via the infundibulum (**Figure 1.11**).

The hypothalamus is responsible for maintaining homeostatic equilibrium, being involved in:

- Pituitary endocrine function
- Efferent output to the autonomic system. It controls the autonomic nervous system

The hypothalamus

Sagittal section

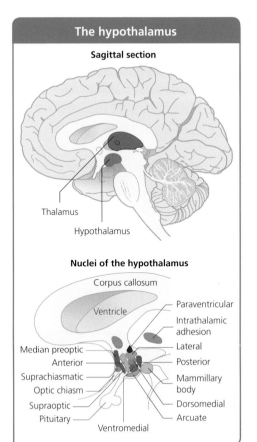

Nuclei of the hypothalamus

Figure 1.11 The hypothalamus.

Hypothalamic axes

Axis	Responses regulated
Hypothalamic–pituitary–adrenal axis (HPA)	Stress responses
Hypothalamic–pituitary–thyroid axis (HPT)	Metabolic rate
Hypothalamic–pituitary–gonadal/ovarian axis (HPG/HPO)	Reproduction

Table 1.6 Hypothalamic axes

Hypothalamic control is important in the maintenance of homeostasis, variations in mood and the stress response. The hypothalamic–pituitary–adrenal axis is a complex set of interactions between the hypothalamus, pituitary and adrenal glands, that controls levels of endogenous steroids and reactions to stress. This may be disturbed in conjunction with significant changes in mood, for example in depression.

> Certain endocrine disorders (Addison's, Cushing's, thyroid and parathyroid disease) precipitate mood disorders such as depression, highlighting the influence of hormones on mental state.

Physiology of stress

Stress has been implicated in the aetiology of many mental health disorders. Any event has the potential to cause an individual to feel stressed. A mild degree of stress is constructive as it prepares an individual to meet everyday challenges such as examinations. Greater degrees of stress are, however, experienced as unpleasant and become harmful. They diminish the individual's ability to perform adequately and may ultimately lead to physical or psychological dysfunction.

The hypothalamic–pituitary–adrenal axis plays a major role in preparing the individual to cope with stressful circumstances. The physiological and psychological responses to stress have three main stages: alarm, resistance or adaptation, and exhaustion (**Table 1.7** and **Figure 1.12**).

and coordinates the autonomic and endocrinological responses in the stress response.

■ Thermoregulation, feeding, thirst, control of the circadian rhythm and memory

Functionally, there are three main hypothalamic pathways that control endocrine function. These are referred to as hypothalamic axes (**Table 1.6**).

> **The hypothalamus can be damaged in thiamine deficiency.** This can occur in Korsakoff's syndrome as part of chronic alcoholism. In this disorder, patients have profound anterograde and retrograde amnesia and a tendency to confabulate (invent facts to fill memory gaps).

The stress response			
Phase	Description	Mechanism	Physiological/psychological consequences
Alarm phase ('Fight or flight' response)	Acute phase response Short-lived	Activation of the sympathetic nervous system mediated by catecholamines	Mobilisation of glucose stores Increase in heart and respiratory rates Increased energy consumption by all cells
Resistance/ adaptation phase	Long-term responses mounted to cope with prolonged stress	HPA activated, resulting in release of cortisol	Lipids released into blood Amino acids/proteins released from muscles Increase in blood glucose. Aldosterone released by adrenal cortex (retention of sodium and water, increased blood pressure) Immunosuppression
Exhaustion phase	Long-term responses no longer sustainable, body becomes unable to function	Prolonged activation and stimulation of HPA results in depletion of body resources and collapse	Prolonged elevated cortisol results in: Muscle breakdown Suppressed immune responses Psychological/psychiatric manifestations, e.g. depression/anxiety/psychosis Impaired insulin production

Table 1.7 Stages of the physiological response to stress. HPA, hypothalamic–pituitary–adrenal axis

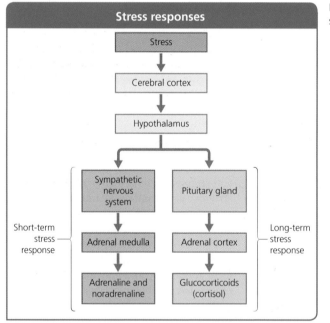

Figure 1.12 Short- and long-term stress responses.

The basal ganglia

The basal ganglia are a group of interconnected nuclei deep in the cerebral hemispheres made up of the:

- Caudate nucleus
- Putamen
- Globus pallidus

They are responsible for the coordination and control of movement. The main neurotransmitter in the basal ganglia is dopamine.

The subthalamic nuclei (below the thalamus) and substantia nigra (in the brainstem) work closely with the basal ganglia to control movement (**Figure 1.13**).

> **Parkinson's disease is a movement disorder caused by decreased dopaminergic transmission in the basal ganglia.** Similar symptoms often appear in patients taking antipsychotic medications, which work by blocking dopaminergic transmission throughout the brain.

Neurophysiology

Neurones communicate via action potentials, which are transient waves of electrical current. These underlie all coordinated mental activity, including emotions, feelings and actions. They are also the basis of the changes that occur in mental health disorders.

The action potential

An action potential is a transient alteration in electrical charge across the cell membrane caused by changing concentrations of sodium (Na^+) and potassium (K^+) ions. It starts at one end of the neurone and is conducted along the membrane to reach the synapses, which are the junctions to the connecting neurones.

Phases of an action potential

The membrane potential (**Figure 1.14**) has five phases:

1. A resting potential of –70 mV: a negative charge inside the cell which is described at this point as hyperpolarised.
2. Depolarisation. A stimulus from another neurone causes a rapid movement of Na^+ and K^+ in opposite directions across the neuronal membrane. Voltage-sensitive Na^+ channels open when depolarisation occurs. Na^+ rapidly enters the cell as its concentration is much higher outside the cell than inside, and there is a negative charge inside. The movement of Na^+ ions into the cells triggers the opening of further Na^+ channels until the net influx of Na^+ is greater than the net efflux of K^+.
3. Firing of the action potential. Once a threshold voltage has been crossed, all the Na^+ channels open. This increases further the inward surge of Na^+. This forms the spike of the action potential. The size and duration of the spike depend on the number of channels present and how long they are open for. A brief period of inactivation then follows as movement of the ions across the channel is blocked.

Figure 1.13 The structure of the basal ganglia.

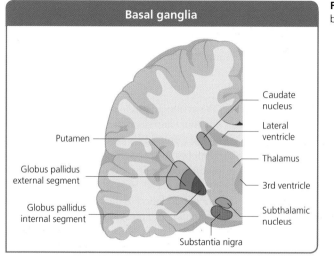

Basal ganglia

Putamen

Globus pallidus external segment

Globus pallidus internal segment

Substantia nigra

Caudate nucleus

Lateral ventricle

Thalamus

3rd ventricle

Subthalamic nucleus

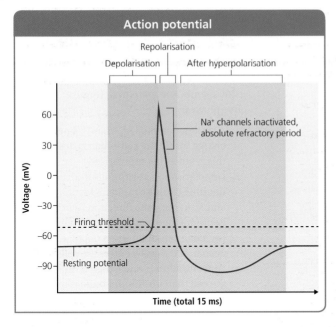

Figure 1.14 The action potential. Initial depolarisation (red) is slow until a threshold is reached that opens the fast Na⁺ channels. Repolarisation (orange) initially overshoots the resting membrane potential (blue).

4. Repolarisation. As the Na⁺ ion channels close, the cell begins to repolarise. Pumps in the membrane have to actively transport Na⁺ out of the cell against the concentration gradient and K⁺ re-enters the cell.
5. Refractory period. The Na⁺ channels are inactivated and the inward K⁺ current is at its strongest. No action potentials can be generated at this point. This phase prevents the neurone from rapid repeat firing and cell death due to cellular depletion.

The action potentials alter the ionic gradient in the next section of membrane, which triggers opening of the voltage-gated Na⁺ channels. This next section then depolarises so that the impulse travels along the neurone.

The synapse

The synapse is the microscopic space between two neurones that are the site of the cell-to-cell communication. The action potentials are transmitted across these gaps via the release of specific chemicals known as neurotransmitters into the synapses (**Figure 1.15**). The following steps take place:

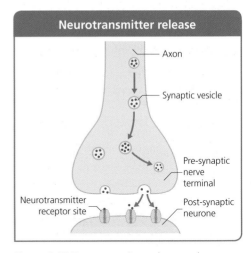

Figure 1.15 Neurotransmitter release at the synapse.

1. The action potential arrives at the nerve terminal and depolarises the presynaptic nerve terminal
2. Depolarisation opens Ca²⁺ channels in the presynaptic terminal, causing an influx of Ca²⁺ ions. This stimulates phosphorylation of the calcium-binding proteins in the presynaptic terminal and allows the presynaptic vesicles that contain

the neurotransmitter to bind with the presynaptic membrane

3. This results in the formation of a small channel through which the vesicles discharge their contents into the synaptic cleft

4. The neurotransmitter diffuses across the synaptic cleft and binds with a postsynaptic receptor. This causes a change in the postsynaptic membrane potential, which generates an action potential in the postsynaptic neurone

Psychiatric medications target different neurotransmitter systems. Blockade and activity at the various neuroreceptors is immediate. However, the therapeutic effect of each psychotropic medication usually takes some weeks to develop fully, i.e. there is a therapeutic delay. This suggests that processes following on from neuroreceptor blockade have to take place for therapeutic effect.

Neurotransmitters		
Size	Class	Neurotransmitters
Small	Acetylcholine (ACh)	Acetylcholine (ACh)
	Biogenic amines	Noradrenaline (NA)
		Adrenaline
		Dopamine (DA)
		Serotonin (5-HT)
		Histamine
	Amino acids	Glutamate (Glu)
		γ-amino butyric acid (GABA)
		Glycine (Gly)
Large	Neuropeptides	Substance P
		Enkephalins/endorphins
		Vasopressin
		Oxytocin
		Somatostatin
		Thyrotrophin-releasing hormone (TRH)

Table 1.8 Major classes of neurotransmitters

Neurotransmitters and receptors

There are more than 100 known neurotransmitters, which can be subdivided into two main types (**Table 1.8**):

- Small molecule neurotransmitters that mediate fast synaptic signalling
- Larger neuropeptides that mediate slower synaptic signalling. These are involved in ongoing background synaptic transmission, in which small amounts of transmitter are continually released without generating action potentials postsynaptically

The nervous system is able to communicate effectively and accurately as different neurotransmitters work specifically on their matching receptor sites to achieve different effects (**Table 1.9**). Changes in many different neurotransmitters have been implicated in psychiatric disorders.

Most neurones can release more than one neurotransmitter. The different neurotransmitters are contained in separate synaptic vesicles within the same nerve terminal. Lower frequency nerve stimulation causes the release of small vesicles alone. High-frequency stimulation causes the release of both small and large vesicles. The pattern of neurotransmitter release thus varies, leading to different effects.

Curare is an acetylcholine antagonist that binds to acetylcholine receptor sites at the neuromuscular junction. It prevents the transmission of impulses across the synapse and results in paralysis. It has been used for centuries by South American tribes as an arrow poison.

Neurotransmitter receptors

The receptors are proteins on the postsynaptic membranes that usually bind specifically to certain neurotransmitters (**Figure 1.16**). This binding results in activation of the post-synaptic neurones. The receptors can only return to an inactive resting state when the neurotransmitter is removed or inactivated. They are then ready to receive further neurotransmitters.

Major neurotransmitter functions			
Neurotransmitter	Location	Role	Clinical relevance
Acetylcholine	Neuromuscular junctions Autonomic nervous system Hippocampus and cerebral cortex	Activation of muscular contraction Learning and memory Sleep and arousal Aggression Thermoregulation Sexual behaviour	Death of cholinergic neurones implicated in Alzheimer's disease
Glutamate	Most excitatory neurones in the CNS, widely distributed throughout the brain	Memory Widespread cerebral excitation	Defective glutamate activity may be implicated in motor neurone disease, epilepsy and Alzheimer's disease
GABA (γ-amino butyric acid)	Most inhibitory neurones in the CNS use GABA or glycine, widely distributed throughout the brain	Active transmitter in one third of all synapses Inhibitory activity via Purkinje cells in cerebellum	Anxiolytics, anti-epileptics (e.g. valium) and alcohol work at GABA receptors
Glycine	Inhibitory, mainly in brain stem and spinal cord	Associated with brain stem nuclei involved in motor and somatosensory systems	Strychnine, a potent poison, blocks glycine receptors and causes convulsions
Dopamine (DA)	Mesolimbic, mesocortical and nigrostriatal pathways	Reinforcement of behaviour (reward systems), planning and movement	Degeneration of DA neurones in nigrostriatal pathways implicated in Parkinson's disease All antipsychotics work by blocking DA activity
Noradrenaline (NA)	Locus coeruleus	Sleep and wakefulness, attention and eating behaviours	Decreased NA implicated in depression and increased NA in mania
Serotonin (5-HT)	Raphe nuclei	Mood, emotional behaviour and sleep	Decreased 5-HT implicated in depression

Table 1.9 The function of major neurotransmitters and their clinical relevance

Neurotransmitters are inactivated by:

■ Detaching from the receptor and diffusing out of the synapse. They are then absorbed by the glial cells
■ Enzyme degradation, in which enzymes break the neurotransmitter down
■ Reuptake, in which the neurotransmitter is taken back up into the presynaptic neurone by transporters that pump it back

Each neurotransmitter has its own specific degradation pathways. Some synapses also have presynaptic autoreceptors that regulate the amount of neurotransmitter released by a process of negative feedback.

Downregulation is responsible for the phenomenon of tolerance and addiction, in which an individual requires increasing doses of a particular drug to achieve the same effect. When the opioid drug heroin is taken repeatedly, the number of receptors at the synapse gradually reduces. The desensitised neurones therefore require increased amounts of heroin to obtain the desired effect.

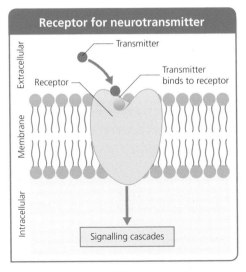

Figure 1.16 Receptors in the nervous system.

Downregulation and upregulation

When a synapse is very active, the receptors become less sensitive to the neurotransmitter in the short term, a process known as desensitisation of the neurone. In the longer term, the number of receptors for the neurotransmitter is decreased due to decreased expression of the genes encoding for them. This is downregulation of the receptors.

Receptors at synapses that are more rarely activated become extremely sensitive to their neurotransmitter. Ultimately, the number of receptors for that neurotransmitter increases. This is known as increased sensitivity and upregulation.

Synapses are relatively inaccessible to investigation in vivo. The effects of individual neurotransmitters can be inferred from an observation of the effects of specific chemicals and their impact upon psychological functioning (**Table 1.10**).

> **Depression may arise in individuals whose post-synaptic receptors have become hypersensitive to neurotransmitters due to a longer term depletion of the underlying neurotransmitter.** Antidepressants correct this by increasing the availability of the monoamine. This results in desensitisation of the receptors over a longer period, relieving the depression.

Neuroplasticity

There are more than 100 trillion synapses in the human brain. They are not rigid unchanging features but undergo frequent remodelling. This is referred to as neuroplasticity and occurs in response to:

- Developmental processes
- External stimuli including stressful experiences
- Hormones, drugs and medications
- Diseases

Neuroplasticity is necessary to encode memory. It facilitates learning and responses to sensory stimuli in the immature brain. It enables the creation of new connections between neurones and deletes old, defective connections.

> **Pathological neuroplasticity has been implicated in the development of some psychiatric disorders,** for example schizophrenia and post-traumatic stress disorder.

Neuroanatomical changes in psychiatric disorders

Neuroanatomical changes are increasingly being identified in specific psychiatric disorders (**Table 1.11**). Structural and cellular change can only be closely examined post mortem. However, functional scanning methods such as positron emission topography, single photon emission CT and functional MRI allow the functioning of different areas of the brain to be studied in individuals with and without psychiatric disorder. Some of these are outlined in **Table 1.11**.

Genetics and psychiatry

Human behaviour and emotion vary enormously from one person to another, and no psychological trait or psychiatric disorder can be explained fully by environment or by inheritance. Multiple genetic and environmental factors, including childhood experience and life events, contribute in different proportions in individual traits to determine a person's behaviour and personality.

Neurotransmitters and psychological symptoms

Psychological symptom	Implicated neurotransmitter	Evidence
Hallucinations and psychotic symptoms	Dopamine (DA)	Amphetamines increase DA release, causing visual and auditory hallucinations
		Dopamine antagonists effective in treating psychosis
		Clinical potency of these drugs correlated to dopamine binding efficacy
		L-DOPA used in Parkinson's disease can cause psychotic symptoms
	Serotonin	LSD (5-HT receptor agonist) causes psychotic symptoms
		Clozapine (antipsychotic for treatment-resistant schizophrenia) acts on dopaminergic and serotonergic receptors, and is more effective than any other antipsychotic
	Glutamate	NDMA antagonists ('party drugs') and ketamine induce psychosis and work on glutamate receptors
		Increased levels of glutamate receptors are found in brains of patients with schizophrenia
Depression and low mood	Noradrenaline and serotonin (monoamines)	Antidepressants increase monoamine levels by inhibiting breakdown or reuptake in the synaptic cleft
		Amphetamines and cocaine increase monoamine levels at synapse and elevate mood
		CSF levels of serotonin metabolites are decreased in depressed individuals
		Reserpine depletes monoamines and depresses mood
Addictive behaviours, pleasure and reward	Dopamine	Cocaine and amphetamine block dopamine reuptake when causing a 'high'
		Alcohol and opiates increase dopamine levels
		Dopamine in the nucleus accumbens mediates the pleasure sensation

Table 1.10 Neurotransmitters responsible for specific psychological symptoms; CSF, cerebrospinal fluid; DA, dopamine; L-DOPA, L-3,4-dihydroxyphenylalanine; LSD, lysergic acid diethylamide; 5-HT, 5-hydroxytryptamine; NDMA, N-nitrosodimethylamine

Neuroanatomical changes in psychiatric disorders

Disorder	Area affected	Noted changes
Schizophrenia	Enlarged lateral ventricles	Decreased neuronal size rather than reduction in numbers of neurones accounts for atrophy
	Atrophy particularly in frontal cortex, temporal lobes and thalamus	
Alzheimer's disease	Atrophy of cerebral cortex, widened sulci and enlarged ventricles, especially in the medial temporal lobes and hippocampus	Extensive loss of pyramidal neurones
		Amyloid plaques and neurofibrillary tangles (clumps of microtubules) in hippocampus and amygdala
		Loss of cholinergic neurones in limbic system
Depression	Prefrontal cortex (ventromedial and dorsolateral areas) and amygdala	Imbalance in activity between areas of the prefrontal cortex on PET scanning during episodes of depression*
Post-traumatic stress disorder	Limbic system (amygdala) and medial prefrontal cortex	Increased activity in amygdala*
		Decreased activity in medial prefrontal cortex*
Addictions	Hypothalamus, mesolimbic dopamine pathways	Increased activity in the pleasure and reward pathways*

* Changes identified via functional scanning techniques

Table 1.11 Neuroanatomical changes in psychiatric disorders

Behavioural and psychological traits that are at least in part inherited include:

- Aspects of personality including degree of sociability, conscientiousness and positivity
- Intelligence
- Artistic ability
- Tendency to addictive behaviours
- Social attitudes

Academic achievement is not only influenced by the genes that determine an individual's intelligence quotient. It is also affected by numerous genes that affect motivation, personality and confidence. Each of these traits is itself complex and influenced by numerous genes.

From epidemiological studies, increased susceptibility to various psychiatric disorders is known to be hereditary (see below). One of the mechanisms for variation in susceptibility may be genetically coded differences in individuals' physiological responsiveness. For example, there may be a variation in the response of the hypothalamic–pituitary–adrenal axis to stress (see page 15).

Studying the genetics of psychiatric disorders

Epidemiological studies

Different types of epidemiological study have helped to identify the contribution of genetics to psychiatric disorders. Family risk studies compare the rate of illness in an affected individual's family against the rate in the wider population. Two other types of study – twin and adoption studies – have provided further information (**Table 1.12**).

In twin studies, the rates of the disorder in identical and non-identical twins are compared. In adoption studies, the rates of illness in the adoptive and biological families are measured. These two types of study provide a kind of natural experiment, allowing the impact of both genes and environment to be considered (**Figure 1.17**).

Even in the 19th century, doctors were trying to establish whether individual patients' psychiatric disorders were hereditary: medical records show that doctors were aware of disorders that ran in families.

Cytogenetic and molecular genetic studies

Cytogenetics is the study of the structure and function of the chromosomes. In molecular genetics, the structure and function of the genes is studied at a molecular level. These types of study have helped characterised specific genes involved in schizophrenia (**Table 1.13**), and identified patterns of inheritance in other disorders.

Pharmacogenetics

This is the study of the inherited differences in drug metabolism that can influence an

Epidemiological studies in psychiatry	
Study design	Method
Family risk	Rates of illness determined in relatives of affected individuals and compared the general population
Twin	Comparison between concordance rates in monozygotic/dizygotic twins: higher rates between monozygotic twins suggest a genetic component
Adoption	Siblings brought up by unrelated adoptive parents studied to make comparisons between:
	Adopted person and biological parents with the disorder versus adopted person and biological person without the disorder (higher rate of disorder in the former indicates a genetic cause)
	Biological parents and adoptive parents of person with the disorder (higher rate of disorder in biological parents suggests genetic cause)

Table 1.12 Epidemiological studies that identify genetic contributions to psychiatric disorders

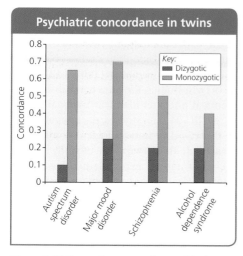

Psychiatric concordance in twins

Key:
■ Dizygotic
■ Monozygotic

Figure 1.17 Concordance rates for psychiatric disorders in monozygotic and dizygotic twins.

individual's responses to medications. For example, genetic coding produces variations in serotonin receptor sites so that people with some genetic subtypes show a poor response to antidepressant medication.

Pharmacogenetics is the study of the inherited differences in drug metabolism that can influence an individual's responses to medications. For example, genetic coding produces variations in serotonin receptor sites so that some genetic subtypes show a poor response to SSRI antidepressant medication.

Psychology

Psychology is the study of normal human behaviour. It helps in explaining and understanding the causes of psychiatric disorders such as anxiety disorders. In addition, it focuses on some of the factors that perpetuate disorders once they have begun (**Table 1.14**). Psychological knowledge is applied to the assessment of mental health disorders to understand the predisposing, precipitating and perpetuating factors that contribute to an individual's experience of mental health problems.

Psychology describes behaviour at both an individual and a societal level. It covers concepts including (**Figure 1.18**):

■ Perception – the organisation, identification and interpretation of sensory information
■ Cognition – thinking, understanding and learning
■ Attention – thinking about, listening to or watching something
■ Emotion – feelings such as sadness, fear, joy and hate
■ Intelligence – the ability to learn and understand things
■ Motivation – the desire to do things, the reasons for people's actions and desires
■ Personality – an individual's characteristic patterns of thinking, feeling and behaving

Genetic inheritance in psychiatric disorders		
Disorder	Epidemiological findings	Molecular genetics
Schizophrenia	Both parents affected = 40% lifetime risk One sibling/one parent/DZ twin affected = 10% lifetime risk 50% concordance rate in MZ twins	Individual genes: dysbindin, neuregulin and G72
Major depressive disorder	One sibling/one parent/parent affected = 15% lifetime risk 46% concordance in MZ twins	Polygenic
Bipolar disorder	One sibling/one parent/parent affected = 10% lifetime risk 79% concordance rate in MZ twins	Polygenic
Alcohol dependence	70% concordance in male MZ twins, 43% in female MZ twins 43% concordance in male DZ twins and 32% in female DZ twins	Unknown

Table 1.13 Genetic inheritance in psychiatric disorders. DZ, dizygotic; MZ, monozygotic

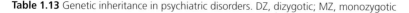

Psychological mechanisms			
Mechanism	Definition	Example	Pathological example
Classical conditioning	Learning by association	A neutral stimulus, like a dinner bell which predicts a meal, provokes a hunger response by inducing involuntary changes in the body as preparation for digestion	Development of anxiety symptoms in crowded places after an initial panic attack in that circumstance
Operant conditioning	Reinforcement of behaviour by its consequences	Positive reinforcement: praising a child for a musical performance will increase the amount the child performs	Care-giving behaviour from relatives re-enforcing the patient's illness behaviour that promoted it
Coping mechanisms	Attempts to cope with stressors	Adaptive: taking up activities to meet new people following a separation or bereavement. Maladaptive: avoiding social company because of shyness	Using drugs or alcohol to diminish symptoms of anxiety or depression

Table 1.14 Psychological mechanisms

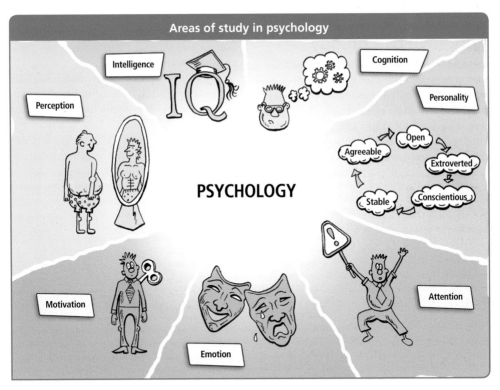

Figure 1.18 Key areas of study in psychology.

Biological psychology

Biological psychology is the study of the biological basis of behaviour and mental activity, including the localisation of specific functions within different regions of the brain. Animal models are often used to study the neural mechanisms underlying specific functions such as memory and learning.

Behavioural psychology

Behavioural psychology focuses on the behaviour of animals and humans, both individually and in societies. This has led to the identification of classical and operant conditioning as mechanisms of learning (**Table 1.14**).

> **Behavioural psychology has led to treatment involving behavioural modification that can be applied to psychiatry.** One example is response avoidance, in which patients with an anxiety disorder are encouraged to identify and discontinue behaviours that are perpetuating their disorder.

Cognitive psychology

Cognitive psychology focuses on the complex processes underlying all mental activity. Cognitive and behavioural psychology together have given rise to the field of cognitive behavioural therapy. This is used in psychiatry for numerous conditions including depression and anxiety.

Sociology

Sociology is the scientific study of social behaviour in terms of its origins, development and organisation. Humans are largely social animals, functioning in relationship to a larger society and influenced in their emotional life and behaviour by societal factors (**Table 1.15**).

Sociologists have played a leading role in identifying and highlighting social events and factors that affect people's mental health. For example, as early as 1897 Emile Durkheim studied variation in rates of suicide, concluding that social isolation contributed significantly to higher rates of suicide in some religious groups and in unmarried people.

Sociological studies have assisted in understanding why the incidence of schizophrenia, which varies between social groups, is higher in poor urban areas. They demonstrated that this is more likely to be a consequence of the social drift into poorer areas of those suffering from schizophrenia rather than these areas being an aetiological factor.

Psychiatric epidemiology and sociology are therefore closely linked. Studies of the impact of stressful life events have contributed to understanding the aetiology of psychiatric disorders. For example, research on the role of neurobiological processes triggered by stressful events has identified changes in cortisol levels and inflammatory responses implicated in the development of anxiety.

Sociological concepts			
Concept	Explanation	Consequence	Relevance in psychiatry
Sick role	The behaviour expected of and attributed to ill people	Confers freedom from onerous responsibilities and expectation of help from others	Exaggerated and reinforced by others and limits progress when the patient is no longer severely ill
Social role	The behaviour attributed to a person as a consequence of the various roles they adopt, e.g. as a parent, an employee/employer	Positive benefits in terms of confidence and status from accepted roles	Challenge to individual's ability to perform that role may further complicate a psychiatric illness
Illness behaviour	The behaviours attributed to a person in the sick role, e.g. seeking help, taking medication, giving up responsibility, consulting doctors	Ability to navigate the challenges of illness productively with help from others	Illness behaviour may be out of proportion to underlying illness, e.g. inability to work with minor ailments
Stigma	Negative and unfair beliefs that may be ascribed to a person by virtue of some characteristic, such as mental illness	Loss of equitable access to social, financial and employment opportunities Vulnerability to bullying and isolation	Reluctance to disclose illness, seek help or accept treatment
Life events	Positive or negative occurrences that have an impact on the health of an individual, e.g. pregnancy, bereavement, loss of a job	Impact upon an individual's ability to function	Significant life events are associated with onset and maintenance of many psychiatric illnesses, e.g. depression, anxiety disorder, psychosis
Social class	Status of an individual within society	Usually defined in terms of job/income	Prevalence of psychiatric disorder varies on the basis of social class, e.g. anorexia nervosa more common in higher social classes
Culture	Approach to life, habits, beliefs and behaviours shared by a group of people	Access to care may be compromised	Impacts upon the presentation of different illnesses and perceptions of illness from others
Social mobility	Change in role or status in society	Social mobility is associated with well-being, self-confidence and access to care	Some psychiatric disorders, e.g. schizophrenia, can lead to downward social mobility
Migration	People moving from one society to another	Social isolation, stigmatisation and loss of status	Implicated as a cause of psychiatric disorder with higher rates of serious mental disorder in migrant populations

Table 1.15 Sociological concepts

Ethical and legal issues in psychiatry

Starter questions

Answers to the following questions are on page 40.

6. Why do we need mental health law?
7. Why is assessment of capacity important?
8. Can people with mental illness take responsibility for their actions?

The ethical practice of psychiatry

Societal attitudes to mentally ill individuals have often shown limited consideration of the ethical elements of psychiatric care. The asylum era, which began in the 18th century in the UK, resulted in institutionalisation of people who were mentally unwell. Care was often poor, with harsh and brutal treatments. In the late 18th century, the first code of practice referring to care of the mentally ill appeared, stipulating that patients should be treated with kindness. This formed the basis for subsequent ethical codes relating to mental illness.

By the 1970s, the World Psychiatric Association had recognised the need for formal guidelines to underpin ethical practice in psychiatry, producing a predecessor of what is now known as the Declaration of Madrid. This outlines the profession's ethical commitments in areas such as informed consent, the right to be treated or to refuse treatment, conflicts of interest, confidentiality and the boundaries of mental illness.

Within psychiatry, particular difficulties are raised by:

- The power imbalance in the professional relationship between psychiatrists and patients. Psychiatrists have the power to institute treatment without the patient's consent, including admission to hospital against their will. This does not occur in any other branch of medicine

- The subjective nature of diagnostic criteria in psychiatry because many diagnoses are founded on clinical observation. This has led to inconsistencies in diagnosis and treatment
- Unclear boundaries between the psychiatric profession and the state. This can result in the sort of abuse that occurred in the Soviet Union with incarceration to suppress political or religious dissent under the false guise of mental illness

Attention-deficit hyperactivity disorder has been implemented differently as a diagnosis in different countries. This has resulted in huge disparities in the rate of prescription of stimulant medication to children. This has been questioned as an inappropriate medicalisation of behavioural variation.

Legal issues in psychiatry

Most patients with psychiatric disorders are able to collaborate with their physician to consider treatment options and give informed consent for treatment. This is called voluntary or informal treatment. For a minority of patients, however, the severity or nature of the illness makes them unable to take part in this process. In this situation, or if the illness presents a risk to the patient or others, treatment without patient consent is necessary. This is called involuntary treatment and usually takes place in an in-patient psychiatric unit.

Mental health legislation exists in most countries to ensure detention for treatment without consent occurs only when strict criteria have been met (see page 30). In addition legislation:

■ Ensures access to effective mental health care
■ Establishes effective mental health facilities and services
■ Develops policy to protect human rights
■ Integrates people with mental disorders into the community
■ Promotes acceptance of mental health issues in society

There is a distinction between law relating to mental capacity to make decisions for oneself, which applies to all patients, and law on detention for treatment, which applies only to patients with psychiatric disorders.

Mental capacity

Mental capacity is the legal term for adults' ability to make decisions for themselves. For a person to have capacity, they must be able to:

■ Understand the relevant information regarding the decision to be made
■ Retain that information for long enough to make a reasoned decision
■ Weigh up the information so that they can make and communicate their decision

Adults are assumed to be able to make a decision unless they have been deemed to be lacking in the capacity to do so. Judgements about capacity are decision-specific: a patient may have capacity for some decisions but not others, because different decisions require different levels of consideration. A patient can be profoundly mentally ill but still have capacity to make some treatment decisions.

Lack of capacity cannot be assumed simply because the patient wishes to make a decision that appears unwise to others. If the patient is deemed to have capacity, their decision must be respected.

In difficult circumstances, more than one clinician is called to assess a patient's competence. Sometimes a law court has to be involved. For example, in England and Wales this is the Court of Protection, under the Mental Capacity Act 2005, and in Scotland it is the Mental Welfare Commission, under the Adults with Incapacity (Scotland) Act 2000. Some countries, such as Northern Ireland, have not yet produced legislation on capacity and competence.

Deprivation of liberty safeguards

These exist to protect people who lack mental capacity. They aim to ensure that people with mental disorders who are in-patients or are living in care homes and supported living do not have their freedom inappropriately restricted. If someone has to be deprived of their liberty, for example preventing a patient with dementia leaving a care home unaccompanied, this must be done safely and only when there is no alternative and it is in the person's best interests. If the same patient was prevented from leaving their room within the care home or from receiving visitors, for example, it is likely that this would constitute an inappropriate deprivation of liberty.

Countries vary as to whether deprivation of liberty safeguards have been written into legislation. In England and Wales, for example, they exist as an amendment to the Mental Capacity Act 2005, whereas in Scotland legislation is in development at the time of writing.

Common law

A third of the world's population lives in countries where common law systems operate. Common law is developed by judges and courts rather than by legislation and therefore it varies between countries.

Under common law in the UK, for example, all adults have a right to refuse treatment even when the consequences of that refusal may be detrimental to them. For competent adults, this cannot be overruled. Conversely, treatment can be administered under common law against a patient's wishes and without their consent in specific circumstance. These include emergencies, situations when a failure to treat might endanger the patient or others, and when it cannot be clearly established that the patient is competent to make relevant decisions.

> **Sometimes it is impossible to assess capacity, for example in an unconscious patient who is presumed to have taken an overdose.** In these circumstances, emergency care is administered in the patient's best interests under common law.

Mental health legislation

All patients should be treated using the least restrictive option. If possible, they should be managed voluntarily and safely with intensive input in the community. However, mental health legislation has to be used when this is not feasible and treatment in hospital is required in the patient's interest or to protect the safety of others. The detail of mental health legislation varies from country to country. However, the principles are not country specific, and the Mental Health Act 2007 of England and Wales is described here to illustrate them.

The Mental Health Act 2007 (England and Wales)

This provides a legal framework for both informal and compulsory care and treatment of people with mental illness, learning disabilities and personality disorders. Commonly used sections relating to admission and detention are outlined in **Table 1.16**. It defines the responsibilities of all people

Mental Health Act 2007 sections relating to admission and detention				
Section	Maximum duration	Patient group	Purpose	Persons involved in recommending the section
2	28 days	Patients in the community Informal inpatients Inpatients under section 5(4) or 5(2)	Admission for fuller assessment than feasible in community and treatment if indicated	Two doctors (one must be Section 12 approved) plus one AMHP or the nearest relative
3	6 months (can be renewed)	Patients in the community Informal inpatients or following use of sections 2, 4, 5 in hospital	Admission for treatment: patient is suffering from a disorder that requires treatment in hospital for the health and/or safety of the patient, or for the protection of others	Two doctors (one of whom must be Section 12 approved), plus one AMHP Nearest relative must consent
4	72 hours	Patients in the community	Admission for emergency assessment when it is not possible to wait for Section 2 to be arranged	One doctor, and one AMHP or nearest relative
5(2)	72 hours	Informal patients in hospital	Emergency order to allow for Mental Health Act assessment to take place	One doctor (in charge of the patient's care)
5(4)	6 hours	Immediate prevention from patient leaving hospital	Detention to allow further assessment for detention by medical staff	Mental health nurse
136	72 hours	Removal to a place of safety	Allows patient with apparent mental illness to be taken to a place of safety (e.g. police station) to be assessed by a medical practitioner	Police officer

Table 1.16 Commonly used sections of the Mental Health Act 2007 (England and Wales) in relation to admission or detention for assessment and treatment. AMHP, approved mental health professional (see Table 1.17)

involved in a patient's care including those listed in **Table 1.17**.

As well as defining criteria for involuntary treatment, the Act states that for any patient being admitted under its provisions, the appropriate treatment must be available in the hospital to which they are being admitted.

> **Mental health law provides only for the compulsory treatment of a psychiatric disorder in a psychiatric hospital.** A patient cannot be detained in a general hospital setting to administer treatment they are refusing for a physical illness.

Definition of mental disorder

The Act defines a mental disorder as 'any disorder or disability of the mind'. This covers mental illness, personality disorder, organic mental disorders such as dementia, eating disorders, intellectual disability and autism spectrum disorders. Psychiatric conditions arising from the abuse of psychoactive substances are also included. However, drug or alcohol abuse in the absence of a psychiatric disorder is not sufficient to allow compulsory admission to hospital.

Discharge from hospital

The Act sets out conditions for the discharge of patients who have been detained for treatment under Section 3. It mandates that local health authorities must provide the patient with suit-able care to support their rehabilitation in the community and prevent further relapses of illness. For patients whose compliance with treatment is poor, this may include a supervised community treatment plan called a Community Treatment Order. This is a form of involuntary outpatient treatment (see below) and requires the patient to meet particular conditions, including return to hospital if they fail to do meet them.

Involuntary outpatient treatment

Since the advent of more effective medication and the closure of the asylums, more patients with psychiatric disorder have been treated as outpatients. Before the 1990s, involuntary treatment could only be administered in a hospital setting. Since then, many countries have introduced legislation that allows outpatient treatment to be provided without patients' consent. This has the advantages of:

- Being less restrictive to patients' liberty
- Reducing the number of admissions to Hospital
- Allowing patients to leave the hospital sooner than would otherwise be the case
- Being more compatible with patients' social inclusion

Involuntary outpatient treatment is, however, only considered when the risks to the patient and to others as a consequence of their mental illness are considered to be low.

Individuals involved in mental health law (England and Wales)	
Official title	**Role**
Section 12 Doctor	Doctor approved to make specific medical recommendations
Approved mental health professional (AMHP)	Mental health worker approved by local authority, e.g. social worker, psychologist, mental health nurse, occupational therapist
Approved clinician	Approved by local authorities to be the responsible clinician
Responsible clinician	Approved clinician with overall responsibility for patient's care, including renewing sections and discharging patient from section
Nearest relative	First relative in the Mental Health Act list
Mental health review tribunal	Panel including a doctor, lawyer and layperson
	who consider appeals against detention and can discharge patients into the community

Table 1.17 Individuals involved in application of mental health law in England and Wales under the Mental Health Act 2007

Advance directives

Advance directives have been in use in psychiatry since the 1980s, particularly for patients with recurrent severe mental illness. When they are well, patients can reach an agreement with their psychiatrist about the appropriate course of treatment if they become ill again. This is then used if they become too unwell to make decisions in their own best interest.

Advance directives may take the form of an explicit list of treatment options to be pursued or an instruction to consult a specific person to make decisions on behalf of the patient.

The term 'advance directives' is being replaced by 'advance decisions'. Advance decisions are legally binding statements that can only be made by persons over the age of 18 with the capacity to make the decision.

Confidentiality

Psychiatrists are bound by the same fundamental principle as other physicians – that they must keep confidential all matters disclosed to them by their patients. Confidentiality is particularly important in psychiatry as many patients make intimate and personal disclosures to their doctor. There are, however, occasions on which confidentiality cannot be maintained, when a patient:

- makes a threat to harm someone else
- insists upon driving when under the influence of alcohol or drugs
- presents a risk that they are unaware of but which may be harmful to others

More subtle conflicts arise when patients are currently extremely unwell and lacking insight. A patient may, for example, be suffering from a psychotic illness and have previously disappeared from the family home. In this case, it may be appropriate to notify the family, even against the patient's wishes, that they are now safe and being cared for in hospital.

Classification of psychiatric disease

Starter questions

Answers to the following questions are on page 41.

9. Why is classifying psychiatric disorders so complex?
10. Why is it necessary to have a classification system for psychiatric disorders?
11. Why are classification systems in psychiatry controversial?

The classification of any group of diseases is usually based on their aetiology.
Classification systems:

- Identify specific groups of signs and symptoms as disorders
- Help to distinguish one diagnosis from another, which allows for specific treatment approaches to be adopted
- Aid communication between health professionals
- Indicate a prognosis
- Are used to focus research on groups of patients with common presentations

The aetiology of many psychiatric disorders remains unclear even where many contributing factors have been identified. This makes it hard to define the boundaries of mental health and mental disorder. In addition, it makes the robust classification of psychiatric disorders difficult.

In medicine, the word 'disease' is used for entries in a classification system. As the pathophysiological basis of many psychiatric presentations remains unknown, the word 'disorder' tends to be used for psychiatric conditions.

The approaches to classification that have been adopted during the history of psychiatry have aimed to represent the differing groups of presenting symptoms.

Organic versus functional disease

In the 19th century, psychiatrists attempted to differentiate between 'organic' and 'functional' diseases. Organic disease was disease that could be shown to be related to pathological dysfunction of the nervous system, whereas functional disease had no identifiable pathological cause. These boundaries have become less clear as more subtle neurological dysfunctions have been demonstrated, for example neurotransmitter abnormalities.

Syndromes

A syndrome is a group of symptoms that consistently occur together or a condition characterised by a particular set of associated symptoms.

Syndromes are the basis of diagnosis in psychiatry and provide a clinical guide to treatment and prognosis.

Psychiatric diagnosis is dependent on detailed careful observation and a description of the patient's mental state. As there may be an overlap between different disorders within the classification of mental illness, a careful consideration of each sign and symptom is vital for appropriate diagnosis and treatment.

Early 19th-century attempts at classification in psychiatry focused on prominent symptoms such as hallucinations that appeared characteristically along with other less remarkable symptoms. From those early origins, modern psychiatry has developed classification systems that detail diagnostic criteria for each psychiatric disorder.

Classification systems

The two widely used classification systems in psychiatry are the International Classification of Disease (ICD) and the Diagnostic and Statistical Manual of Mental Disorders (DSM). Both systems describe explicit diagnostic criteria but there are minor descriptive differences between the two. Both are reviewed and updated periodically by a panel of experts. Each new edition is denoted by a number: for the ICD classification these are ordinary numbers and for the DSM they are roman numerals.

The DSM employs operational criteria to establish diagnostic validity and is used in both clinical and research work. The ICD focuses on clinical usefulness and diagnostic prototypes. It has two distinct versions, one for clinical practice and a separate version that is more restrictive in its detail and is used for research purposes. In general, the ICD is mainly used for clinical purposes and the DSM is preferred for research.

International Classification of Disease

The ICD is a list produced by the World Health Organization to outline an agreed and meaningful framework that can be used internationally as a common language for all physical and psychiatric disorders (**Table 1.18**). It is the most widely used system. This framework facilitates the comparison of data from different populations at any time and from the same population over time, allowing a wide comparison of international data.

Diagnostic and Statistical Manual of Mental Disorders

This is published by the American Psychiatric Association and is also widely used,

Categories in the ICD-10 classification	
ICD-10 category	Description
F0–F9	Organic disorders including delirium, dementia
F10–F19	Mental and behavioural disorder related to psychoactive substance misuse
F20–F29	Schizophrenia and related disorders
F30–F39	Affective disorders
F40–F49	Anxiety, stress-related disorders and somatoform disorder
F50–F59	Behavioural syndromes associated with physiological disturbances and physical factors
F60–F69	Personality disorders
F70–F79	Learning disabilities
F80–F89	Developmental disorders, e.g. autism spectrum disorder
F90–F98	Childhood emotional and behavioural disorders

Table 1.18 Main categories of mental disorder in the ICD-10 classification

particularly in the USA and Canada. It covers all psychiatric disorders in conjunction with the known causes of these disorders, demographic information and the evidence base for appropriate current treatment.

> **The inclusion of 'temper dysregulation disorder' in DSM-V has provoked widespread controversy.** Many are citing this as an example of the medical profession overmedicalising what would otherwise be recognised as a normal variation of behaviour in children – temper tantrums.

The DSM adopts a multiaxial approach to diagnosing mental illness, recognising the other factors in a patient's life that impact on their mental health (**Table 1.19**).

Limitations of classification systems

There are limitations with any classification system in which diagnoses are based upon groups of symptoms rather than pathological

Axes in the DSM		
Axis	Content	Explanation and examples
I	Clinical syndromes	Diagnosis, e.g. depression, schizophrenia
II	Developmental and personality disorders	Autism spectrum disorder and intellectual disability apparent from childhood
		Personality disorders impacting on an individual's interaction with the world
III	Physical conditions which contribute to development of or continue Axis I and II disorders	Brain injury
		HIV resulting in symptoms of mental illness
IV	Life events impacting on an individual's function	Bereavement
		Change or loss of employment
V	Patient's level of functioning	Current level of functioning is rated and compared to their best level in the last 12 months to assess impact

Table 1.19 Axes in the Diagnostic and Statistical Manual of Mental Disorders (DSM)

findings. Cultural factors may result in different diagnoses being made in different contexts. In addition, scientific research may produce findings that refute the nature of a diagnosis. Such classification systems can, however, provide a useful framework for understanding and communicating the nature of a patient's problems.

Internal hierarchy of diagnoses

There is also an internal hierarchy of diagnosis in psychiatry that ranks the five major categories of psychiatric disorder according to their severity. Patients often present with symptoms that fit into more than one category of disorder and, in treating any individual patient, disorders at the top of the hierarchy are considered before those lower down.

Organic disorders are ranked at the top of the pyramid (**Figure 1.19**). Therefore, organic disorder must be excluded and/or treated first. Psychotic symptoms with an organic cause, for example, will not respond fully to treatment if there is an underlying physical cause.

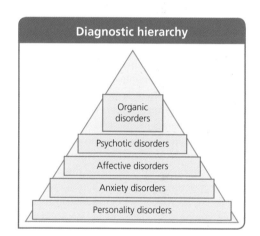

Figure 1.19 The diagnostic hierarchy of psychiatric disorders.

Delirium is an acute, transient condition that presents with confusion, agitation and often hallucinations. It is an organic condition with numerous physical causes including infection, endocrine abnormalities, drugs and alcohol. Treatment of the underlying cause should resolve all the symptoms.

Global mental health

Starter questions

Answers to the following questions are on page 41.

12. Why is global mental health increasingly being recognised as a major issue?
13. Why are global rates of mental illness higher in women than in men?
14. Why is so little money spent on mental health disorders internationally, compared to physical disorders?

Together, psychiatric and substance use disorders contribute to more than 10% to the global burden of disease, which is more than all cancers (8%). Four of the ten diseases with the highest global burden are psychiatric disorders: depression, schizophrenia, substance abuse and bipolar disorder.

Many affected people live in low-income countries where there is limited provision of treatment for these disorders. Around 75% have no access to mental health services (**Table 1.20**) both as a result of inadequate provision of service and remote, inaccessible living conditions. In these countries, innovations in the diagnosis and treatment of psychiatric illness are often neglected, the priorities being infectious diseases, famine, drought and war. Mental health disorders double in prevalence in the aftermath of natural disasters. In addition to the trauma experienced in these situations, access to mental health services is severely compromised.

Global variation in mental health disorders

The major psychiatric disorders, including schizophrenia, depression and dementia, occur in all cultures but there is some variation in their prevalence between different countries (**Tables 1.21**, **1.22**, and **Figure 1.20**). Around 25% of all people have a psychiatric diagnosis at some point in their lives. About 20% of all patients consulting in primary health care settings have a psychiatric disorder, many of which go unrecognised.

Globally, women have a 1.5–2.0 times greater risk of becoming mentally ill than men, partly as a consequence of social disadvantage and abuse.

Some disorders, for example eating disorders, are seen nearly entirely in developed cultures and are almost unheard of in low-income countries. Establishing the prevalence

Prevalence of mental health disorders		
Mental health disorder	Global prevalence	Proportion not receiving treatment
All mental health disorders	450 million	75%
Depression	350 million	90%
Schizophrenia	24 million	50%
Completed suicide	1 million per annum	N/A
Dementias	35.6 million (will double by 2030 and triple by 2050)	Huge variation between countries; global figures not available

Table 1.20 Global prevalence of mental health disorders

Comparative rate of suicides	
Suicide rate (annual no. of suicides per 100,000)	Country
High (>16)	Eastern Europe (Lithuania, Belarus, Kazakhstan, Hungary), Russia, Japan
Medium (5–16)	USA, Brazil, UK, Germany, Thailand
Low (<5)	Peru, Italy, Saudi Arabia, Egypt, Israel

Table 1.21 Suicide rate in different countries

Global variation in mental disorders		
Country	Global comparison	12 month prevalence (%)
USA, Ukraine	Highest	27
Colombia, New Zealand, Lebanon, France	Medium	20.4–18.9
Japan, China, Nigeria, Israel	Lowest	7.4–6.0

Table 1.22 Global variation in the prevalence of all mental disorders. Identified in national surveys using ICD/DSM criteria

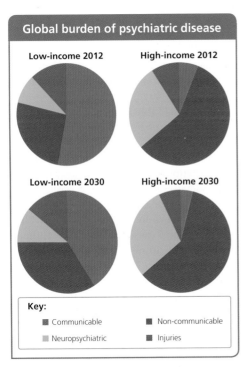

Global burden of psychiatric disease

Low-income 2012   High-income 2012

Low-income 2030   High-income 2030

Key:
■ Communicable   ■ Non-communicable
■ Neuropsychiatric   ■ Injuries

Figure 1.20 The contribution of psychiatric disorders to the global burden of disease in 2012 and the projected figures for 2030 (% of cases). (a) Low-income countries in 2012. (b) High-income countries in 2012. (c) Low-income countries in 2030. (d) High-income countries in 2030.

of individual mental disorders in different cultures is complicated by:

■ The lack of data from some areas, particularly in low-income countries

■ Variations in the methods used to collate the data
■ Variations in the approach to diagnosis
■ The cultural impact of mental disorder, resulting in different rates of presentation in different cultures

Depression

Depression is more common in high-income countries. It is now so commonly diagnosed in the USA that it is considered a 'luxury disorder' – one that is seen in more affluent societies. However, global estimates suggest that as few as one in 10 people receive adequate, effective treatment for their condition. This is due to variations in attitudes to depression and access to mental health care.

Schizophrenia

Schizophrenia affects around seven in every 1000 adults globally. It remains unclear whether it is more common in particular ethnic groups.

People with schizophrenia who are medically treated have a better prognosis in some lower income countries than in well-developed countries. This appears to result from a better reintegration into family life and better support after illness. However, more than 90% of untreated people with schizophrenia live in developing countries, and lack of early recognition and treatment for these people leads to chronic disabling illness.

Suicide

Suicide is one of the top 20 causes of death globally for all ages:

- Suicide rates have increased by 60% in the last 45 years
- Worldwide, suicide represents around 2% of the global burden of disease. This is equal to the burden caused by war and homicide, and twice the burden for diabetes
- Around 86% of the world's annual suicides occur in low- and middle-income countries
- In China and India, rates of suicide are equal in men and women. Otherwise suicide is more common in men, especially young men

Many people who commit suicide are mentally ill (**Table 1.23**). However, in some countries, such as Japan, it is socially acceptable to commit suicide, for example to avoid bringing shame on the family.

Dementia

The prevalence of dementia is rapidly increasing in line with the ageing population.

Lifetime risk of suicide	
Disorder	Lifetime suicide risk (%)
Mood disorders (mostly depression)	6–15
Alcohol dependence syndrome	7–15
Schizophrenia	4–10

Table 1.23 Lifetime risk of suicide by underlying disorder

It is now the leading cause of older people requiring care. This has a devastating effect on the families of the caregivers, emotionally, socially and financially.

The awareness of dementia is now increasing, and it is beginning to be included in the health agendas of many low- and middle income-countries. However, services will have to expand massively to cope with the disability produced by this disorder.

Global variation in access to mental health care

Almost half of the world's population lives in countries where there is fewer than one psychiatrist per 200,000 people (**Table 1.24**) Such shortages of skilled professional staff are one of the main barriers to accessing care in low-income countries. Access to treatment is highly correlated with a country's level of development (**Table 1.24**).

Some cultures believe that mental disorders are not treatable conditions, or that these conditions arise from possession from spirits. This sometimes leads to them being secluded from society, either cared for within their family structure or, in the worst cases, restrained unlawfully to contain them. They are thus denied access to their basic human rights, hidden from society and sometimes abused.

Many countries do not have an adequate legal system to protect the rights of patients with mental health disorders. This results in them being cared for in inadequate institutions in poor conditions.

Provision of mental health care		
Provision	High-income countries	Low-income countries
Number of psychiatrists per 100, 000 population	8.6	<0.5 (0.05 in Africa)
Spending per capita on mental health services	US$2	US$0.25
Provision of psychosocial interventions	Available at 60% of mental health services	Available at 14% of mental health services
Proportion of national health budget spent on mental health services	5.1%	0.5%
Covered by mental health legislation	92%	<35%

Table 1.24 Provision of mental health care

In addition, mental health is often not considered a public health priority in low-income countries, communicable diseases being the focus of health-care funding. Mental health services are often poorly organised and badly led.

Global mental health initiatives

Mental health disorders often start early in life, impairing learning and social functioning and increasing the chance of other physical health problems developing. Psychiatric disorder increases the risk of many communicable and non-communicable diseases, such as cardiovascular disease, endocrine disorders or infections, and vice versa, which is particularly relevant in low-income countries.

As a result, the impact of mental health disorders in terms of a patient's health, employment and relationships is considerable. In addition, there is a significant impact on the health-care systems, especially where disorders are poorly treated. This results in greater disability and a greater requirement for care.

The financial resource required to improve mental health care significantly is relatively modest, at US$2 per capita per annum. The majority of countries allocate less than 2% of their health budget to mental health (**Table 1.25**); doubling this to 4% would make a substantial impact.

Allocation of resources	
Area	Allocation of health budget on psychiatric/neuropsychiatric illness
Europe	>5%
South-east Asia	>50% of countries allocate <1%
Africa	>70% of countries allocate <1%

Table 1.25 Allocation of health care resources to mental health disorders

The WHO has instituted a Gap Action Programme to increase mental health services, especially in low- and middle-income countries. This aims to reduce the global burden of psychiatric disease so that people can live healthier lives and contribute to the further development of their own countries.

The aims of the programme include:

■ Improving access to mental health services
■ Offering treatment by suitably skilled health workers in appropriate settings
■ The reorganisation, delivery and evaluation of services
■ Greater access to government aid, including disability benefits, housing and work programmes to improve community life
■ Numerous initiatives, including the institution of mental health treatment guidelines and standards are underway

Answers to starter questions

1. Compared with other areas of medicine, psychiatry has always had great overlap with religion and popular culture, and psychiatric disorders have been stigmatised for centuries. Associations of mental illness with violence in films and literature play a strong role in creating stigma, and media reporting often exacerbates this by focusing on the negative aspects. The unique use of compulsory confinement of patients in psychiatry adds to this.

2. In psychiatry, diagnosis depends on a detailed psychiatric assessment; few disorders are identified by tests or investigations and the scientific basis of many disorders is not immediately evident. Decision making involves collaboration between doctor and patient, and does not necessarily adhere to detailed algorithms. Each individual requires a different approach, which can result in a perception of subjectivity.

3. Serious physical illness has a higher incidence and occurs at a younger age among psychiatric patients. Lifestyle factors such as smoking, alcohol and substance misuse, lack of exercise and obesity worsen the prognosis of these physical illnesses. Patients with comorbid physical and psychiatric illness are less likely to access screening programmes and comply with medication and treatment regimes. Suicide also contributes to the lower life expectancy, but to a lesser extent.

4. Early classification systems made a distinction between disorders known to be caused by physical/anatomical changes in the nervous system and those in which no physical basis could be demonstrated. This has become less meaningful with increasingly sophisticated research that has demonstrated genetic contributions, biochemical and endocrinological changes, and neurotransmitter changes underling many of these 'disorders of the mind'.

5. Observing the effects of different medications and illicit substances helps identify the neurotransmitters involved in different psychiatric disorders. For example, amphetamines cause both dopamine release and psychosis, and antipsychotic medications cause dopamine blockade, with the degree of blockade directly related to the antipsychotic efficacy of the drugs. This suggests that dopamine over-activity is the underlying neurotransmitter change in the aetiology of schizophrenia.

6. Mental Health Law is often thought to exist solely to allow the compulsory treatment of dangerous patients in hospital. However, it also ensures patients receive the treatment they require, legislates that care should always be available, and mandates the establishment of appropriate facilities for this. It protects patients' human rights and seeks to integrate them back into their community when this might otherwise be difficult.

7. Assessing capacity allows medical professionals to judge if an individual is capable of making decisions about different aspects of their treatment. All adults are assumed to be competent unless a judgement has been made to the contrary.

8. Many profoundly mentally ill patients still have the capacity to make certain decisions and be responsible for their actions. Judgements regarding capacity are specific; different decisions require different levels of consideration and understanding. So a patient may be unwell, but able to fully understand and agree to an aspect of their treatment, while being unable to understand that they are too unwell to look after themselves.

Answers *continued*

9. The simplest way to classify disorders on the basis of their aetiology, which is difficult in psychiatry where the aetiology of most disorders is not known. A lack of clear diagnostic tests and investigations, as well as huge variations in individual patient presentations, further complicate this. Classification in psychiatry relies upon indentifying groups of co-occurring symptoms.

10. Having a classification system allows specific treatments to be offered for each disorder. This becomes increasingly important as more specific treatments become available. It aids communication between professionals and allows doctors to advise patients more accurately regarding prognosis and treatment.

11. The classification of psychiatric disorders is periodically updated and societal changes are reflected in this. As knowledge increases, new conditions are included in classification systems which have previously been considered to be variants of normal behaviour, such as attention deficit hyperactivity disorder and temper dysregulation disorder. Critics are concerned about the over-medicalisation and potential over-treatment of behavioural variations.

12. Mental health disorders contribute to 14% of the global burden of disease, but the majority of countries allocate less than 2% of their health budget to mental health. As these disorders are often chronic, especially if untreated, their impact in terms of burden of care, loss of income and emotional distress is immense and is becoming increasingly recognised.

13. Women are twice as likely to develop mental health problems. Factors contributing to this include societal disadvantages, lack of employment, abuse and poor living conditions, which are more likely to affect women and can result in mental illness.

14. A lack of funding partly reflects the social position of psychiatry compared with physical disorders and the stigma that is still associated with mental disorders. Much psychiatric morbidity is hidden globally, and a lack of recognition has led to under-reporting and underestimation of the global burden of psychiatric disorders. The role of the media in driving awareness of physical conditions is also partly responsible for psychiatric disorders not being prioritised, with healthcare campaigns often focusing on physically evident disorders such as heart disease and cancer.

Chapter 2
Clinical essentials

Introduction 43
How to take a history 44
Psychiatric examination 53

Investigations 72
Management options 74

Introduction

Psychiatry is a unique medical specialty in which a broad knowledge of psychology and neuroscience is combined in diagnosis and management. A wide variety of psychiatric disorders present in every medical setting, from post-surgical acute confusional disorders to severe depressive disorder in patients with Parkinson's disease. Excellent communication skills lie at the heart of psychiatric practice, and more emphasis is placed on clinical assessment and observation than in any other branch of medicine.

Psychiatric assessment starts with a detailed history and mental state examination (MSE) in which all aspects of a patient's psychological and social functioning are explored. This may be supplemented by psychological assessments, investigations and imaging. Unique to psychiatry is the use of compulsory treatment for patients who are unwilling or unable to consent to necessary treatment. The legal framework for this is discussed in Chapter 1.

Psychiatric treatments include neuropsychopharmacology, psychotherapy and psychosocial interventions, which must be carefully integrated to meet the needs of each individual patient.

How to take a history

Starter questions

Answers to the following questions are on page 95.

1. How do you ask patients personal questions?
2. Why is the family history so important in psychiatric interviewing?
3. What is the difference between a psychiatric history and the mental state examination?
4. What are the three Ps and why are they important?

This section focuses on taking a careful and complete history to provide a detailed account on which a differential diagnosis can be based.

The elements of psychiatric history taking are:

- History of the presenting complaint
- Past psychiatric history
- Past medical history
- Family psychiatric history
- Personal history
- Significant relationships
- Social history
- Forensic history
- The patient's premorbid personality
- Collateral history

In psychiatry, a distinction between symptoms and signs would be artificial because they are inextricably linked. This chapter does not make this distinction.

> **Make your patient feel at ease as early as you can in the interview.** Ensure the environment makes them feel safe and allows them to discuss private information. However, do not forget your own safety: ensure you are able to call for help if needed.

Skills for successful history taking

Many students have concerns about interviewing patients in psychiatry (**Table 2.1**), most of which are unfounded and based on inaccurate media portrayals. However, safety must always be the first consideration in interviewing any patient (**Table 2.2**).

Environment

The first psychiatric interview is vital for both information gathering and establishing a strong therapeutic relationship. Psychiatric assessments take place in a wide variety of settings such as general hospital wards, emergency departments, police stations and patients' homes. Wherever possible, the interview should take place in a safe, private, comfortable room with no interruptions.

If possible, see the patient alone first to allow them to tell their story freely. However, bear in mind that having a close relative can help the patient to feel secure, especially if the patient is particularly anxious or distressed.

Communication skills

Good communication skills (**Table 2.3**) are of paramount importance. Patients are more likely to relax and describe their experiences fully if they are at ease and feel that the interviewer is listening to and understanding them. Non-verbal communication is particularly important: being distracted, hurried or tense is apparent to the patient.

> **Tailor your note taking to the content of the interview;** when the patient is discussing difficult, disturbing or distressing areas, avoid taking notes as it interferes with building rapport.

Student fears about psychiatric patients	
Student fear	Reality
'Psychiatric patients are dangerous; they might attack me'	Most are not violent. Patients who are violent are usually known to be so and students do not interview them alone
'Mentioning suicide is dangerous; it might put ideas into their head'	Mentioning suicide does not cause patients to harm themselves if they had not thought of it before
'I might make them worse by talking to them'	Most patients benefit from talking about their problems to someone who is interested and understanding
'I won't be able to communicate with them'	Patients usually respond well to a genuine, kind and compassionate approach; getting the questions exactly right is less important
'I won't know whether they are telling the truth or not'	Establishing good rapport and getting a detailed description of the problems is more important than knowing whether they are true
'I'll upset them if I ask all these personal questions'	Most questions can be carefully worded to avoid any upset; apologise and move on if the patient is distressed

Table 2.1 Student fears about psychiatric patients

Safety considerations for psychiatric interviews	
Safety factors	Appropriate considerations
Environmental	Choose a private but not isolated room where you can be seen
	Place the patient furthest away from the door with a clear path for you to access the door first if necessary
	Arrange the furniture to allow comfortable personal space for you and the patient and remove any objects which could be used as weapons (including things the patient has brought with them)
	Know where the panic buttons are and how to access rapid support
Your behaviour	Dress appropriately; do not wear anything which could be used against you (scarves, neckties, necklaces) and avoid sexually provocative clothing
	Tie up long hair
	As students, interviewing in pairs is preferable
	Tell staff where you are and who you are with; never undertake an interview without having checked it is appropriate with staff first
	Always be clear and open about who you are and your purpose
	Mention that you will be taking notes but be prepared not to if this agitates the patient
	Be calm; many mood states are infectious and changes in your behaviour will also affect the patient
	Take everything the patient is saying seriously
	If particular subjects are causing the patient to become agitated or threatening, avoid them until an easier rapport can be established
	Apologise and politely end the interview if it appears to be unduly upsetting or agitating for the patient
	Make staff aware if an interview has been difficult
Patient	If violence is likely, do not interview the patient unless in the company of a member of staff
	Do not continue to interview a patient if it becomes apparent they have a weapon
	If the patient is becoming increasingly threatening or intimidating end the interview
	If the patient does not speak the same language as you, arrange for an interpreter (preferably not related to the patient) to be present

Table 2.2 Safety considerations for psychiatric interviews

Communication skills for psychiatric interviews

Communication skill	Application	Example
Introduction	Calm, clear, polite and respectful; withdraw if the patient clearly does not want to speak	'Hello. My name is Alex Lewis and I'm a fourth year medical student. Would it be possible for me to ask you some questions today about how you are feeling?'
	Let the patient know how long the interview will last	'It will probably take about half an hour. Is that okay?'
Non-verbal communication	Body language must match verbal communication; conveying reticence, anxiety, disinterest or lack of empathy will destroy the rapport	Sit still, look interested and establish non-confrontational, attentive eye-contact without invading the patient's personal space
Open questions, use of silence and active listening	Some patients are reticent about telling their story again. Don't overwhelm them with a barrage of questions; use open questions and leave pauses to encourage them to tell their story	'Tell me more about that'
	Show interest by responding non-verbally	'Go on. . .' Offer small prompts, nod and make encouraging noises
Clarification	Ask for clarification if you don't understand something. Patients sometimes use unfamiliar terms (e.g. relating to drug misuse) and it becomes obvious if you don't understand	'Can you tell me what heavenly blue is please? I've never heard of that'
	Ask patients to expand on areas they have not fully explained	'I didn't quite understand what you meant when you said. . .'
Empathy	Pay close attention to your patient's body language and respond to what you see	'It looks as though that really upset you'
	Avoid stating phrases that state the obvious or for which you should be able to make a reasonable guess	Avoid: 'That must be really difficult for you' 'How does that make you feel?'
	Express your empathic feelings non-verbally	Lean forward, change your expression or lower your tone of voice
Using patient's own words (short summaries)	Show you have been listening by picking up short stretches of the patient's speech and reflecting them back to them; this may prompt them to say more	'You said you haven't been able to go out of the house recently. . .?'
Tolerance	Do not demonstrate disapproval, or phrase questions in a way which imply judgment	Avoid: 'Surely you wouldn't think of killing yourself when you have two small children?'
Flexibility	Keep a mental note of various issues to link and return to later in the history; following a rigid history format is unlikely to be successful	'You mentioned earlier that you had left your job a couple of months ago. Why was that?'
Genuine interest	Patients tell you extraordinary things; respond naturally and appropriately, and ask all the questions which come to mind	'You mentioned that you noticed your mother had been replaced by someone else. Tell me more about that'. 'How did you know that was the case?'
Signposting	Make the patient aware when you are about to introduce a difficult topic	'These next questions may seem a little personal but I do need to ask you about your personal life'

Table 2.3 Communication skills for psychiatric interviews

Patients' stories are all very different, requiring flexibility in the interview. Using the following headings will ensure that all areas are considered.

History of the presenting complaint

The history starts with a detailed description of the presenting complaint. An open question allows the patient to start explaining what has been happening. Then use the patient's own words to expand on the nature of what has been happening.

- 'Tell me a little about why you have come to see us today.'
- 'So, you've noticed that people have been treating you differently these last few weeks; tell me more about that.'

As with any physical condition, the presenting complaint must be clarified. Patients often volunteer much of the information in their spontaneous account but closed questions are also necessary to get a clearer picture.

- 'How long has this been going on?'
- 'Did anything set this off?'
- 'Does anything make it better or worse?'
- 'Since this started, has it been getting worse, getting better or staying much the same?'
- 'Have you noticed any other problems or symptoms?'
- 'This problem has been happening for some time; what in particular made you come to see us today?'
- 'How is this affecting your everyday life?'

Specific questions are triggered by the nature of the presenting symptom. For example, if the patient's presenting complaint appears to be related to hallucinations, ask in detail about the hallucinations. Further enquiry should identify and relevant associated symptoms, for example delusions in the case of hallucinations (see Chapter 4).

> **Ask questions that occur to you naturally in response to the patient's problems.** For example, if a patient tells you they are hearing someone speaking to them when no one is around, ask what the voice sounds like, whether the patient recognises it and whether it is always the same person. This makes it clear that you are genuinely interested in the patient's experiences.

Past psychiatric history

The past psychiatric history can usually be connected to the presenting complaint quite naturally.

- 'Have you experienced anything like this in the past?'
- 'Have you had to see a doctor about this kind of problem before?'

If the patient confirms they have had previous episodes, find out what these were like. This includes a description of:

- When they happened
- What was happening in the patient's life at the time
- How long they lasted
- Whether they needed treatment in hospital
- What that treatment consisted of
- Whether the patient knows the diagnosis of those episodes

This is more difficult if the patient has no insight into their condition or does not connect current illness with previous episodes. In such instances, more general questions can be used.

- 'Have you ever experienced any problems with your mental health or stress-related problems in the past?'

Past medical history

Ask about other illnesses which have required medical or surgical treatment. Treatments for many medical conditions can affect the treatment of a mental health condition. In addition, many psychiatric illnesses present in conjunction with or as a consequence of a physical disorder and the medical history often gives clues to the aetiology of the mental health presentation.

The past medical history must include a clear list of any medications the patient is or has recently been taking.

Family psychiatric history

Many psychiatric illnesses, such as depression and schizophrenia, have some degree of genetic inheritance. Asking about the patient's own past history leads naturally on to asking about the health of other family members. This includes a general enquiry about illnesses that run in the family and a more specific enquiry about any family history of mental health disorders.

- 'Has anyone else in your family had any problems similar to this?'

- 'Has anyone in your family had problems with their nerves or needed to see a doctor because of problems with their mental health?'

Draw a family tree to indicate the key family members, significant medical events and family psychiatric history (**Figure 2.1**).

Personal history

Ask the patient to describe their life more broadly: you are trying to build up a picture of them, their experiences and the events that have had a significant impact on them. Start with general questions and then move to more specific ones.

- 'Tell me more about your early life and childhood.'

Many patients need specific prompts about their birth, their early years and development and their experience growing up in their family. Ask them about their early relationships: who were they close to, did they experience any difficulties and was their childhood happy? What were they like as a child?

As with all areas of the psychiatric history, respond, as you would to a colleague or friend, with interest and curiosity to know more about the events that shaped them as a person.

Ask specifically about the person's education.

- 'Tell me about your time at school; what was that like?'
- 'Did you have any problems at school? How did you get on with your teachers and your peers?'
- 'How did you get on academically? Did you take any exams before you left school?'

Then ask about their further education and occupation after leaving school. List significant events in their occupational history chronologically. Find out how they have got on at work, their successes and failures and the reasons for these.

Significant relationships

Note all the patient's significant relationships and the significant events relating to these. Include breakdowns of relationships and the patient's response.

Don't shy away from talking about the patient's relationships. Although this feels difficult, personal and intrusive, relationships are central to the patient's life and experience. It is helpful to adopt a matter-of-fact approach to broaching difficult subjects, followed by empathic responses to sensitive information the patient reveals.

A sexual history should be included, including the age of menarche for women, the age of first intercourse and the number of partners

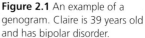

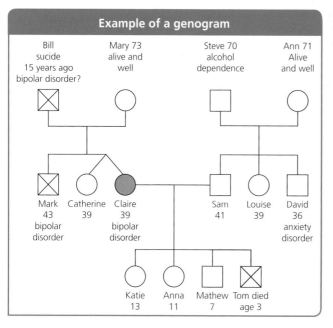

Figure 2.1 An example of a genogram. Claire is 39 years old and has bipolar disorder.

after this. Ask about the patient's sexual orientation and what their relationships have been like. Ask specifically about any experiences of physical or sexual abuse, although this is sometimes deferred until a later interview as the patient may be too acutely unwell to address such sensitive areas.

It helps to 'signpost' this part of the history to introduce very personal questions.

> ■ 'Forgive me, but I need to ask you a few more detailed questions that are important but may seem a little personal.'

In particular, find out about the patient's current relationship and any problems they are experiencing, including any possibility of physical or sexual abuse.

Always adopt a flexible approach to interviewing patients with mental health disorders. For example, it is sometimes inappropriate to ask a patient who is very agitated or overaroused about the details of their sexual history. Use your judgement to prioritise the most important areas of the history for immediate assessment.

Social history

This explores the social context of the patient's life. Occupation will have been covered earlier in the personal history, but ask here about the patient's financial circumstances. Ask about their housing, who lives with them and whether they have responsibility for others either at home or elsewhere. Outline whether they have interests, activities and friendships outside the home (**Table 2.4**).

Substance misuse

No history is complete without a detailed history of the patient's use of drugs and alcohol, both past and present. Do not make assumptions, based upon for example the patient's appearance, age, gender and profession, about whether they misuse drugs or alcohol. Start with an open screening question.

> ■ 'Can I ask you whether you drink any alcohol or use any recreational drugs?'

You can then follow up with specific questions about each of these. Different patients use very different expressions to describe drug use. For example, older patients may need an explanation of what a recreational

Questions in a social history	
Category	**Questions to ask the patient**
Family	What support do they receive from their family and what is their family's attitude to their problems
	Situation at home: who is there, how is the atmosphere?
	Other social support?
Friendships	Are there people in whom the patient can confide?
	What other support does the patient receive, e.g. groups, charities?
	Any negative influences, e.g. people who encourage substance misuse, encourage stigma?
Housing	Details of accommodation: e.g. owned/ rented, state of repair, space, any problems?
Self-care	Any problems coping with activities of daily living?
	Do they receive any support for this?
Finances	Any problems?
	Do they receive any support for this?
Activities	What does the patient do in a typical day?
	What are their interests and hobbies?

Table 2.4 Core questions to ask a patient when taking a social history

drug is and younger patients are often more familiar with a wide range of expressions describing popular drug use. Expand on your questions if the patient does not understand them, and ask for clarification if the patient uses a term you do not understand.

> **Do not be frightened to ask a patient the meaning of any words you do not understand.** There are many street names for illicit drugs that you may not recognise. If you do not ask for clarification, it both hinders your understanding and risks making you looking stupid when this comes to light!

For any alcohol or drug use volunteered, ask for details in a matter-of-fact fashion. Clarify what the patient uses, what quantities they use and how long they have used it. Avoid phrasing questions in a judgemental manner and do not show surprise even if the patient discloses remarkable facts.

Forensic history

A forensic history is a history of contact with the police and/or criminal justice system. This should be included in every history.

> ■ 'Have you ever been in trouble with the law or the police?'

If this is met with an emphatic 'no', no further enquiry is necessary. If the patient tells you they have a criminal record, it must be recorded in detail. This should include the nature of the offences, when they occurred and what the consequences were for the patient.

Link this to the rest of the patient's history, establishing when these incidents occurred and whether they were linked to episodes of mental illness or substance abuse.

Premorbid personality

It is easy to make false assumptions about a person's character and personality when they are acutely unwell as acute illness often has a profound effect on behaviour. The patient's previous history has provided a certain amount of information but this area invites the patient to describe how they feel they are as a person.

Patients find this quite difficult and it is often necessary to offer a few attempts with reworded questions depending on the individual patient. Specific prompts are needed if the patient struggles to describe themselves.

> ■ 'Tell me a little bit about what you are like as a person when you are well?'
>
> ■ 'Do you feel you are very different from your normal self at the moment? If so, in what way?'
>
> ■ 'How would your family and friends describe you?'
>
> ■ 'Are you the kind of person who worries a lot, copes well with pressure, socialises easily, etc.?'

Linking elements of the patient's history flexibly in response to the presenting complaint always gains a higher grade at examination stations than rigidly following the same scheme for every patient. It is better to take a flexible patient-centred approach even if it means you miss one or two elements out.

Collateral history

Even the most experienced interviewer does not always get the full story, especially if the patient is acutely distressed, uncooperative or confused. A collateral history from someone who is related to, or knows, the patient is helpful in filling in gaps, giving a better indication of the patient's personality when they are healthy and the events leading up to the current illness.

Many patients are accompanied by a relative and can give consent for a discussion to take place with that relative. If they are on their own, always gain the patient's consent before contacting a relative for further information in all but the most extreme circumstances; not doing so is a breach of confidentiality.

The biopsychosocial model and the three Ps

The biopsychosocial model is a way of categorising a presenting illness in terms of the biological, psychological and social factors that have contributed to its aetiology, pathogenesis and continuation (**Figure 2.2**). Identifying and addressing all of these factors ensures that treatment includes all available approaches to manage the patient's problems.

The biopsychosocial model for mental illness includes the following factors:

- Biological – defective physiological functioning of the mind and body
- Psychological – the underlying psychological causes of a problem such as negative thinking or chronic emotional distress
- Social – including culture, poverty and socioeconomic status

Biopsychosocial factors are all closely interlinked. Life events present discrete trigger factors for psychiatric illness but it is likely that the effects of such stressors are mediated through biological mechanisms.

The aetiology of a psychiatric presentation is further understood by characterising factors as predisposing to, precipitating and perpetuating the patient's illness (**Table 2.5**):

- **Predisposing factors** – what factors have made this patient more likely to develop a psychiatric illness?
- **Precipitating factors** – what factors have made this patient ill right now?
- **Perpetuating factors** – what factors are stopping this patient from getting better, sometimes despite adequate treatment?

Establishing these helps to explain and understand the patient's illness at this specific time and directs treatment appropriately (**Table 2.6**). Failing to address these factors can prevent recovery.

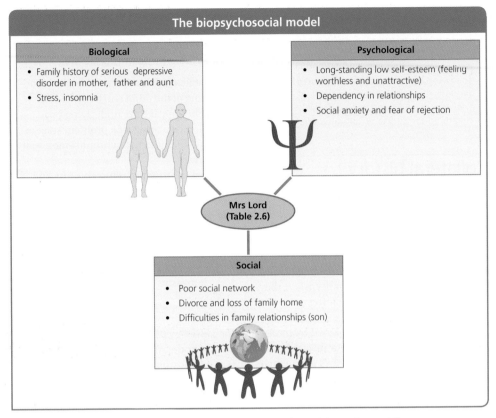

Figure 2.2 The biopsychosocial model: factors contributing to the aetiology of mental illness.

Factors affecting psychiatric disorder aetiology			
3 Ps	Biological	Psychological	Social
Predisposing factors	Organic conditions	Cognitive distortions	Childhood abuse/bullying
	Genetic factors	Maladaptive behaviours	Poor social support
	Family history	Psychodynamic factors	Housing issues
	Substance abuse	Personality factors	Unemployment
		Poor parenting	
Precipitating factors	Organic conditions	Grief	Life events
	Substance abuse	Stress	
	Non-compliance		
	Treatment resistance		
	Disordered sleep		
Perpetuating factors	Organic conditions	Poor insight	Stigma
	Substance abuse	Personality traits	Poor social support
	Non-concordance	High expressed emotion	Poor housing
	Treatment resistance	Lack of confiding relationships	Unemployment
	Sleep pattern	Maladaptive behaviours	

Table 2.5 The biopsychosocial model and the three Ps of psychiatric disorder aetiology: examples of common factors

| | Using the three Ps | | |

Mrs Lord is 54-year-old woman with a family history of depression who develops a depressive illness after her divorce. She was very dependent upon her husband and feels she cannot manage without him. She has always felt unattractive and worthless. She moved house following the break-up of her marital home and now has a poor relationship with her oldest son who blames her for the breakdown in relationship. She has never had close friends and does not discuss her problems at work because she fears it will annoy her workmates.

Category	Predisposing factors	Precipitating factors	Perpetuating factors
Biological	Family history of depression	Stress, lack of sleep, loss of appetite	Lack of sleep
Psychological	Dependency upon husband Feeling of unattractiveness and worthlessness	Feeling she cannot manage without the immediate support of her husband	Social anxiety and fear of rejection from friends and neighbours
Social	Lack of network of close friends	Divorce and loss of house and family home	Isolation and loss of family bonds

Table 2.6 Using the three Ps to understand all of the factors that have contributed to a patient's illness

Psychiatric examination

Starter questions

Answers to the following questions are on page 95.

5. Is there a difference between illusions and hallucinations?
6. Are hallucinations always 'abnormal'?
7. Why are physical examinations carried out on patients with apparent mental illness?

The psychiatric history provides relevant information regarding the patient's symptoms and experiences, but full assessment of a psychiatric condition also requires a mental state examination (MSE) to be performed. This systematically identifies and records all the patient's psychiatric signs and symptoms.

The MSE is equivalent to the physical examination in other specialties and plays a major role in establishing the patient's diagnosis. A physical examination is also performed in psychiatric illness but in this context provides supporting information by assessing the patient's baseline health and screening for underlying physical illness.

The mental state examination

The MSE is the cornerstone of a psychiatric assessment, and describes aspects of the patient's psychological functioning at a specific point in time in a structured, organised way. Its framework ensures that all aspects of the patient's psychopathology are covered.

The assessment begins as soon as the interviewer meets the patient. For example, a careful note should be made of the patient's presentation. Focused observation allows the interviewer to produce a detailed account of the patient's expression, movements and behaviour, which contributes to the differential diagnosis. Less evident signs are identified by specific questioning.

Also key to the examination are:

- A use of descriptive psychopathology – having a good understanding of the terminology used to describe any psychopathology observed
- Empathy – establishing a positive and empathic rapport
- Caution – keeping an open mind regarding the diagnosis

> A 'normal' MSE does not necessarily mean you have got it wrong. Patients demonstrate different symptoms at different times, appearing quite well at one point in the day but floridly disturbed at another. This is important and should be noted.

Do not be daunted by the psychiatric examination. Listening carefully, picking up subtle cues and using sensitive non-verbal and verbal skills encourages the patient to tell their story. This then helps to produce a clear and detailed account of their experiences.

Descriptive psychopathology

Descriptive psychopathology is the detailed and precise description of abnormal experiences, as related by the patient or observed by the examiner during the psychiatric interview. It does not explain the signs and symptoms but allows them to be described and communicated to all members of the mental health-care team.

Empathy

Empathy is the capacity to understand or feel things from another person's point of view, or the ability to put yourself in another person's shoes.

Being empathic can be challenging if the patient's experiences appear to be so extraordinary or unusual that it is difficult to really imagine or understand them. Remember how real and compelling these experiences are to the patient. Showing disbelief or contradicting the patient damages your rapport and could make them reluctant to tell their story.

Keep an open mind

Remember that one sign or symptom does not create a diagnosis. Making assumptions on the basis of a single symptom results in a failure to carefully assess and describe all the features of the patient's presentation. This is as potentially misleading as making a physical diagnosis on the basis of a single finding in a clinical examination.

> Although the components of the MSE should initially be memorised, do not try to force the structure on an interview. With experience, it becomes second nature to cover all the areas that are relevant to the individual patient with a natural dynamic.

Components of the mental state examination

The MSE is structured to encompass observations in seven categories:

1. Appearance and behaviour
2. Speech
3. Mood and affect
4. Perceptions
5. Thoughts
6. Cognition
7. Insight

> Use the information that the patient provides during the history to focus on relevant areas of the MSE. Personalising your approach avoids undue repetition, which may make the patient think you have not been listening.

Appearance and behaviour

This information is based on observations made throughout the interview rather than direct questioning. Keep a careful mental note of any relevant features to record later (**Figure 2.3**).

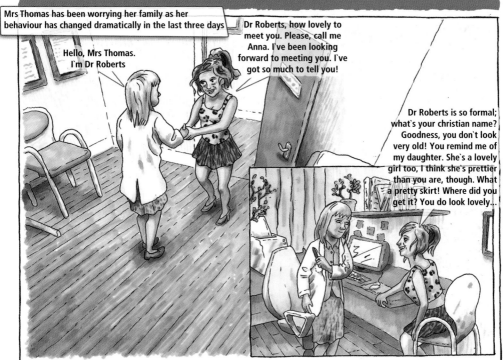

Appearance and behaviour

Mrs Thomas has been worrying her family as her behaviour has changed dramatically in the last three days

Hello, Mrs Thomas. I'm Dr Roberts

Dr Roberts, how lovely to meet you. Please, call me Anna. I've been looking forward to meeting you. I've got so much to tell you!

Dr Roberts is so formal; what's your christian name? Goodness, you don't look very old! You remind me of my daughter. She's a lovely girl too, I think she's prettier than you are, though. What a pretty skirt! Where did you get it? You do look lovely...

Figure 2.3 Appearance and behaviour.

General appearance

The patient's general appearance provides vital clues to their mental state (Figure 2.3):

- Do they look physically unwell? – be alert to physical signs during the assessment as some psychiatric presentations (e.g. delirium) have an underlying physical cause (e.g. infection)
- Are there physical problems such as blindness or deafness, which you need to make adjustments for in your interview?
- Is the patient alert, oriented and fully conscious?
- What is their build? – note whether they are underweight or overweight, as weight changes are common in psychiatric disorders such as depression
- Self-care – how does their personal grooming and level of hygiene appear? This could be a sign of significant self-neglect, e.g. in depression and schizophrenia

- How are they dressed? – a manic patient may be dressed inappropriately for the weather, e.g. wearing inadequate, brightly coloured, chaotic summer clothing in the winter. Oversized baggy clothing is used to conceal weight loss in anorexia nervosa. Particular styles of dress or wearing of unusual garments such as a military uniform should be noted
- Are there physical signs of addictive behaviours such as needle marks and tracks on the arms, breath smelling of alcohol, pinpoint pupils or slurring of speech
- Are there physical signs of an eating disorder? – e.g. self-induced vomiting can cause calluses on the knuckles (Russell's sign) or damaged teeth
- Are there signs of deliberate self-harm?

Expression

The patient's expression often provides vital information on their emotional state.

Are they:

- Expressionless and unresponsive to the conversation?
- Labile in expression, e.g. moving rapidly from weeping to laughing?
- Smiling continuously, appearing elated?
- Gesturing and animated, or lifeless and still?
- Weeping throughout the conversation, or looking angry or afraid?

Attitude

The patient's attitude to the interviewer provides further information regarding their mental state. Are they:

- Cooperative in establishing an open rapport, making it easy to engage in conversation?
- Hostile, evasive or suspicious, suggesting underlying paranoid thoughts?
- Apathetic, as in chronic psychotic conditions or profound depression?
- Easily distracted and unable to focus on the conversation, suggestive of hypomania or a psychotic disorder?

- Overfamiliar, asking personal questions and invading the interviewer's personal space, which is often seen in hypomanic patients?

Psychomotor function

This focuses on the patient's level of motor activity relating to their underlying mental processes. Concentrate on what they are doing during the interview:

- Are their movements slowed due to the psychomotor retardation of depression?
- Are they agitated and physically restless because of anxiety?
- Are they moving rapidly around the room, singing, picking up objects and struggling to focus on the conversation, which is suggestive of hypomania?
- Are they displaying any abnormal movements? Many patients display abnormal movements (**Table 2.7**) as a consequence of psychotropic medications, particularly antipsychotics

Other abnormal movements can be deliberately elicited during the examination (**Table 2.8**).

Spontaneous abnormal movements		
Abnormal movement	Description	Associated conditions
Tremor	Involuntary rhythmic, muscle contractions. Most common involuntary movement. Frequently occurs in the hands	Parkinson's disease Side-effect of many psychotropic medications
Tic	Involuntary, repetitive, non-rhythmic, purposeless movement or vocalisation	Neurological disorders
Mannerism	Repetitive, odd, idiosyncratic movements that appear goal-directed, e.g. endless tie straightening.	Schizophrenia Personality disorders
Stereotypy	Repetitive, odd, non-goal directed movement, e.g. rocking	Intellectual disability Schizophrenia
Dystonia	Sustained muscle contractions. Twisting and repetitive movements or abnormal postures. Most commonly affects neck, eyes and upper trunk, e.g. grimacing, torticollis, blepharospasm	Acute side-effect to some antipsychotic medications Schizophrenia
Akathisia	Subjective, unpleasant feeling of physical restlessness. Patient wants to move the legs, fidget or shuffle	Side-effect of psychotropic medications
Dyskinesia	Involuntary, repetitive, rhythmic, purposeless movements of tongue, face, limbs or trunk. Most typically affects orofacial muscles with repeated tongue protrusion, chewing or grimacing	Long-term side-effect of psychotropic medication

Table 2.7 Spontaneous abnormal movements and their associated conditions

Speech

Note the structure and form of a person's speech (**Figure 2.4**). The content (ideas and beliefs) is considered later, with thoughts and perceptions (see page 60).

- Rate
- Quality and form
- Volume and tone

'Normal' speech is highly variable but is generally spontaneous, logical, coherent and relevant.

Abnormal movements elicited during examination	
Movement	Description
Forced grasping	Repeated shaking of the interviewer's hand each time it is offered, despite being asked not to
Echopraxia	Patient copies everything the interviewer does, despite being asked not to
Perseveration	Repetition of previous response to stimulus which is not appropriate to second stimulus; e.g. patient is asked to touch nose with right forefinger and does so correctly but when asked to put their left hand on their right ear they again touch their nose with their right forefinger. Can also be demonstrated in speech
Automatic obedience	Patient carries out all requests, irrespective of consequences, like an automaton
Obstruction	Patient suddenly stops unpredictably in the course of what they are doing; they may continue after a pause or move on to a different action
Ambitendency	Alternation between co-operation and opposition
Mitgehen	Interviewer can move the patient's limbs with only fingertip pressure (like moving an anglepoise lamp)
Negativism	Patient resists the interviewer's requests

Table 2.8 Abnormal movements elicited during examination

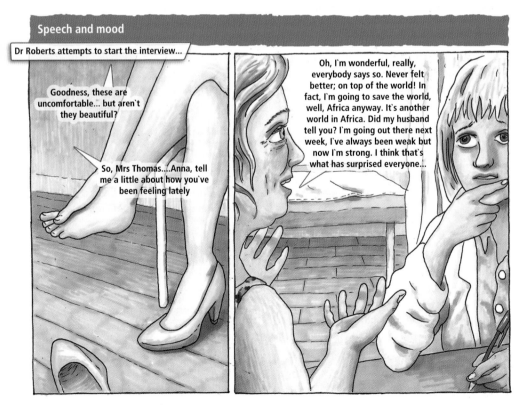

Figure 2.4 Speech and mood.

Rate

Variations in the rate of production of speech include the following:

- Pressure of speech is an increase in the amount and speed of spontaneous speech. This occurs in very anxious or agitated patients and, characteristically, in hypomanic patients. This speech is difficult to interrupt or stop
- Retardation of speech is seen in depressed patients who demonstrate long pauses in their speech
- Poverty of speech is a decrease in the amount of spontaneous speech. This accompanies retardation of speech in depression. It is also seen in patients with chronic schizophrenia
- Elective mutism is a complete absence of spontaneous, voluntary speech due to an underlying psychogenic cause

Quality and form

Abnormalities in the quality and form of speech are shown in **Table 2.9**.

Volume and tone

The volume and tone can be:

- Monotonous and soft, with a loss of variation in inflection and stress. This is seen in depressed patients and those with severe frontal lobe damage
- Loud and angry, as in agitated or acutely disturbed or psychotic patients
- Shouting and sarcastic in anger
- Weak and soft in anxiety

Mood and affect

Mood and affect are distinct:

- Mood is the patient's prolonged, subjective emotional state, which prevails over a period of time and which they can describe to the interviewer
- Affect is the emotional state as observed (objectively) by the examiner and judged from the patient's expressions

Affect is therefore a more transitory state that is observed from the outside. Many features of a subjective mood change are noted in the history, for example changes in sleep, appetite and diurnal variation of mood. This allows the interviewer to build up a picture of the patient's own subjective experience of their mood.

Affect

Observing the patient's posture, facial expression, speech and emotional reactivity allows their affect to be objectively described as:

- Euthymic – an apparently normal mood
- Irritable – demonstrating reduced control over their feelings of anger or frustration
- Angry
- Anxious – demonstrating a sense of fear or apprehension
- Agitated – physical restlessness as a consequence of underlying worry
- Perplexed – baffled or bewildered about something
- Suspicious – appearing mistrustful of someone or something
- Depressed – low in mood
- Elated – euphoric, 'high' with an elevated mood
- Guilty
- Frightened

How does the patient make you feel?
This is often relevant as it reflects their mental state. For example, depression in your patient can make you feel sad and an anxious patient sometimes makes you feel agitated.

Range of affect

Affect is described as being reactive, labile, blunted, flat or incongruous (**Figure 2.5**):

- Reactive affect is the normal range of affect that people express. A range of emotions is visible, with changes of expression, speech and gesture in accordance with what the patient is saying. Many patients' affects vary markedly during the clinical interview
- Labile affect is a rapid alternation between extremes of expression, such as moving quickly from laughter to tears and back again. This is seen with bipolar affective disorder and in many neurological

conditions including traumatic brain injuries, stroke, dementias, multiple sclerosis and brain tumours

■ Blunted affect describes a noticeable reduction in the range of emotion displayed. Patients appear unresponsive in conversation and display little variability and intensity in their emotions. This is most commonly associated with the negative symptoms of schizophrenia

■ Flat affect describes the reduced expression of emotion that is seen in severe depressive disorders

■ Incongruous affect is entirely inconsistent with the circumstances or the patient's subjective mood, for example if a patient laughs when describing the recent death of a close relative. This is seen in patients with chronic schizophrenia

Speech abnormalities		
Form of speech	Description	Associated conditions
Circumstantial speech	Organised speech with excessive detail and irrelevancies, delaying the patient from getting to the point	Schizophrenia Obsessive compulsive disorder Stable personality characteristic
Tangential speech	Organised speech skirts around the topic and never reaches the point of the conversation	Schizophrenia Bipolar disorder Organic brain disorders
Flight of ideas	Accelerated flow of speech Logical connection between sequential ideas Rapid speed of movement from one subject to another Ideas linked by normal connections or through word puns and rhymes	Hypomania
Neologism	A new word with an idiosyncratic, personal meaning	Schizophrenia
Clang association	Linking words together based on coincident sound rather than meaning, e.g. rhyming words used in succession	Manic phase of bipolar affective disorder
Word salad	Recognisable words arranged completely meaninglessly in incoherent sentences	Schizophrenia
Paragrammatism	Disorder of grammatical construction, e.g. dog for taken I have a walk	Organic disorders including Wernicke's aphasia Schizophrenia
Logoclonia	Repetition of the last syllable of every word	Parkinson's disease Alzheimer's disease
Palilalia	Repetition of patient's own word when it is no longer appropriate	Seen in numerous conditions including Tourette's syndrome, autism spectrum disorder, following strokes, epilepsy
Echolalia	Repetition of the examiner's words and speech	Autism spectrum disorder and Asperger's syndrome Tourette's syndrome Alzheimer's disease Schizophrenia
Coprolalia	Involuntary shouting of obscenities	Tourette's syndrome

Table 2.9 Speech abnormalities and their associated conditions

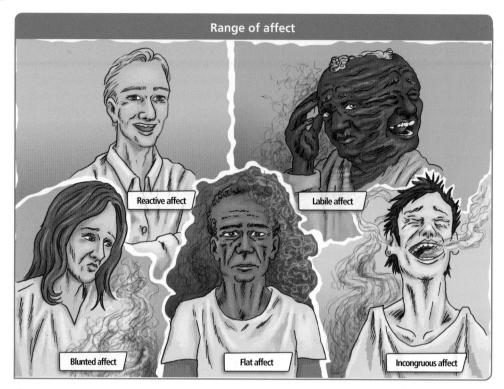

Figure 2.5 Descriptive terms for range of affect.

Suicidal ideation

Ideas of suicide or self-harm. may have been described spontaneously during the history. If not, ask directly about them here. A thorough description of the patient's ideas of self-harm or suicide is necessary to assess the level of risk presented by the patient. Any ideas of harm to others should also be noted.

Perceptions

Perception is the process by which people interpret and organise sensations to make sense of the world around them. Central to this are sensations received from the sensory pathways (visual, auditory, olfactory, gustatory, kinaesthetic and proprioceptive). Perception requires the processing of this raw sensory input. It is influenced by many interrelated factors including context, memory, previous experiences, cultural expectations and personal views and opinions.

Disordered perception can occur in any of the five sensory modalities and should be identified and recorded during the MSE (**Figure 2.6**).

Illusions

An illusion is a sensory distortion – a misperception of a real, physical stimulus. The most common illusions are visual. Illusions may occur in healthy individuals. They arise more readily where attention is reduced or during heightened emotional states, for example misperceiving a shape as an intruder in the semi-darkness when anxious. Illusions most commonly in occur patients whose levels of concentration and attention are impaired, for example in acute confusional states.

Hallucinations

A hallucination is unlike an illusion in that no external stimulus is required to produce it. It arises spontaneously in the absence of a real stimulus, alongside ordinary, real perceptions. The most obvious example is hearing a clear voice speaking when no one has actually spoken: an auditory hallucination.

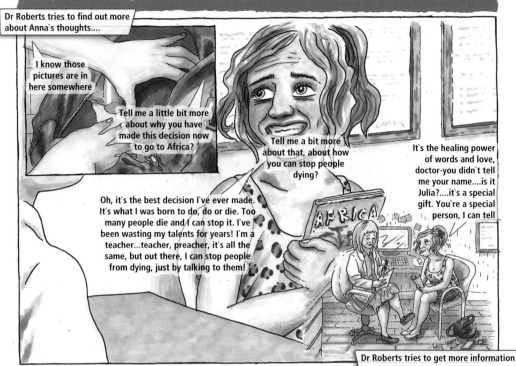

Figure 2.6 Perceptions and thoughts.

Hallucinations often signify severe mental illness (**Table 2.10**). However, they also occur in healthy people, in whom they are usually brief and relatively simple. Examples are hypnopompic and hypnagogic hallucinations: the brief sensation of hearing or seeing something (such as hearing one's name shouted out) on waking or falling asleep, respectively.

> **Telling patients their hallucinations are not real is unlikely to be helpful.** This usually prevents them from discussing them further. Patients experience hallucinations as a normal sensory experience.

Thoughts

Three characteristics of thought should be considered:

- Stream or flow of thought
- Form of thought
- Content of thought

Stream or flow of thought and form of thought are best considered by careful attention to the patient's speech. In addition to the abnormalities of thought identified during history taking, further abnormalities of the form and stream of thought can be observed in conversation with the patient (**Table 2.11**).

Disorders of content of thought

This focuses on the patient's beliefs and ideas. It includes eliciting and carefully describing any:

- Phobias – specific fears of an object or situation
- Obsessions – persistent ideas dominating the patient's thoughts
- Preoccupations and worries
- Delusions

Delusions

A delusion is a fixed, false, unshakeable belief that is out of keeping with the patient's religious, cultural or educational background. It is held with strong conviction and cannot

Hallucinations and associated conditions		
Type of hallucination	Description	Associated illness
Auditory hallucinations	Sophisticated, organised sounds, most commonly speech or music	Severe mental illness, particularly functional psychoses
Gedankenlautwerden (audible thoughts)	Hears their own thoughts spoken aloud as they are thinking them	
Echo de la pensée (thought echo)	Hears their own thoughts spoken out loud immediately after they have thought them	
Second person auditory hallucinations	Voices address the patient directly, e.g. 'You are evil. Everybody hates you'	
Third person auditory hallucinations	Voices speak about the patient, referring to them as she/he. They may discuss the patient, argue about them or describe everything they are doing as they do it (running commentary)	
Visual hallucinations	May be complex images of objects and people and the background surrounding them (panoramic), tiny animals or people (Lilliputian hallucinations) as in delirium tremens	Organic states including drug induced conditions
Charles Bonnet syndrome	Complex visual hallucinations in people with significantly reduced vision	No other associated psychopathology
Olfactory hallucinations	Often unpleasant smells with personal significance. May develop false beliefs, e.g. that someone is pumping gas into their house	Schizophrenia, epilepsy and other organic states
Gustatory hallucinations	May co-exist with olfactory hallucinations. Often unpleasant	Schizophrenia Temporal lobe epilepsy
Hallucinations of bodily sensation	Superficial: abnormal perception of heat or cold, e.g. 'my body is on fire'	Schizophrenia Addictions
	Sensation of being touched, e.g. formication, the sensation of little insects crawling on or just under the skin	Schizophrenia Cocaine addiction and alcohol withdrawal
	Kinaesthetic: abnormal sensations of muscle or joint sense, feeling that limbs are being bent or rocked about	Benzodiazepine withdrawal and alcohol intoxication
	Visceral: false perceptions of inner organs, e.g. 'I can feel mucus collecting around my brain'	Schizophrenia

Table 2.10 Hallucinations and their associated conditions

be swayed by appealing to reason. Delusions are often, but not always, bizarre ideas that feel as real to the patient as any other thought or idea. They usually indicate serious mental illness (Table 2.12).

Delusions can be primary or secondary according to the context of their stimulation (Table 2.13).

Cognition

This focuses on the patient's global intellectual functioning, as perceived throughout the history and MSE. It can also be assessed formally, although this is not always necessary or feasible. Many patients will have demonstrated that they are cognitively intact during the history from the clarity and detail of the account they are able to give.

Notice the following in the course of the interview:

- Level of consciousness
- Orientation in time, place and person – does your patient know who they are, where they are and what time, day, week or year it is?
- Level of attention and concentration – can they keep their mind on what is being discussed?

Disorders in the stream and form of thought		
Disorder	Description	Associated conditions
Stream of thought		
Pressure of thought	Pressure of speech, abundant, varied thoughts flowing through the mind at increased speed	Hypomania
Poverty of thought	Poverty of speech (little spontaneous speech), thoughts diminished in frequency and speed	Severe depression Schizophrenia
Thought blocking	Sudden break in conversation, experiences a sudden loss in train of thought, in mid-sentence, which cannot subsequently be picked up	Schizophrenia
Form of thought		
Loosening of associations	Rapid movement from one subject to another in conversation. Links between topics are difficult or impossible to see. Speech appears muddled and illogical (Knight's move thinking)	Schizophrenia
Over-inclusive thinking	Excessively detailed, largely irrelevant speech (circumstantiality). Conceptual boundaries of thought are weakened	Schizophrenia Some personality disorders Obsessive compulsive disorder
Concrete thinking	Inability to understand metaphors and abstract ideas; tested by asking the patient to interpret a proverb or saying	Chronic schizophrenia Intellectual disability

Table 2.11 Disorders in the stream and form of thought and their associated conditions

Delusions		
Type	Description	Associated conditions
Control	Belief that thought, feeling or action is being controlled by an outside agency Thought interference (insertion, withdrawal or broadcasting) Control of affect, volition and actions	Schizophrenia
Persecution	Belief that someone or something means to do them harm, e.g. following them/spying on them	Schizophrenia
Reference	Belief that ordinary objects or events have special significance for the person, e.g. news reports on TV refer to them specifically	Schizophrenia
Grandeur	Belief that they have extraordinary special gifts or qualities, e.g. knowing something that will save us all from climate change	Mania/hypomania
Nihilistic	Belief that the patient, or other important things, no longer exist, a form of extreme negativity, e.g. the patient believes that their internal organs are rotting away, or that they are homeless	Depressive psychosis
Guilt	Belief that a terrible wrong, sin or crime has been committed, e.g. death of a partner or the economic recession	Depressive psychosis
Jealousy	Delusions centred on the belief that a partner is cheating on them, based on false evidence	Psychotic disorders Pathological jealousy
Hypochondriacal	Belief that something is terribly wrong with the body	Hypochondriasis
Infestation	Belief that the skin is infested by parasites	Ekbom's syndrome Schizophrenia

Table 2.12 Delusions and their associated conditions

Primary and secondary delusions			
Type	Context	Associated disorders	Example
Primary delusions (rare)	Spontaneously	Schizophrenia	A delusional perception: the attachment of a delusional idea to an ordinary perception, e.g. patient sees a red car parked at a strange angle and suddenly knows they are being pursued by religious fanatics
Secondary delusions	Arise from an existing predisposing mood state or experience	Depression Psychosis	Delusional beliefs to explain a hallucinatory voice in patients with any psychotic disorder or development of delusions that the patient is going to die in the context of depression

Table 2.13 Primary and secondary delusions

- Memory – are they struggling to remember details in response to questions?
- General level of intellectual functioning (some information will have been gained from the patient's school and occupational history).

Mini-mental state examination

A mini-mental state examination (MMSE) is used to formally assess cognitive functioning: the intellectual processes of perception, thinking, reasoning, and remembering. It is not always appropriate to do an MMSE; some patients are too agitated to co-operate with the testing, such as when acutely psychotically unwell. Patients with an intellectual disability may find it distressing and patients with significant communication disorders or severe hearing disability may find it hard to comply. It is also likely to produce misleading results in patients who are acutely physically unwell or suffering from a current depressive disorder because the illness has a transient impact upon cognition which resolves when the patient recovers.

A standard widely used test is Folstein's MMSE, a 30-question checklist with a maximum score of 30 points (**Table 2.14**). Scores of 25–30 are considered to be in the normal range. Although it is not a diagnostic test, scores of 18–24 indicate mild to moderate cognitive impairment and scores of 17 or less indicate severe impairment.

Insight

Insight is the patient's awareness of, and ability to understand the origins and meaning of their current feelings, behaviour and symptoms. It is not simply present or absent. A patient may have partial insight, for example understanding that the voices they are hearing are unusual but attributing them to an outside source.

Consider whether the patient:

- Thinks that anything about their experience is seen and understood as abnormal by others, and is understood by the patient to be abnormal
- Understands these abnormal experiences arise as a consequence of mental illness
- Accepts that this illness requires treatment

> **Level of insight carries significant implications for treatment.** A patient who cannot accept that the voices they hear are unreal is unlikely to accept medical treatment for these symptoms.

Although a patient may understand that something is wrong and that their current experiences could be a form of illness, they may not believe that any treatment is appropriate for them.

A patient who is completely lacking in insight will have no understanding that illness can account for their symptoms and wholeheartedly believes that their current symptoms are entirely real. Persuading these patients that they are ill and that treatment is both beneficial and necessary usually requires a great deal of negotiation.

Some patients do develop good insight into the symptoms experienced in a previous episode of illness but consider their current

The mini-mental state examination (MMSE)		
Section	Content	Total points
Orientation	Ask what is the day, date and time	10
	Ask for information about their current location	
Registration	Say three unlinked words to the patient, e.g. sheep, car, wall, giving each clearly and slowly	3
	Ask them to repeat them back	
	Award one point for each correct word	
Attention	Ask them to complete a task that requires them to maintain attention for a few moments, e.g. repeatedly subtracting a number from a given starting point or spelling something backwards.	5
	Observe 5 stages	
Delayed recall	Ask them to recall the objects named earlier	3
Language, comprehending and following instructions	Ask them to complete a number of tasks, including naming specific objects, repeating brief phrases, following an instruction in three parts, reading, writing and copying (**Figure 2.7**)	9

Table 2.14 Key sections of the Folstein mini-mental state examination (MMSE). Points are allocated for correct answers within each section to a total score of 30 points

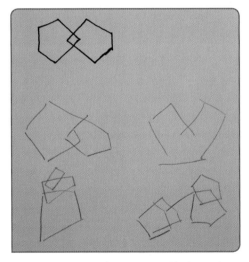

Figure 2.7 Attempts by a patient with dementia to copy two pentagons (top left).

symptoms to be different and unrelated to that illness, and therefore remain difficult to engage in treatment.

> Learn all the definitions of the different features of the MSE: they frequently appear in multiple choice examinations.

How to carry out a mental state examination

Record the MSE under the seven headings described on page 66 (**Table 2.15**). Some areas require only careful observation during the interview, whereas others benefit from a proactive approach to elicit the signs.

> Begin your MSE as soon as you meet the patient, observing their appearance and how they relate to other staff, relatives and yourself.

Appearance and behaviour

Describe the patient's appearance and behaviour in some detail. They may seem impolite but terms used to describe poor grooming and hygiene include unshaven, unkempt, unwashed or tangled hair, malodorous and dishevelled. Comment on the rapport established with the patient, their eye contact and cooperation with the interview process. Describe any abnormalities of gait and movement.

Certain signs are sometimes subtle and only relevant if they indicate a change. For example, wearing no make-up is likely to be of significance in a woman who normally takes enormous pride in her appearance and is usually immaculately made-up.

Assessing speech

Comment on the patient's speech in terms of quantity, rate, volume and fluency using the descriptors from the section on speech on page 57.

The mental state examination	
Category	**Description**
Appearance and behaviour	Describe the patient's: ■ General appearance ■ Expression ■ Attitude ■ Rapport with the interviewer ■ Psychomotor function/abnormal movements
Speech	Consider: ■ Rate of production of speech ■ Quality and form of speech ■ Volume and tone of speech
Mood	Describe: ■ Affect (the patient's apparent mood as perceived by the interviewer) ■ Mood (the patient's persistent mood state as described by the patient) ■ Range of affect ■ Suicidal ideation
Perceptions	Identify any illusions or hallucinations For any abnormal perceptions identify: ■ Modality (which of the five senses does it affect?) ■ Clear details of the abnormal perception ■ Any delusions arising out of the false perception which the patient uses to explain it
Thoughts	Consider : ■ Stream or flow of thought ■ Form of thought ■ Content of thought. Describe each delusion clearly giving verbatim examples
Cognitions	Note the patient's: ■ Level of consciousness ■ Orientation in time, place and person. Does the patient know who they are, where they are and what time/day/week/year it is? ■ Level of attention and concentration. Can they keep their mind on what you are discussing? ■ Memory. Are they struggling to remember details in response to your questions? ■ General level of intellectual functioning. You will have gained some detail of this from the patient's school/occupational history ■ Carry out a complete MMSE if there is any suspicion of cognitive impairment
Insight	Consider the three aspects of insight: 1. Does the patient think that that any of their experiences are abnormal, or would be seen as abnormal by others? 2. Does the patient understand that these abnormal experiences arise as a consequence of mental illness? 3. Does the patient accept that this illness requires treatment?

Table 2.15 Summary of the mental state examination

Assessing mood

Describe the patient's mood subjectively and objectively and make a note of the range of affect demonstrated throughout the interview. Patients often spontaneously describe their mood during the history. If not, ask direct questions to assess this.

- 'How have you been feeling recently?'
- 'Have you noticed any change in your mood or spirits?'
- 'Have you noticed any change in your energy levels recently?'
- 'Are you able to enjoy things as you usually do?'

Depending on the answers to these opening questions, ask relevant follow-up questions to elicit further symptoms of a mood disorder. For example, ask about sleep, appetite, concentration, diurnal variation of mood and libido.

Affect

Comment on the patient's mood state as it appears during the interview. Terms used include sad, angry, hostile, indifferent, euthymic, dysphoric, perplexed, elated, euphoric, anxious, animated and irritable.

Range of affect

Comment on the patient's range of affect. Are they are appropriately expressive during the consultation, laughing when something is funny or weeping when it is sad? Alternatively, is their affect restricted, for example if they are uniformly sad with little animation? Comment on whether their affect is appropriate to the discussion or whether there is any evidence of incongruence.

Suicidal ideation

When a patient has been discussing recent distressing events, ask an opening question to elicit suicidal ideation, relating your question back to the information the patient has already given you.

- 'Sometimes, when people are really struggling with difficult things as you have been doing, they get desperate and think about ending their own life. Has that been happening for you?'
- 'Do you ever feel hopeless about the future, or do you ever feel that life isn't worth living?
- 'Have you ever thought you would like to end your own life? '

If the patient admits to experiencing suicidal ideas, ask for a detailed account. Include any plans such as timing, the method they might use and actions taken such as hoarding tablets.

Eliciting abnormal perceptions

If the patient has already volunteered information on abnormal perceptions during your interview, ask for more details. If not, ask about this now. To avoid awkwardness in raising the subject of hallucinations, use a tactful opening statement .

- 'Do you ever hear strange noises or voices when there is no one around?'
- 'When people are feeling stressed, they can sometimes hear or see things that other people don't notice. Has that ever happened to you?'
- 'Have you ever heard your own thoughts as if they were being spoken aloud?'

If the answer is clearly no and you have no reason to suspect that the patient is experiencing abnormal perceptions, there is no need to pursue this. However, for any hallucinations described, obtain a clear picture of their nature and effect on the patient.

- 'Who do you think it is'?
- 'Is the voice male or female?'
- 'Is there more than one voice?'
- 'What does the voice say?'
- 'Does the voice speak to you directly or does it speak about you, commenting on what you are doing?'
- 'Does the voice give you commands? Does it tell you to do things you don't want to do?'
- 'Does the voice speak your thoughts out loud?'
- 'How often does it happen? How long does it last? Is it associated with any particular circumstances?'
- 'What effect is having on you? How does it make you feel?'

Assessing thoughts

The flow and form of the patient's thoughts can be observed from their speech without any specific questioning. Note any abnormalities (Table 2.11).

If the patient has not already volunteered information on any unusual ideas or beliefs, open a tactful enquiry to explore this.

- 'Some of the questions I'm going to ask you might seem a little bit strange; don't let that worry you – they're questions we ask everyone.'
- 'Has anything strange or unusual been happening to you lately?'
- 'Is anyone giving you a hard time or trying to harm you in any way at the moment?'
- 'Have you noticed anything strange or suspicious lately?'

Judge how to proceed depending upon the patient's answers, responding sensitively

and exploring any positive replies. It is helpful to get a detailed account of the patient's experiences. To encourage this, show an interest in what your patient is saying without disagreeing even when they are describing something that clearly cannot be real. Above all, do not engage in arguments about the reality of their experience.

If the answer to the screening questions is very definitely no, do not persist in asking minutely detailed questions on all of the different types of delusion you can think of.

Assessing cognition

If your patient can give a good account of themselves, it is often unnecessary to undertake more formal cognitive testing. Carry out a full MMSE with older patients as a screen for dementia and those who appear to have disordered cognitive functioning.

Assessing insight

You may have gained a clear impression of the patient's level of insight during the interview. Direct your questions to assess exactly what the patient understands about their current condition.

- 'Do you think there is anything wrong with you at the moment? Do you think you are your normal self at the moment?'
- 'What do you think is wrong? What do you think is causing it? Do you think you are unwell in any way?'
- 'Do you think we could help you with your problems at the moment? Would you be happy for us to offer you some treatment for this problem?'

Try to weave these questions into your discussion at appropriately sensitive moments when they relate well to what the patient is saying (**Figure 2.8**).

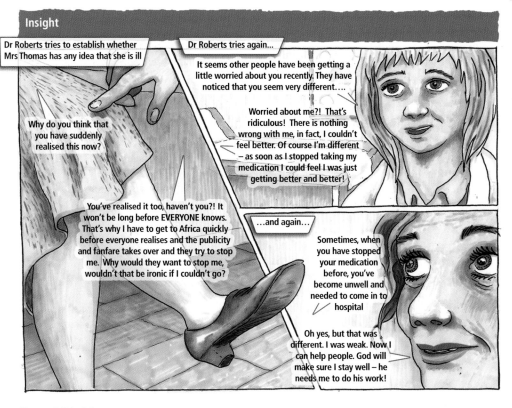

Figure 2.8 Insight.

> **Some patients are unwilling or unable to describe their thoughts, feelings and experiences.** It is still useful to follow the MSE systematically, making detailed notes on what you can describe. A relative or carer can often supply further details to give a more complete picture.

Physical examination

For all patients presenting with mental health issues, a full physical examination should also be carried out. This is important for a number of reasons:

- Coexisting physical disorders (such as Parkinson's disease and endocrine disorders sometimes contribute to the onset of psychiatric disorder. Conversely, if the patient has become too unwell to take their medications properly the physical disorder also demands attention

- Organic disorders sometimes present for the first time with psychiatric symptoms, e.g. brain tumours presenting with behavioural or mood changes, and hypothyroidism presenting with depressive symptoms
- Physical complications of psychiatric illness are often present, such as undisclosed deliberate self-harm, falls or injuries
- Psychotropic medication may need to be prescribed for the first time, requiring the patient's baseline physical health to be assessed. Existing physical conditions mean some medications are inappropriate; e.g. antipsychotic medication can cause extrapyramidal side effects in a person with Parkinson's disease
- Side-effects of psychotropic medications may arise; establishing the patient's baseline physical health allows for the monitoring of development of medication side-effects that the patient may be unaware of
- The physical health of people with sometimes chronically debilitating

psychiatric disorders is also often poor. Lifestyle factors such as poor diet, smoking and substance abuse have further detrimental effects. Patients' contact with medical services is sometimes sporadic and unpredictable, so presentation to the psychiatric services is a good opportunity to reassess the physical condition and treat any apparent physical disorders.

The physical examination includes an assessment of the patient's vital signs and an examination of the cardiovascular, respiratory and gastrointestinal systems. A full neurological system examination is also necessary as there is considerable overlap between neurological and psychiatric presentations.

Tailoring examination to history and presentation

More specific examination is indicated by details in the history:

■ A diagnosis of alcoholic liver disease may be supported by spider naevi, palmar erythema, jaundice and an enlarged liver
■ Side effects such as parkinsonism, tremor, rigidity, dystonia and tardive dyskinesia occur in patients on long-term antipsychotic medication.

Investigations

For most new patients there will need to be some basic laboratory investigations. Other investigations will be indicated by the history and MSE. If there is any indication of a serious underlying neurological cause for the presentation, or the symptoms presenting do not clearly fit any particular disorder, brain imaging is sometimes required to exclude central neurological lesions. Investigations are described in more details on pages 72–74.

Formulation of the case

Formulation describes the process of pulling together all the information from the history, MSE and physical examination into a succinct summary. This allows the findings to be

clearly communicated both verbally and in the clinical records.

> **A formulation is a structured, clear description of all the relevant information.** It must paint a clear picture of the patient's problems for other mental health workers.

The formulation consists of the following:

■ Case summary
■ Differential diagnosis
■ Risk
■ Aetiology
■ Management
■ Prognosis

Case summary

Describe the patient, including name, age, occupation, ethnicity, marital status and social circumstances. Then detail the history of the current episode of illness, followed by a concise summary of the relevant points of the history, MSE and physical examination.

Differential diagnosis

For each differential diagnosis, describe the evidence and reasons for and against it.

The differential diagnoses are presented according to the diagnostic hierarchy (see page 35). Organic states take precedence over all other diagnoses and must be ruled out before diagnosing a psychiatric disorder.

Ranking of disorders

Where two psychiatric disorders coexist, such as psychosis and drug abuse, note both. Describe the relationship between the two. When multiple disorders are present, they are ranked in the following order of precedence:

1. Psychosis
2. Affective disorders
3. Neuroses
4. Personality disorders

This order reflects the hierarchy of diagnosis (see page 35), which is based upon the severity of the disorders and directs treatment to the most severe disorders first. For example, if a patient meets the diagnostic criteria for schizophrenia but also has symptoms of anxiety, the diagnosis of schizophrenia will be prioritised for treatment. Successful treatment of the psychotic symptoms usually also results in a reduction of anxiety.

Risk

Describe risk in terms of the risk of harm the patient presents both to themself and to others. Include not only deliberate self-harm and suicidal ideas, but also self-neglect and exploitation by others as a consequence of mental state.

Risk to others arises as a direct result of violent acts carried out by the patient and also from the patient's inability to care for their dependents as they usually do. Describe the risk as low, moderate or high and give supporting evidence. Many psychiatric services also use risk assessment tools to quantify risk formally.

Aetiology

This is usually a complex mix of different factors that contribute to the patient being unwell at this particular time. It is sometimes frustratingly difficult to identify.

Consider the aetiological factors in terms of the biopsychosocial model and the '3 Ps' (see page 51, Table 2.5 and Figure 2.2). This provides a broader understanding of an individual's illness and a clearer picture of all of the contributory factors.

Management

This part of the formulation includes all aspects of a patient's care. Start with any special investigations on the basis of the history, MSE and physical examination. This may include consulting those closely involved in the patient's care and looking at medical records.

The management plan should address the issue of risk. It should, for example, ensure that a patient who is unable to look after themselves properly or has plans to harm themselves is cared for in an environment where that risk can be safely contained. Rather than focusing on just the medical management, refer to the elicited contributing factors of the biopsychosocial model to ensure that all the patient's needs are addressed. Consider both the immediate and longer term care needs.

Prognosis

Finish the formulation with a consideration of the patient's prognosis. Base this on the established evidence base for each disorder and on the features in the patient's own history and social circumstances that may affect the prognosis, such as a patient's refusal to take medication or attend for treatment. Consider both the immediate prognosis for this current episode of illness and the longer term consequences of the presenting condition.

Using the biopsychosocial approach in your formulation in your clinical examinations not only demonstrates that you are thinking about all aspects of a patient's problems, but also reminds you to cover areas you might forget under pressure.

Learning to synthesise and present a formulation takes practice, particularly in terms of knowing what information to leave out. Practise by using the headings given here. For each, focus only on the key information to give a clear picture of the presenting problem and management plan.

Investigations

Starter questions

Answers to the following questions are on page 96.

8. How do you decide which investigations to do for a patient with a psychiatric disorder?
9. Should all new patients with a psychotic illness have a CT scan of their brain?

Clinical skills and judgement are of paramount importance in psychiatry. They are supplemented by laboratory or imaging investigations as indicated by the findings of the psychiatric and physical examination. However, most new patients should undergo some basic laboratory investigations, as a basic health screen and to check for underlying disturbances that may contribute to a mental health disorder, e.g. hypothyroidism. It is also necessary to establish baseline cardiovascular, liver and renal function, and glucose and lipid levels, before commencing any medication which may impact upon these. Brain imaging may be required to exclude central neurological lesions, especially if the presenting symptoms do not clearly fit specific disorders or there are physical neurological symptoms.

Blood tests

Psychiatric indications for a blood test are summarised in **Table 2.16**.

Infection screening

This must be considered in all patients with confusion, delirium or dementia who may not be able to describe their symptoms. It includes, when indicated by the symptoms:

- A midstream urine sample, which is cultured or analysed for microorganisms
- A chest X-ray to seek lung infections
- Blood cultures to assess for sepsis
- Wound swabs to identify infections
- Sputum and stool specimens

Imaging and electrocardiography

Radiological scanning for neurological lesions is not a matter of routine but is performed where indicated, the presentation could have a physical rather than a psychiatric cause (**Table 2.17**).

An electrocardiogram (ECG) is indicated for patients with cardiovascular signs and those who are taking or are likely to be prescribed medications that have cardiovascular side effects.

Rating scales

Rating scales are sets of questions drawn together to elicit information about particular attitudes, attributes or disorders. They allow values to be assigned to specific items. They are useful for quantifying particular qualities and, in some cases, identifying the presence of a particular disorder such as depression. Examples include scales to detect psychiatric symptomatology in broad patient populations, and scales designed to assess and identify specific personality disorders or the degree of dementia.

Screening scales

Scales can be used in populations without psychiatric conditions to identify patients

	Blood and urine tests used in psychiatry	
Presentation	Test	Reason for performing investigation
Mood changes Psychotic symptoms Major psychiatric disorders	FBC	Check haemoglobin for anaemia
		Check WCC for infection
		Check MCV for macrocytosis with alcohol abuse
	U&E	Check renal function before prescribing
		Check for changes caused by medication
	LFTs	Check for raised γGT in alcohol misuse and establish baseline prior to prescribing
	TFTs	Check for hypo - or hyperthyroidism causing presenting symptoms, such as hypothyroidism causing cognitive dysfunction, depression or psychosis (myxoedema madness)
		Check for prescribed lithium, as it causes abnormal thyroid function
	Calcium and phosphate	Check for hypo - and hypercalcaemia causing presenting symptoms, such as pins and needles in the hands and feet
	B12 and folate	Check, if indicated, due to malnutrition/alcohol misuse/family history
	Urine drug screen	Check for any illicit substance misuse causing presenting symptoms (particularly likely with visual hallucinations).
	Syphilis serology (VDRL)	Check for syphilis if risk factors present
	Fasting glucose	Check for hypo- or hypoglyacaemia, which may be causing confusion and as baseline before commencing medications
	CRP	Check for raised CRP, which may indicate inflammatory or autoimmune conditions causing presenting symptoms
Memory loss	FBC	Check haemoglobin for anaemia
		Check WCC for infection
	U&E	Check for dehydration, renal failure, hyponatraemia
	LFTs	Check for alcohol misuse
	TFTs	Check for hypothyroidism causing memory impairment
	Calcium and phosphate	Check for hypercalcaemia causing confusion, impaired concentration and memory loss
	B12 and folate	Check for deficiencies as these cause reversible dementia
	Glucose	Check for undiagnosed or poorly controlled diabetes
	VDRL	Check for neurosyphilis
Eating disorders	FBC	Check for anaemia associated with chronic undernutrition
	U&E	Check Na^+ and K^+, especially where self-induced vomiting an issue
	LFTs	Check as part of initial metabolic assessment, including albumin level as sign of malnutrition
	TFTs	Check for hyperthyroidism in significant weight loss
	ESR	Check to exclude inflammatory/autoimmune disorders presenting with anorexia
	Phosphate	Check as baseline to guide treatment and refeeding, and in the assessment of general metabolic condition

Table 2.16 Blood and urine tests used in psychiatry and reasons for their use. CRP, C-reactive protein; ESR, erythrocyte sedimentation rate; FBC, full blood count; γGT, gamma-glutamyl transferase; LFTs, liver function tests; MCV, mean cell volume; TFTs, thyroid function tests; U & E, urea and electrolytes; VDRL, venereal disease research laboratory test; WCC, white cell count.

Indications for radiological investigations and ECG	
Investigation	Indication
EEG, CT, or MRI	Suspected intracranial pathology, e.g. haemorrhage, epileptic focus or space occupying lesion
	Focal neurological signs
	First onset of psychotic symptoms late in life (especially with any symptoms suggesting an organic basis to presentation, e.g. confusion or visual hallucinations)
	Prior to starting medication in dementia
ECG	Patients with a cardiac history Medications that affect QT interval, e.g. lithium and tricyclic antidepressants
	Patients with eating disorders who are likely to have bradycardia, arrhythmias, long QT interval
DEXA bone density scanning	Anorexia nervosa (bone density is likely to be low in chronic anorexia)

Table 2.17 Indications for radiological imaging and electrocardiography (ECG) in psychiatric presentations. CT, computed tomography; EEG, electroencephalography; MRI, magnetic resonance imaging

with undiagnosed mental illness. They include the Patient Health Questionnaire 9, widely used in general practice in the UK. They can also be used recurrently to monitor the progress of a disorder.

Detailed assessment

More sophisticated rating scales such as the Hamilton Anxiety and Depression scale and the MMSE offer more detailed assessments that are useful for diagnosing and monitoring the progress of psychiatric conditions.

Psychologists use detailed rating scales in patient assessments, including:

■ Personality inventories
■ Intelligence tests
■ Neuropsychological tests
■ Behavioural rating scales

Management options

Starter questions

Answers to the following questions are on page 96.

10. In what situations are psychological therapies used?
11. Can children take antidepressants?
12. Are all antipsychotic medications equally effective?

Psychiatric treatment includes psychological therapies such as counselling, and physical treatments such as medication. These are often used in combination. For example, psychotropic medications are usually prescribed with basic supportive counselling or a more complex psychological therapy.

Good psychiatric care offers a holistic approach to the patient, addressing all aspects of a patient's physical, psychological and social needs. This can be challenging, particularly in areas where psychiatric services are not well-established and limited options are available.

Psychological treatments

Psychological treatments are structured approaches to working with patients to address their difficulties using a variety of techniques. They are effective for many disorders, particularly anxiety and depression.

This section describes all forms of psychological treatment (**Table 2.18**). In practice psychotherapy is often seen as quite separate from other psychological treatments. In part, this is a because of the different scientific backgrounds of those practising each. Psychologists study all aspects of human behaviour, with an

Psychological therapies			
Type	Delivery	Underlying concepts	Indications
Counselling or supportive psychotherapy	Variable, usually brief	Explanation, reassurance, support and education. Identifies and resolves difficulties in everyday life	Minor mental health problems, mild anxieties and depression usually in primary care setting
Interpersonal therapy (IPT)	Weekly, 3–4 months	Improves skills and functioning in interpersonal relationships	Depression Eating disorders
Psychodynamic psychotherapy	At least once per week, prolonged periods	Makes unconscious processes conscious, i.e. addresses underlying conflicts that result in symptom formation Various orientations and approaches	Anxiety and inability to deal with stress, some depressions, difficulty sustaining relationships Sexual problems, bereavement, eating disorders, self harm, obsessional behaviour, panic attacks, phobia and addictions Personality disorders
Dialectical behavioural therapy	Weekly, variable periods	Incorporates components of CBT and mindfulness: teaches individuals skills of mindfulness, distress tolerance, emotion regulation and interpersonal effectiveness	Borderline personality disorder
Group psychotherapy	Weekly, months/ years	Helps patients identify maladaptive behaviours in supportive social setting and addresses emotional difficulties via group feedback	Relationship difficulties, some personality disorders, depression, anxiety and obsessive compulsive disorder, bereavement groups
Family therapy	From one session to many, over months	Directed at family as whole unit, improves family dynamic to improve the patient's condition	Wide range of presentations, mainly in children and adolescents
Therapeutic communities	9–18 months	Resident patients working together on social/emotional functioning, taking increasing responsibility for themselves	Severe personality disorders (antisocial and borderline)
Behaviour therapy	Weekly, 6–12 weeks	Changes maladaptive behaviours, based on learning theories (classical/operant conditioning)	Phobias, post traumatic stress disorder, anxiety, depression, obsessive compulsive disorder
Cognitive behavioural therapy (CBT)	Weekly, 6–12 weeks	Addresses negative thoughts, focusing on automatic thoughts and dysfunctional assumptions, feelings and behaviours (**Figure 2.9**) Goal-oriented, focuses on here and now rather than on development of problems	Depression Anxiety Eating disorders Some personality disorders

Table 2.18 Psychological therapies and their indications.

emphasis on measuring qualities and on the validity of specific behavioural and cognitive interventions. Psychotherapists come from a broad range of backgrounds and largely rely on the use of analytic approaches to working with a patient, with a strong theoretical background to their work but limited evidence.

The choice of psychological therapy depends on:

- The patient's diagnosis
- Their personal circumstances and beliefs regarding the different treatments
- What is available in their locality

Counselling

Counselling – supportive psychotherapy – refers to a range of basic psychological treatments for minor mental health problems. It is usually offered in primary care settings, is brief in duration and emphasises helping patients to manage their own difficulties.

It can be helpful with patients experiencing:

- Mild anxiety or depression
- Bereavement or an adverse life-event
- A new treatment that may have delayed efficacy, such as an antidepressant, which can take 2–3 weeks to have an effect
- Life crises that will not immediately resolve, such as illness in a close relative

Interpersonal therapy

Interpersonal therapy is based upon the central assumption that psychological symptoms, such as depressed mood, are understandable as responses to current difficulties in relationships. These responses in turn affect the quality of the relationships. It tends to be brief (around 12 sessions) and focuses on current problems rather than childhood or past incidents.

Interpersonal therapy can be useful with:

- Role disputes and conflicts, e.g. difficulty working with others
- Role transitions, e.g. following separation or divorce
- Deficits in interpersonal communication
- Dealing with loss and grief

Psychodynamic psychotherapy

Freud originated the model of psychoanalysis, which has subsequently developed into a variety of approaches (see page 6). Its central aim is to address long-standing difficulties, exploring behaviours and thinking patterns that contribute to the patient's current difficulties (**Table 2.19**). It is a specialised approach that requires lengthy training.

Techniques used in psychodynamic psychotherapy	
Technique	Description
Free association	Patient encouraged to allow their thoughts to wander freely from a relevant starting point to stimulate recall of repressed memories
Dream interpretation	Dreams discussed to unlock their meaning
Interpretation of transference	Transference is when a patient inappropriately transfers feelings from a previous, significant relationship onto the therapist, e.g. patient feels angry with the therapist who unconsciously reminds patient of cold, distant father
	Used to explore patient's feelings towards significant individuals in their past
Interpretation of counter-transference	Counter-transference occurs when the therapist experiences feelings from a significant previous relationship and transfers them onto the patient
Analysis of defence mechanisms	Analysis of mechanisms patients use to deal with unpleasant emotions which are unacceptable to the them and pushed into the unconscious mind by repression

Table 2.19 Techniques used in psychodynamic psychotherapy

To benefit patients need to be able to reflect and explore their own feelings and thoughts in some depth. They must be willing to explore difficult and upsetting issues in their past life.

Psychodynamic treatment can be brief, lasting just a few weeks, or long-term over months or years. Classically, patients were seen several times per week for an hour at a time, as it was thought that this frequency was required to maintain adequate momentum in exploring the patient's problems. More realistically, patients are seen weekly for a year or more.

Brief psychodynamic therapy is indicated for patients with:

- Low self-esteem
- Difficulties making relationships
- Eating disorders
- Sexual dysfunctions

Longer term psychotherapy, which may continue for a number of years, is indicated for patients with more entrenched problems that significantly impair their functioning in social and interpersonal contexts and in conjunction with a psychiatric disorder.

> Many of Freud's theories focusing on sexual drives have been refuted as too narrow in their explanation. Modern psychotherapy considers a much broader range of experiences which contribute to of the feelings, ideas and drives that underlie human behaviour, including many other early-life experiences.

Group psychotherapy

Group psychotherapy is used for many of the same purposes as individual therapy, including support, problem solving and psychodynamic psychotherapy. Similarly, its approach and method are varied according to the purpose of the treatment. It allows participants to observe their own responses to others in a group setting and to share experiences and gain support from others in similar circumstances. It is particularly helpful for those whose problems are related to their interactions with others, for people with personality disorders and for groups of patients with the same problem, such as self-harm.

Most groups meet once a week for an hour, with one or two therapists in the group. The group sometimes has a specific focus, for example bereavement, eating disorders or addictions. In the case of personality disorders, it aims to address a range of interpersonal and relationship difficulties as they present.

> The best known group therapy is Alcoholics Anonymous (AA). Founded in 1935 in the USA, AA has spread across the globe to diverse cultures. It offers a group therapeutic approach run for and by people who struggle with alcohol addiction.

Therapeutic communities

These are an intensive form of group psychotherapy that aims to modify personality and engrained behaviours. Participants live in a community together for 9–18 months, sharing structured daily activities and attending small and large groups in which they discuss problems and issues. Residents are encouraged to take increasing responsibility and help each other to identify their maladaptive responses and behaviours.

This approach is expensive, however, and is generally reserved for patients with antisocial or borderline personality disorders for whom other approaches have failed.

Behaviour therapy

Behaviour therapy treats symptoms and behaviours that are reinforced and maintained by the actions that the patient undertakes in an attempt to control their symptoms and diminish their own distress (**Table 2.20**). The therapies are based on classical learning theory (see page 25) and are usually delivered by clinical psychologists over a brief series of weekly sessions (i.e. 6–12 weeks).

Behaviour therapy techniques		
Technique	Description	Indication
Relaxation training	Lowers muscle tone and autonomic arousal using: ■ Relaxation of different muscle groups in turn ■ Slowing breathing ■ Emptying mind of worrying thoughts Taught in sessions, practised at home using relaxation tape	Anxiety disorders Some physical disorders, e.g. hypertension
Exposure	Gradual exposure in incremental fashion to feared and avoided situations (desensitisation) Rapid, sudden exposure to feared situation/stimulus (flooding)	Phobic disorders
Response prevention	Obsessional rituals diminish with prolonged attempts to resist them Rituals are suppressed until attendant anxiety has diminished, e.g. preventing patient from ritualistic hand-washing until anxiety subsides	Obsessional disorders
Thought stopping	Sudden, intrusive stimulus interrupts obsessional thought stream, e.g. sharply twanging an elastic band around wrist Patient eventually interrupts the thoughts without the band	Obsessional thoughts
Assertiveness training	Responses to social situations analysed and new techniques for managing difficult situations taught	Social anxiety Excessive shyness
Self-control	Increasing control over destructive behaviours Self-monitoring used with self-reinforcement, awarding self-rewards when goals are successfully reached	Over-eating Smoking Eating disorders
Contingency management	Control of abnormal behaviours reinforced by others Identifies and reduces reinforcers of abnormal behaviours, and rewards desirable behaviours	Temper tantrums Aggressive behaviour in children
Activity scheduling	Assist in overcoming negative behavioural responses in context of low mood Patients schedule particular activities, gradually increasing activity and stimulation	Depression Chronic schizophrenia

Table 2.20 Behaviour therapy techniques and their indications

Cognitive behavioural therapy

Cognitive behavioural therapy (CBT) combines behavioural and cognitive techniques to address disorders in which abnormal behaviours and negatively reinforcing cognitions (thoughts and thought patterns) occur together.

CBT was originally developed by the psychiatrist Aaron Beck in the 1960s. It has become increasingly popular in the last 20 years as a way of addressing:

■ Anxiety disorders
■ Mild to moderate depression
■ Eating disorders

■ Chronic schizophrenia, as an adjunctive treatment

CBT is based on the central assumption that how individuals think about things affects their feelings and behaviours (**Figure 2.9**).

Cognitive techniques include identifying:

■ Automatic thoughts – the thoughts that enter a patient's mind in response to specific situations
■ Dysfunctional assumptions – the faulty beliefs and rules by which people live, e.g. 'If I fail this exam, I am a useless person'

CBT is undertaken by trained professionals working with individuals or small groups

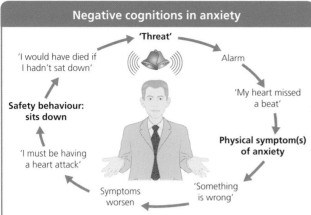

Negative cognitions in anxiety

'Threat'

'I would have died if I hadn't sat down'

Alarm

Safety behaviour: sits down

'My heart missed a beat'

'I must be having a heart attack'

Physical symptom(s) of anxiety

Symptoms worsen

'Something is wrong'

Figure 2.9 Negative cognitions in anxiety.

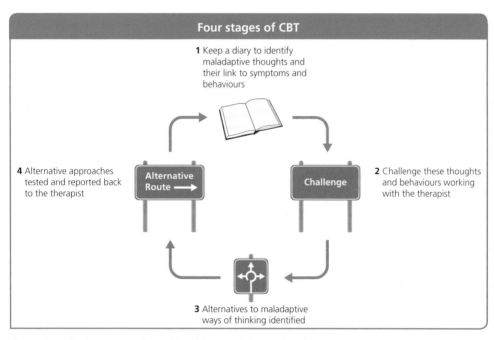

Four stages of CBT

1 Keep a diary to identify maladaptive thoughts and their link to symptoms and behaviours

4 Alternative approaches tested and reported back to the therapist

Alternative Route →

Challenge

2 Challenge these thoughts and behaviours working with the therapist

3 Alternatives to maladaptive ways of thinking identified

Figure 2.10 The four stages of cognitive behavioural therapy (CBT).

and is generally relatively brief (6–12 sessions on a weekly basis). There are four stages of CBT therapy (**Figure 2.10**).

Other psychological techniques are used alongside CBT, including teaching the patient techniques to distract them from their thoughts and routines, relaxation training, graded exposure to difficult situations and stimuli, and activity scheduling (in which patients are encouraged to establish a more productive daily routine to break negative patterns of behaviour).

Dialectical behaviour therapy

The psychologist Marsha Linehan developed dialetical behaviour therapy from the principles of CBT for patients with borderline personality disorder. Linehan observed that patients with a borderline personality disorder cannot identify their own emotional experiences and have a low tolerance for rejection and frustration.

The technique aims to help patients to cope with self-destructive behaviours such as deliberate self-harm, substance abuse and eating disorders. Patients are seen weekly. They are encouraged to learn strategies for coping with distressing situations, improving their relationships with others and decreasing their self-destructive behaviours. Approaches used include giving advice, using metaphor and story telling, and confrontation.

Pharmacological therapy

Antidepressant and antipsychotic medications have had a major impact on the practice of psychiatry, with millions of prescriptions being issued each year for depression alone. While psychotropic medication has undoubtedly had a positive impact in psychiatry, the fact that it is an easier option than lengthy psychological treatments creates its own problems. This is especially the case where specialist psychiatric provision is poor. In these circumstances, there is a risk that medications are over-prescribed, and other beneficial approaches to treatment are being tried. Furthermore, if supervision of patients is poor, prescriptions continue unchanged for many years. This results in over-treatment, and potentially in under-treatment as patient concordance is often poor in these circumstances.

> Psychotropic medications are drugs that have their principal effect on psychological symptoms.

Psychotropic medications are divided into groups according to their primary action. Several have secondary actions, making them useful for other purposes. For example, benzodiazepines are used in anaesthesia, the treatment of epilepsy and alcohol and drug detoxification.

Prescribing in psychiatry requires much more than simply knowing the facts and figures about the relevant drugs. Patients require a clear explanation of a medication's purpose and anticipated side effects, and should be told that it will not work immediately.

The main groups of psychotropic medications are:

- Antidepressants
- Antipsychotics
- Anxiolytics and hypnotics
- Mood-stabilising drugs
- Cognition-enhancing drugs

> Prescribing for patients with psychiatric disorders is an art as well as a science. Simply providing a prescription without a clear explanation and exploration of the patient's views is unlikely to be effective.

Concordance

Many patients do not take their medications as prescribed and do not fully appreciate the need to do so. Factors influencing concordance include level of insight, motivation, side effects and education (**Table 2.21**).

Patients may have concerns about taking medication (see Table 3.8). These must be identified and addressed to improve concordance. Patients must understand the reasons for taking their psychotropic medications and must have the opportunity to raise their concerns, explore their fears and understand all of the relevant facts.

> Make sure you know the name and major properties of one common drug from each of the categories described in this section, rather than trying to know minute details about all of them.

Antidepressant medications

The first antidepressant medication was imipramine, marketed as Tofranil in 1958. It was quickly followed by dozens of rivals, also tricyclic antidepressants, so-called because of their triple benzene ring molecular structure.

There is now a wide variety of antidepressants, in five main groups:

- Tricyclic antidepressants (TCAs)
- Selective serotonin reuptake inhibitors (SSRIs)

- Serotonin and noradrenaline (norepi-nephrine) reuptake inhibitors (SNRIs)
- Noradrenergic and specific serotonergic antidepressants (NaSSA)
- Monoamine oxidase inhibitors (MAOIs)

Most antidepressants have a long half-life, are given once a day and take around 2 weeks to begin to establish a therapeutic effect effect. They work by raising the concentrations of monoamine neurotransmitters (e.g. noradrenaline and serotonin) in the synaptic cleft (see page 18). It is not known why there is a delay in clinical effect when the neurochemical effect is almost immediate. Selectivity of the drug to target noradrenaline or 5-HT varies between groups of drugs and between compounds in the same group.

Withdrawal effects

Although they do not cause tolerance (requiring increasing doses to achieve the same effect) in the way that drugs of addiction do, antidepressants often provoke unpleasant withdrawal symptoms and must be withdrawn slowly at the end of the treatment period. Sudden withdrawal causes restlessness, insomnia, anxiety and nausea. Withdrawal effects are less problematic with fluoxetine as it has a very long half-life, and worse with some newer preparations such as paroxetine and venlafaxine.

> **All antidepressants should be tapered off slowly, gradually reducing the dose over many weeks.** Withdrawal effects, including gastrointestinal disturbances, headache, agitation, dizziness and insomnia can emerge with any antidepressant.

Serotonin syndrome

Serotonin syndrome (or toxicity) is a set of symptoms caused by excess serotonin levels. It can occur with high doses of a single drug or with multiple drugs that affect serotonin levels. It typically occurs when starting or increasing an antidepressant medication. It is also seen when switching to another antidepressant without a 'washout' period in between treatment courses.

Symptoms can develop rapidly and include:

- Agitation and restlessness
- Gastrointestinal symptoms including nausea, vomiting and diarrhoea
- Tachycardia and hypertension, with rapid changes in blood pressure
- A raised body temperature
- Poor coordination and hyperreflexia
- Hallucinations

Serotonin syndrome can be difficult to diagnose in the early stages because some of the symptoms can be confused with extreme anxiety. Physical causes of the presenting symptoms and neuroleptic malignant syndrome (see page 87) must always be ruled out first.

When serotonin syndrome is diagnosed, the offending medication(s) should be withdrawn. Some patients require observation and treatment in hospital. This may include treatment with benzodiazepines to decrease the agitation, restlessness and neurological symptoms, and intravenous fluids to restore and maintain hydration whilst the patient is acutely unwell. Acute treatment usually resolves the symptoms rapidly, i.e. within 24 hours.

> **Serotonin syndrome is potentially fatal.** It is best avoided by tapering and withdrawing antidepressant medications slowly, with a clear interval before starting the next.

Tricyclic antidepressants

These have largely been replaced by newer agents with less side-effects but they are the most effective treatment for some patients with severe depression.

TCAs should always be started at a moderate dose, gradually building up over 2 weeks; this minimises the side effects. Elderly patients and those with liver or kidney problems, in whom the metabolism of TCAs is decreased require lower doses.

Drugs in this group

Amitriptyline, clomipramine, imipramine and dothiepin are the most widely used compounds in this group.

Lofepramine is a modified TCA with fewer side effects and is less sedating.

Trazodone is a modified TCA with fewer anticholinergic side effects but is more sedating.

> **TCAs are the potentially most dangerous antidepressants in overdose**, as fatal arrhythmias develop in some cases.

Mode of action

TCAs block the reuptake of amines by competition for the binding site of the amine transporter (**Figure 2.11**). This raises monoamine concentrations in the synaptic cleft, increasing the stimulation of the postsynaptic receptors.

Indications

- Depression
- Anxiety disorders
- Obsessive compulsive disorder
- Nocturnal enuresis
- Chronic pain
- Prophylaxis of migraine
- Narcolepsy

Contraindications

- Agranulocytosis (exacerbated by TCAs)
- Severe liver damage (poor metabolism leads to toxicity)
- Glaucoma (exacerbated by anticholinergic side effects)
- Prostatic hypertrophy (exacerbated by anticholinergic side effects)

Adverse effects

Among the many adverse effects of TCAs is toxicity towards the cardiovascular system in overdose.

These include:

- Toxicity in overdose, causing ventricular fibrillation, conduction problems in the heart, low blood pressure, respiratory depression, convulsions, hallucinations and coma
- Antimuscarinic side effects producing a dry mouth, constipation, blurred vision, urinary retention, especially in patients with prostatic hypertrophy, and confusion in the elderly
- Antihistamine effects causing sedation
- α-Adrenoceptor blockade leading to hypotension
- Seizures, especially in patients with pre-existing epilepsy

Interactions

TCAs interact with:

- Antihypertensive medications, increasing the hypotensive effect of

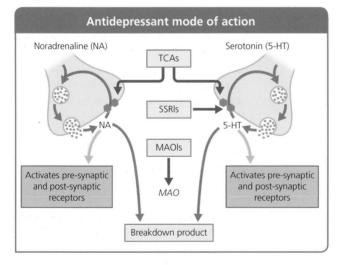

Figure 2.11 Mode of action of antidepressant drugs. MAO, monoamine oxidase; MAOIs, monoamine oxidase inhibitors; SSRIs, selective serotonin reuptake inhibitors; TCAs, tricyclic antidepressants.

angiotensin-converting enzyme inhibitors such as captopril
- MAOIs, potentially causing a hypertensive crisis
- Phenytoin, as they share a metabolic pathway – phenytoin levels may increase
- Adrenaline (epinephrine) and noradrenaline, as together they can cause severe hypertension

Selective serotonin reuptake inhibitors

These were developed to provide a safer medication than tricyclic TCAs. Their antidepressant efficacy is similar but they have fewer anticholinergic side effects. They are now more commonly prescribed than TCAs as they are also useful in a number of other psychiatric conditions, such as anxiety and eating disorders.

Drugs in this group

Fluoxetine, fluvoxamine, paroxetine, sertraline, citalopram and escitalopram are included in this group.

Mode of action

These drugs selectively inhibit the reuptake of serotonin into the presynaptic neurone, raising synaptic levels.

Indications

- Depression
- Anxiety disorders
- Obsessive compulsive disorder
- Bulimia nervosa

Adverse effects

These include:

- Nausea and vomiting
- Diarrhoea
- Sexual dysfunction
- Insomnia
- Tremor
- Headache

SSRIs should be used with caution in children as the adverse events may outweigh the benefits, for example some studies have suggested that antidepressants increase the risk of suicide in adolescents.

Interactions

SSRIs should not be prescribed with MAOIs as this can produce serotonin syndrome (see page 81).

Serotonin and noradrenaline reuptake inhibitors

Drugs in this group

Venlafaxine and duloxetine are included in this group.

Mode of action

SNRIs block presynaptic reuptake pumps for noradrenaline and serotonin. They have little effect on muscarinic, histaminergic or α-adrenergic neurones.

Indications

- Major depression
- Generalised anxiety disorder
- Diabetic neuropathy (duloxetine)
- Urinary stress incontinence (duloxetine)

Higher doses of venlaxfaxine (above 150 mg daily) are prescribed only via psychiatry services with regular outpatient supervision.

Contraindications

SNRIs are contraindicated in patients with:

- A high risk of cardiac arrhythmias
- Uncontrolled hypertension

SNRIs are not recommended in children because they may increase the suicide rate.

Adverse effects

The side effects are similar to SSRIs and include:

- Nausea and vomiting
- Diarrhoea
- Sexual dysfunction
- Insomnia
- Tremor
- Headache

Venlafaxine lacks the sedative and antimuscarinic side effects of TCAs but has a higher risk of withdrawal effects than most other antidepressants. It must always be withdrawn gradually over several weeks.

Noradrenergic and specific serotonergic antidepressants (NaSSAs)

These specifically target central serotonergic synapses so have fewer peripheral side effects seen with SSRIs. Unlike SSRIs, NaSSAs cause sedation, which can be useful in treating patients with insomnia as a symptom of their depression.

Drugs in this group

Mirtazapine is one of the drugs in this group.

Mode of action

NaSSAs antagonise presynaptic α_2-adrenoceptors, which increases central noradrenergic and serotonergic transmission.

Indications

NaSSAs are used to treat major depression.

Adverse effects

These include:

■ Increased appetite and weight gain
■ Postural hypotension
■ Peripheral oedema
■ Sedation, tiredness and drowsiness

Rarely, mirtazapine may cause blood disorders; patients should be advised to report fevers or sore throats or other signs of infections during treatment.

Monoamine oxidase inhibitors

These were discovered around the same time as TCAs. In practice, MAOIs are rarely used as a first-choice because of their side effects and interactions with food and medications. They are occasionally used for patients who have responded well to them in the past or in whom other antidepressants have failed.

They are usually prescribed by psychiatrists rather than general practitioners. Patients must be made fully aware of the lists of interactions and must be highly motivated to adhere to a diet that excludes certain foods.

Drugs in this group

Phenelzine, isocarboxazid and tranylcypromine are all irreversible MAOIs, which means that they permanently bind covalently to monoamine oxidase.

Moclobemide is a reversible MAOI.

Mode of action

MAOIs inhibit the mitochondrial enzyme monoamine oxidase. In the neurones, this decreases the breakdown (via oxidation) of monoamines and raises their levels in the synaptic cleft increasing monoaminergic.

The effect of the early irreversible MAOIs continues until new enzyme is produced, which is up to 2 weeks after they have been discontinued.

Indications

■ Depression, especially atypical depression that has not responded to other antidepressants
■ Anxiety disorders

Contraindications

MAOIs are contraindicated in patients with:

■ Liver disease
■ Cerebrovascular disease
■ Phaeochromocytoma
■ Congestive cardiac failure
■ Conditions that require the prescription of any of the drugs listed in the interactions section.

Adverse effects

These include:

■ Hypotension
■ Tremors, insomnia
■ Increased appetite and weight gain
■ Tyramine–cheese reaction

Interactions

MAOIs interfere with the enzymes responsible for the breakdown of:

■ Barbiturates
■ Phenytoin
■ Antiparkinsonian drugs
■ Insulin and oral hypoglycaemics
■ Morphine, pethidine and cocaine
■ Alcohol

The effect of these drugs is therefore potentiated by MAOIs so they should not be prescribed together.

In addition, a number of drugs with a hypertensive effect are metabolised by monoamine oxidase. These should also be avoided as they will produce an exaggerated hypertensive effect in combination with MAOIs. They include:

- Adrenaline and noradrenaline
- Amphetamine
- Fenfluramine
- L-Dopa and dopamine

Combination with TCAs can lead to serotonin syndrome.

MAOIs also inhibit the metabolism of tyramine, which is present in various foods. If large amounts of tyramine are consumed in conjunction with MAOIs, blood pressure rises rapidly leading to a hypertensive crisis that potentially results in a cerebral haemorrhage.

> **Patients being prescribed MAOIs must be advised to avoid all foods containing tyramine, such as:**
>
> - Most cheeses
> - Meat (Bovril) and yeast (Marmite) extracts
> - Smoked or pickled fish
> - Hung poultry or game
> - Some red wines and beer

Antipsychotic medications

Antipsychotic drugs reduce the purposeless overactivity, hallucinations, delusions and abnormal perceptions that are associated with schizophrenia, mania and other psychotic disorders, including organic psychoses.

The first antipsychotic, chlorpromazine, was discovered in the early 1950s. It had a huge social impact, allowing patients who had previously been held for many years in large asylums to be looked after in the community (**Figure 2.12**).

Antipsychotic drugs block dopamine receptors to varying degrees. This variation in blockage probably underlies their different therapeutic effects and variable extrapyramidal side effects. The original, or 'conventional', antipsychotics were limited by the severity of these side effects, leading to the push to develop a second generation of 'atypical' antipsychotics. Atypical antipsychotics are also active as serotonin-2A receptor antagonists and have a different side effect profile from the original antipsychotics.

> **National Institute for Health and Care Excellence guidelines** recommend that atypical antipsychotics should be the first-line treatment for newly diagnosed schizophrenia ('first-episode schizophrenia', FEP)

Prescribing antipsychotics

Antipsychotic medication is usually initiated as a new prescription by specialist psychiatric practitioners. Because of the severity and frequency of their side effects, weight, fasting blood sugar, full blood count, lipids, urea and electrolytes and liver function tests should be checked as baseline measurements before

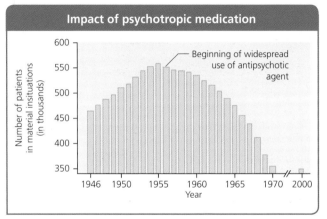

Impact of psychotropic medication

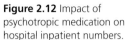

Figure 2.12 Impact of psychotropic medication on hospital inpatient numbers.

medications are started. These must be rechecked at least annually, depending on the drug used and the patient's health.

Patients often have to take these medications for many months or years so the side effects may limit their acceptability (**Table 2.22**). The minimum effective dose should therefore be used. Patients should be regularly monitored to assess their mental state and the presence of side effects.

There is a high risk of relapse if antipsychotic medication is stopped suddenly. Withdrawal should always be done slowly and under close monitoring by outpatient psychiatric services.

> **Patients must be warned about weight gain as a side effect of antipsychotic agents.** They must be given appropriate support and dietary advice to avoid significant weight gain.

Conventional antipsychotics

These are the first-generation antipsychotic preparations, also called 'typical' antipsychotics. They bind very strongly to dopamine receptors.

Side effects of antidopaminergic medication		
Symptom	Description	Management
Acute dystonia	Occurs early in treatment, presents with: ■ Torticollis ■ Tongue protrusion ■ Grimacing ■ Blepharospasm ■ Arching of the spine	Anticholinergic medication (e.g. biperiden)
Akathisia	Unpleasant subjective sensation of needing to keep limbs constantly moving Appears within 2 weeks of starting treatment	Reduce dose
Parkinsonian symptoms	The most frequent EPSE. Appear after weeks of treatment with: ■ Akinesia ■ Stooped posture ■ Rigidity in the muscles ■ Coarse tremor	Reduce dose May require antimuscarinic drug (e.g. procyclidine) for treatment (but should be avoided in the long term as it increases the risk of tardive dyskinesia)
Tardive dyskinesia	Late side-effect in 15% of patients on long-term antipsychotic medication: ■ Chewing and sucking movements ■ Grimacing ■ Akathisia ■ Choreoathetoid movements	May take months, or never improve after medication is stopped Prescribe at lowest effective dose to avoid development Limited effective treatment Very stigmatising
Hormonal changes	Dopamine blockade in the tuberoinfundibular pathway causes: ■ Raised prolactin levels ■ Amenorrhoea ■ Galactorrhoea ■ Gynaecomastia	Reduce dose or change to an atypical antipsychotic (e.g. olanzapine)

Table 2.22 Side effects of antidopaminergic medication. EPSE, extrapyramidal side effect

Drugs in this group

Chlorpromazine, thioridazine, trifluoperazine, haloperidol and sulpiride are included in this group.

Mode of action

Conventional antipsychotic medications work by blocking D_2 receptors in the mesolimbic system of the brain (see page 20). Unfortunately, they also block D_2 receptors in the rest of the brain. This causes:

- Motor symptoms (extrapyramidal symptoms, Figure 4.3) in the nigrostriatal pathway
- Hormonal symptoms (Figure 4.3) via blockade in the tuberoinfundibular pathway

They also have some activity at muscarinic, histaminergic and α-adrenergic receptors, causing further side effects by their blockade (**Figure 2.13**).

Indications

- Schizophrenia and schizoaffective disorders
- Acute psychotic disorders
- Depressive illness with psychotic features
- Mania with psychotic symptoms
- Organic psychoses
- Acute confusional states
- Severe anxiety (for a few days only, in addition to psychological treatment)
- Psychomotor agitation or excitement (adjunctive treatment for a few days only)

They are also used in non-psychiatric disorders such as motor tic disorders (Gilles de la Tourette syndrome), nausea and vomiting, (especially in palliative care) severe pruritis, intractable hiccoughs.

> **Neuroleptic malignant syndrome is a rare, potentially fatal complication of antipsychotic drugs.** It begins suddenly, usually within the first 10 days of treatment. The patient has fluctuating levels of consciousness, hyperthermia, muscular rigidity and autonomic disturbance with rapidly fluctuating pulse and blood pressure. It is fatal in about 20% of cases. Treatment is supportive by cooling the patient, maintaining hydration and preventing secondary complications such as respiratory or renal failure.

Contraindications

These include:

- Myasthenia gravis
- Addison's disease
- Glaucoma
- Past or current bone marrow depression

They should also be used with caution in patients with cardiovascular disease, Parkinson's disease and liver disease. Patients should be assessed by a specialist at least annually.

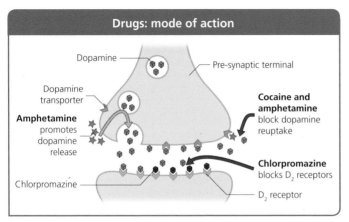

Drugs: mode of action

Dopamine

Pre-synaptic terminal

Dopamine transporter

Cocaine and amphetamine block dopamine reuptake

Amphetamine promotes dopamine release

Chlorpromazine blocks D_2 receptors

Chlorpromazine

D_2 receptor

Figure 2.13 Mode of action of antipsychotic drugs. D_2, dopamine type 2.

Adverse effects

These are related to the different receptor systems that are blocked:

- Antidopaminergic effects are the most troublesome and frequent side effects (**Table 2.17**)
- Weight gain is a common feature of all antipsychotic medications, probably due to serotonergic blockade in the hypothalamus
- Antiadrenergic effects include postural hypotension, sexual side effects (including decreased arousal and impotence), a dry mouth, urinary symptoms, constipation, blurred vision and precipitation of glaucoma
- Neuroleptic malignant syndrome due to dopaminergic blockade
- Demotivation, lack of interest and apathy – dose-dependent consequences of long-term treatment due to mesolimbic dopaminergic blockade. Patients may be unable to motivate themselves to work, form relationships or even look after their own basic needs

Miscellaneous other effects include:

- Sedation
- Sexual side effects
- Cardiac arrhythmias
- Hypothermia
- Exacerbation of epilepsy
- Photosensitivity
- Abnormal pigmentation of the skin

Atypical antipsychotics

These second-generation or 'atypical antipsychotics were developed with the aim of producing effective drugs that have fewer extrapyramidal side effects than the conventional medications. As a result, they are generally better tolerated than the conventional drugs. They may also perform better than conventional antipsychotics in reducing the negative symptoms of schizophrenia.

Drugs in this group

Olanzapine, risperidone, aripiprazole, quetiapine , lurasidone and paliperidone are included in this group.

Mode of action

These agents vary in the extent to which they bind to D_2 and D_4 dopamine receptors. They also have a range of activities at 5-HT$_2$, α_1-adrenoceptors and muscarinic receptors. Although the precise mechanism of action is unclear, the balance between their D_2 and 5-HT$_2$ activity may contribute to their therapeutic actions.

Indications

- Schizophrenia
- Mania
- Agitation and acutely disturbed behaviour (in psychotic disorders)
- Organic psychoses

Adverse effects

Atypical antipsychotics are much less likely to cause movement disorders and hormonal disorders than conventional antipsychotics. However, they vary considerably in the other side effects they cause (**Table 2.23**). More than 50% of people with schizophrenia are overweight or obese. Atypical antipsychotics, especially olanzapine and clozapine, contribute to weight gain more significantly than other antipsychotics. Weight is monitored carefully in all patients prescribed these medications. Weight management programmes and exercise are introduced soon after prescription, and ultimately a change of medication is required if weight gain is excessive.

> **In elderly patients suffering from dementia, antipsychotic drugs have a small increased risk of stroke or transient ischaemic attack.** They should only be used in elderly patients to treat severe psychotic symptoms and only be prescribed in small doses, usually less than half the recommended adult dose.

Clozapine

This atypical antipsychotic was originally trialled in the 1960s. Some patients suffered fatal hyperthermia and others developed fatal agranulocytosis, so it was withdrawn. Reintroduced in the 1980s for use only in

Adverse effects of atypical antipsychotic medications

Side effect	Adverse effect	Causative agents
Weight-gain	Can be extreme Viewed as the most significant negative effect	Most likely with olanzapine and clozapine
Hormonal changes	Less problematic than with conventional antipsychotics Raised prolactin levels causing problems such as loss of libido and breast enlargement (in men and women)	Least likely with clozapine and quetiapine Most likely with risperidone
Hypotension	Caused by sympathetic blockade Particularly noticeable if medication started at too high a dose	Most likely with quetiapine, olanzapine and clozapine
Sedation	Can be a useful side-effect for patients with troublesome insomnia	Most likely with olanzapine, quetiapine and clozapine
Epilepsy	Rare but all antipsychotics can trigger it in susceptible patients	Most likely with clozapine
Extrapyramidal effects	Extremely limiting and distressing movement problems	Least likely with quetiapine and clozapine Most likely with risperidone
Bed-wetting	Starts early in treatment in 50% of patients	Clozapine only
Hyperglycaemia and hyperlipidaemia	Likely in patients with high risk of developing diabetes	Greatest with olanzapine and clozapine

Table 2.23 Adverse effects of atypical antipsychotic medications

treatment-resistant schizophrenia, it is only dispensed directly to patients specifically registered for its prescription, and regular white cell counts are required.

Around 30% of patients who have not responded to other antipsychotic medications respond to clozapine.

Mode of action
Clozapine has mixed receptor activity, with potent action on serotonergic receptors in addition to dopamine blockade. It is a less potent dopamine blocker than many other antipsychotics so is less likely to cause extrapyramidal side effects.

Indications

- Treatment-resistant schizophrenia: schizophrenia that has failed to respond adequately to at least two other antipsychotic medications (at least one of which being atypical) despite adherence to the correct regimen and in the absence of substance abuse)
- Psychosis in Parkinson's disease

Contraindications
Patients with a history of:

- Neutropenia
- Severe cardiac disorders
- Bone marrow disorders
- Paralytic ileus
- Uncontrolled epilepsy
- Alcoholic psychosis

Adverse effects

- Agranulocytosis – neutropenia and potentially fatal agranulocytosis due to the risk of severe infections and septicaemia
- Myocarditis and cardiomyopathy, sometimes fatal (usually in the first 2 months). Reduced blood pressure and increases in heart rate also occur
- Gastrointestinal obstruction
- Hypersalivation
- Weight gain
- Hyperlipidaemia, hypercholesterolaemia, hyperglycaemia (and occasionally diabetes)

Monitoring

It is mandatory to monitor the white cell count weekly for 18 weeks, then fortnightly for 1 year and at least monthly thereafter. Clozapine must be discontinued if WBC <3000/mm³.

Depot antipsychotic medications

These are administered by intramuscular injection every 2–4 weeks. They are reserved for patients who are unable to maintain a regular commitment to oral medication and therefore have a significant risk of relapse. Although most of these drugs are typical antipsychotics, atypical antipsychotics are now also available in this form. The chemical effects of these preparations are the same as the oral compounds.

Anxiolytics and hypnotics

Anxiolytics and hypnotics work on the central nervous system to treat anxiety and insomnia. They should be used sparingly and ideally in conjunction with a psychological approach aimed at addressing the root cause of the anxiety. Treatment should be brief, i.e. less than a few days and certainly under 3 weeks, due to the risk of tolerance and dependence. This is, especially important with benzodiazepines.

Benzodiazepines

As benzodiazepines are extremely addictive; an alternative should be considered wherever possible. However, they are still prescribed for a few days immediately after traumatic events. Some antidepressant medications are now licensed for use in anxiety and are frequently used instead, particularly in chronic anxiety.

Withdrawal effects occur on discontinuation if benzodiazepines have been prescribed continuously for more than a few weeks. They include:

- Apprehension and anxiety
- Insomnia
- Tremor
- Muscle twitching
- Rarely, seizures

Short-acting compounds (half-life <6 hours) are prescribed for intermittent anxiety or initial insomnia and used in anaesthesia,

particularly as a sedative before surgery. Longer acting compounds (half-life 10–30 hours) are prescribed for constant anxiety and alcohol withdrawal, but only for short periods of time. They are metabolised more slowly and have increased half-lives in elderly patients due to the diminished metabolism of drugs.

Benzodiazepines should be tapered gradually to minimise withdrawal symptoms:

- Switch to a long-acting preparation first

- Taper the dose off slowly over 6–8 weeks

Drugs in this group

These include long-acting compounds, for example diazepam, nitrazepam and chlordiazepoxide, and short-acting compounds such as temazepam and lorazepam.

Mode of action

Benzodiazepines attach to specific binding sites on γ-aminobutyric acid (GABA) receptors in the central nervous system. This binding increases (i.e. potentiates) the inhibitory effect that results when GABA binds to its receptor (**Figure 2.14**).

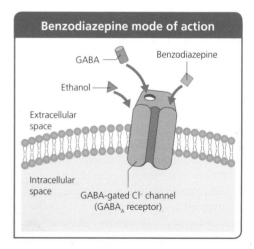

Benzodiazepine mode of action

GABA

Benzodiazepine

Ethanol

Extracellular space

Intracellular space

GABA-gated Cl⁻ channel (GABA$_A$ receptor)

Figure 2.14 Mode of action of benzodiazepines. GABA, γ-aminobutyric acid.

Indications

- Anxiety
- Sedation or sleep induction
- Muscle relaxation
- For its anticonvulsant effect
- Anterograde amnesia
- Rapid tranquillisation (in acute psychiatric disturbance)
- Mania
- Detoxification from alcohol

Adverse effects

- Drowsiness
- Confusion
- Forgetfulness
- Impairment of motor control (at higher doses)
- Tolerance and dependence
- Respiratory depression in conjunction with alcohol

Short-acting hypnotics

These drugs aim to induce sleep with less hangover and without dependence. However, dependence has been reported and they are therefore not licensed for long-term use.

> The ideal hypnotic would increase the length and quality of sleep, maintain the normal structure and pattern of sleep and cause no hangover. No current drugs achieve this. Side effects and dependence are problematic so no hypnotics should be prescribed continuously for longer than a couple of weeks.

Drugs in this group

Zopiclone and zolpidem are included in this group.

Mode of action

The mechanism of action of these hypnotics is very similar to that of benzodiazepines. They bind to the benzodiazepine-binding sites on the GABA receptors, increasing the inhibitory effect of GABA in the central nervous system. However, they appear to have less affinity for the GABAergic synapses involved in cognitive functioning such as memory.

They have a short duration of action and therefore do not accumulate, particularly in elderly patients.

Indications

They are used for the short-term treatment of insomnia (up to 2 weeks).

Adverse effects

These include:

- A metallic taste
- Heartburn
- Daytime drowsiness
- Rebound insomnia on withdrawal

5-HT1$_A$ agonists

Azapirones are 5HT1$_A$ agonists with an anti-anxiety effect. They do not appear to lead to tolerance or dependence. Their actions are slower and less powerful than those of benzodiazepines, taking a couple of weeks to become effective in relieving anxiety.

They are not an effective sedative or muscle relaxant.

Drugs in this group

Buspirone is a member of this group.

Mode of action

5-HT1$_A$ agonists work by activating the pre-synaptic 5-HT1$_A$ autoreceptors, which are autoinhibitory, especially in the dorsal raphe nucleus which has a role in arousal, and patterns of sleep and wakening.

Indications

These drugs reduce anxiety without sedation or motor incoordination.

Adverse effects

- Nausea
- Giddiness
- Restlessness
- Headache

β-Adrenergic antagonists

β-Adrenergic antagonists (beta-blockers) are primarily used in the treatment of hypertension, angina and cardiac arrhythmias as well as in chronic anxiety disorders. They have no central effect on anxiety so do not relieve its psychological component. However, they can relieve the peripheral manifestations such as palpitation and tremor.

Drugs in this group

Propranolol and atenolol are included in this group.

Mode of action

β-Adrenergic antagonists act by blocking the effect of endogenous mediators at the β-adrenoceptors, functioning at these receptors as competitive antagonists.

Indications

These are used in chronic anxiety disorders (where the physical symptoms predominate) and performance anxiety (as in performing arts and sports).

Contraindications

- Asthma
- A history of bronchospasm or obstructive airways disease
- Cardiac failure
- Heart block
- A low systolic blood pressure (below 90 mmHg)
- A low pulse rate (below 60 bpm)

Contraindications

These include:

- Shortness of breath
- Reduced circulation to the extremities (cold fingers and toes)
- Insomnia and nightmares
- Tiredness, lassitude and muscle weakness

Mood stabilisers

Mood stabilisers are used to prevent the recurrence of episodes of bipolar disorder. The medications within this group are not a discrete pharmacological class.

The most frequently used mood stabilisers are lithium and various anticonvulsant medications.

Lithium

Lithium has been used since 1949 for treating and preventing recurrences of mania.

Mode of action

Lithium affects a huge range of physiological processes but it is unclear which is responsible for its therapeutic effects in affective disorders. It is a monovalent cation that mimics the role of sodium in excitable tissues. It appears to affect the neurotransmitter-induced activation of second-messenger systems in the cell. Lithium had a very narrow therapeutic window and requires weekly to monthly monitoring of blood levels (see below).

> **The sudden withdrawal of lithium usually provokes a rapid deterioration in mental state.** Some patients show irritability and emotional lability, and a rapid relapse into a manic mood state. Lithium should be discontinued gradually and avoided in patients whose compliance is so erratic that they frequently miss or discontinue their medication.

Indications

- Acute mania
- Prophylaxis of bipolar disorder
- Treatment-resistant depression

Contraindications

- The first trimester of pregnancy (because of increased rates of heart abnormalities in the fetus)
- Renal failure
- Cardiac failure or recent myocardial infarction

Adverse effects

These include:

- Nausea and vomiting
- Tremor

- Thirst, polydipsia and polyuria
- Renal effects
- Thyroid dysfunction
- Weight gain
- Central nervous system (especially cerebellar) toxicity

> **Lithium toxicity is potentially fatal.**
> It is usually provoked by drugs that interfere with its excretion, including non-steroidal anti-inflammatory drugs and diuretics. It is also caused by lithium overdose and the significant changes in homeostatic salt balance that arise with vomiting or diarrhoea. Urgent medical care is required for rehydration. In severe cases, dialysis is used to rapidly remove the lithium from the blood.

Monitoring

Monitoring of all patients taking lithium is essential to maintain a therapeutic level and minimise its potential adverse effects, particularly on the kidneys and thyroid. Basic investigations prior to commencing treatment include:

- A full blood count
- Renal function tests
- Thyroid function tests
- A pregnancy test where appropriate
- An ECG

These establish baseline renal and thyroid function, and exclude cardiac problems, including recent infarcts, which may be exacerbated by lithium.

Once the patient has started lithium, blood assays are done weekly to monitor the lithium level. When the level has stabilised, it is checked every 3 months, with an annual assay of renal and thyroid function. Therapeutic levels are in the range of 0.4–0.8 mmol/L. Symptoms of toxicity start to appear above 1.5 mmol/L.

> **Any patient started on lithium must be given a clear explanation of several factors:**
>
> - The common side effects
> - The necessity of taking the exact dosage prescribed
> - The toxic effects the patient should look out for and report
> - Advice about when it is justifiable to stop taking lithium and contact their medical practitioner
> - The importance of regular blood monitoring
> - Factors that can cause an increase in lithium levels, e.g. gastroenteritis or dehydration, renal infections and use of commonly available medications such as non-steroidal anti-inflammatory drugs
>
> With the patient's consent, it is often wise to include a close family member in this discussion.

Interactions

Lithium concentrations may be increased by:

- Haloperidol
- Thiazide diuretics
- Muscle relaxants – if possible, lithium should be tapered off before surgery requiring the use of these agents as they will be potentiated by lithium
- Non-steroidal anti-inflammatory drugs
- Some antibiotics, e.g. metronidazole
- Some antihypertensive drugs, e.g. angiotensin-converting enzyme inhibitors

Anticonvulsants

These are widely prescribed to prevent seizures in epilepsy but they are being increasingly used as mood stabilisers. The first to be used for the prophylaxis of bipolar affective disorder was carbamazepine, followed by sodium valproate. Newer anticonvulsants, such as lamotrigine, appear to be more antidepressant than antimanic. These compounds do not share a common mode of action and are only prescribed with regular psychiatric outpatient follow-up.

Cognition-enhancing drugs

Cognition-enhancing drugs were first introduced in the 1990s and are primarily used to treat mild to moderate Alzheimer's disease. In the UK, they are currently only prescribed for patients in the care of specialist psychiatric services. Their benefit in individual patients is evaluated by regular cognitive assessments. Up to 50% of patients show a slower rate of cognitive decline. The drugs is discontinued in patients who continue to decline rapidly.

Drugs in this group

Donepezil, galantamine, rivastigmine and memantine are included in this group.

Mode of action

They are reversible inhibitors of acetylcholinesterase, leading to an increased level and duration of action of acetylcholine, the neurotransmitter which is deficient in this disorder. Galantamine is also an agonist at the nicotinic receptor.

Memantine is an antagonist at the N-methyl-D-aspartate receptor, affecting glutamate transmission.

Indications

- In mild to moderate dementia in Alzheimer's disease: donepezil, galantamine or rivastigmine
- In moderate dementia in Alzheimer's disease: memantine is prescribed to patients who cannot tolerate anticholinesterase inhibitors
- In severe dementia: memantine

There is currently no good evidence that these days are effective in frontotemporal dementia (including Pick's disease) and the evidence for use in Lewy body dementia remains inconclusive.

Adverse effects

These include:

- Anorexia

- Nausea and vomiting
- Diarrhoea
- Insomnia
- Fatigue

Physical treatments

Physical treatments in psychiatry have largely been discontinued since the introduction of psychotropic medications. Historic treatments, such as insulin coma treatment for schizophrenia, had limited efficacy and unacceptable side-effects, including neurological damage. Electroconvulsive therapy is the only physical treatment currently in regular use.

Electroconvulsive therapy

Electroconvulsive therapy (ECT) involves the administration of a short-acting anaesthetic followed by the induction of a controlled, modified seizure. An electrical charge is applied via electrodes to the patient's temples. ECT is usually administered two or three times per week for between four and 12 treatments.

ECT has retained a negative reputation in the media, as most portrayals are based on the early decades of its administration. Modern anaesthesia and carefully controlled administration of electrical charge have made modern ECT a much safer and less frightening treatment. Its use is nowadays more strictly controlled. For example, procedures relating to consent have been tightened up and accreditation schemes for centres administering ECT have been developed. ECT retains a role in psychiatry in the treatment of:

- Severe depression, particularly psychotic depression
- Treatment-resistant depression
- Depression in which there is a significant suicide risk
- Puerperal psychosis
- Acute treatment-resistant mania
- Acute schizophrenia with catatonic or affective features

It is only used after adequate attempts with other treatments have failed or if the disorder is life threatening.

Although its mode of action remains poorly understood, the efficacy of ECT equals that of antidepressants and its onset of action is faster, which can be particularly important where there is a high risk to the patient.

Functional MRI studies suggest that ECT decreases frontal cortex perfusion, metabolism and functional connections to other areas, and increases hippocampal volume and neuronal chemical metabolites.

Adverse effects include:

- Headaches post-treatment
- Transient memory impairment
- More rarely, long-term loss of some memories

ECT is contraindicated in:

- Patients for whom anaesthetics are contraindicated
- Conditions where the rises in blood pressure and heart rate that occur during treatment are dangerous, such as raised intracranial pressure for any reason, cerebral aneurysms or recent myocardial infarction

Answers to starter questions

1. Tact and judgement are always required when asking personal questions and sometimes, for example with a very agitated or disturbed patient, it would not be appropriate to ask at all. Signposting questions and asking permission is helpful, alerting the patient to the fact that you are going to ask some difficult questions.

2. Many psychiatric disorders have a genetic contribution to their aetiology, so a family history will provide important information about the patient's background, helping to identify any disorders which run in their family.

3. The psychiatric history covers everything of relevance to the patient and their life up to and including the time of their presentation. The mental state examination (MSE) describes the patient's psychological functioning at the specific moment of assessment in a structured way. The MSE is equivalent to physical examinations in other specialties and plays a major role in establishing the patient's diagnosis.

4. The three Ps are the predisposing, precipitating and perpetuating factors in a patient's history. They describe the factors which have made the patient more likely to develop a certain illness, caused the illness to appear at a specific time and prevent the patient from getting better, respectively. Identifying these aetiological factors and addressing them with appropriate treatments helps the patient to recover and prevents further episodes of illness.

5. Hallucinations have no evident external stimulus for their creation, whereas illusions focus on a real physical stimulus that is misperceived or misinterpreted by the patient.

6. Hallucinations are not always abnormal. Healthy people can also experience them, such as when we hear something shouted out at the point when we are falling asleep or waking up.

7. Disorders which appear to be psychiatric often have an underlying physical cause, for example depression arising as a consequence of thyroid disorder or secondary to Parkinson's disease. The physical health of patients with chronic psychiatric disorders is also poorer than for the rest of the population, partly because of lifestyle factors such as poor diet, lack of exercise and smoking. Many psychotropic medications cause physical side effects, such as the extrapyramidal effects of antipsychotics or the thyroid dysfunction that occurs with lithium.

Answers *continued*

8. Investigations are undertaken for a number of reasons:
    - to identify underlying organic causes for the psychiatric presentation
    - to assess the patient's general health
    - to investigate any co-occurring physical illness
    - to establish baseline levels before initiating treatments which may impact upon the patient's health.

    Choosing an investigation is therefore determined by the patient's presentation, history and relevant findings on physical examination.

9. Not necessarily: for example it may be clear that the psychosis has been precipitated by drug misuse or that the presenting symptoms are entirely typical of schizophrenia. However, for patients whose symptoms that could indicate an organic cause for the psychosis, patients with unusual presentations and first presentations in older patients, a CT scan should be undertaken to rule out an underlying intracranial pathology.

10. Psychological therapies should be considered for all psychiatric patients, often in conjunction with medication. They are also indicated for a wide range of disorders from minor mental health disorders to behavioural disorders, anxiety, depression and phobias.

11. Children can take antidepressants. For example, anti-depressants are prescribed in small doses, for conditions such as nocturnal enuresis. However, they should be prescribed with caution, particularly selective serotonin reuptake inhibitors, as they are associated with increased suicide rates in patients under 18 years of age.

12. All antipsychotic medications are similarly effective against the positive symptoms of schizophrenia. Atypical antipsychotics are more effective against the negative symptoms. One antipsychotic medication, clozapine, is more effective than all others but is only used for treatment-resistant schizophrenia because of its side-effect profile.

Chapter 3
Affective (mood) disorders

Introduction. 97
Case 1 Low mood. 98
Case 2 Overactivity 102
Depressive disorders 105
Bipolar affective disorder 115
Persistent mood disorders. 121

Starter questions

Answers to the following questions are on page 122.

1. Should all patients with depression be treated with antidepressants?
2. Why do we still use electroconvulsive therapy when we have so many antidepressants?
3. Does everyone with a depressive illness have further episodes?
4. Can antidepressants cause mania?
5. Is depression a curable illness?
6. Is mania fun?
7. If antidepressants aren't addictive, why can't they be suddenly discontinued?

Introduction

Feeling a complex range of emotions is a normal part of human experience. Mood changes occur in response to day-to-day events and also occur naturally without obvious specific triggers. Mood or 'affective' disorders occur when the range of these emotional experiences becomes significantly disturbed compared with the normal variation. People suffering from mood disorders experience prolonged periods of extremes of mood that affect their daily functioning and activity levels.

Mood disorders are divided into:

- disorders of low mood (depression), and
- elated mood (mania).

Many patients do not recognise their own depression so do not seek medical treatment. Others feel ashamed of it and avoid consulting the doctor, fearing the impact of a diagnosis on work and relationships.

Depression frequently occurs as a single episode but many people experience further episodes. Bipolar affective disorder is a serious recurrent mood disorder in which patients experience episodes of both depression and mania.

Depression is the most common psychiatric disorder and the fourth leading cause of disease and disability worldwide. Population estimates may underestimate its prevalence as it often goes undiagnosed and untreated. This is especially true when it arises alongside physical illnesses.

Case 1 Low mood

Presentation

Angela Bailey, aged 55, presents to her general practitioner (GP) having felt tired all the time for the last couple of months. She is in trouble at work due to an increasing number of days off sick. She has lost interest in her hobbies and feels very sad and alone.

Initial interpretation

Feeling tired all the time is a common, vague symptom that can indicate various underlying physical problems (e.g. anaemia, thyroid disease or malignancy).

Angela's loss of interest in her activities (anhedonia) and her persistent low mood, in combination with her loss of energy, also raise the possibility of a depressive illness. The duration and impact of her symptoms suggest a mood disorder rather than an ordinary fluctuation in mood.

History

Angela is a secretary in a busy accountancy firm. She is usually fit and well,

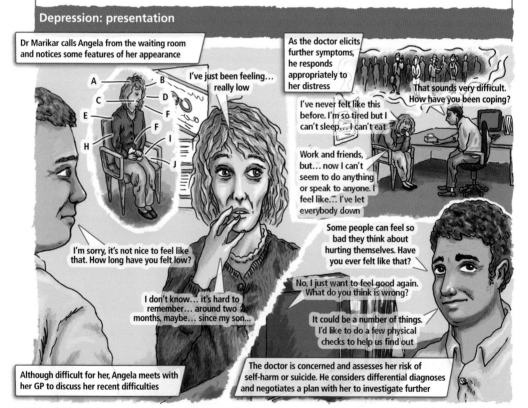

Depression: presentation

A. Disheveled hair B. Downcast eyes and poor eye contact C. Frown/worried expression D. Tearfulness E. Weight loss/loose-fitting clothes F. Dry lips and mouth G. Closed body posture H. Dirty clothes, unkempt appearance I. Dirty nails J. Poor personal hygiene/body odour

has no medical problems and does not take regular medication. She was divorced 6 years ago and her two children, aged 18 and 21, are both away at university; her younger son left three months ago. Until recently, she was very active, regularly attending the gym and hobby groups.

For the last 2 months, she has been feeling very down with little motivation to do anything. She feels as if there is a 'dark cloud' over everything. She has stopped seeing friends and no longer looks forward to talking to her children as she fears she will be tearful.

Angela feels ashamed of her inability to cope and thinks she is a failure, ruminating on thoughts that she has been a poor mother and wife. She is worried about losing her job but finds it increasingly difficult to face her employment. At work, she makes frequent mistakes and struggles to focus on simple tasks. When asked, she admits that she sometimes feels there is no point in going on.

She lies awake in the early hours unable to go back to sleep. She cannot be bothered to cook for herself, particularly as her appetite is poor, and does not bother with housework as it seems pointless. She feels very 'slowed-down'.

Angela has never experienced this before and has never seen a psychiatrist. She is not sure if she has a family history of mental illness. However, she recalls that her father drank excessively and was absent for long periods during her childhood. Her family never discussed this. Her father died of pneumonia in his 70s.

Angela's mother and grandmother both had thyroid problems.

Full systems enquiry does not suggest any underlying physical illness. In particular, she has not noted any skin changes, breathlessness, palpitations, change in heat tolerance or change in her bowels which would have indicated thyroid disorders or anaemia.

Use the interview to explore the patient's perspective and understanding of depression. Stigma, a lack of knowledge about depression and the negative cognitions that depressed patients experience all affect their willingness to engage in treatment. Ensuring the patient feels heard, understood and supported through this time can improve their immediate prognosis.

Interpretation of history

Angela's history is suggestive of a depressive episode, possibly triggered by her last child going to university. She has become socially isolated and no longer feels central to family life.

She takes no medications, making an iatrogenic (disorder caused by medical treatment) cause for her mood unlikely. Alcohol misuse must also be considered. She has a family history of alcohol misuse and many people use alcohol to 'self-medicate' their mood or sleep problems. Her history does not suggest thyroid disease or another physical cause for her symptoms.

Examination

Full systems physical examination is normal. A full mental state examination is undertaken (**Table 3.1**).

Investigations

Blood tests include renal function, thyroid function and liver function tests, calcium and blood glucose levels and a full blood count (**Table 3.2**).

Interpretation of findings

Angela's further history, examination and blood tests do not strongly suggest any underlying physical condition. She denies excessive alcohol use.

Case 1 *continued*

Category	Description
Angela Bailey's mental state examination	
Appearance and behaviour	Middle-aged, Caucasian lady, wearing no make-up, with slightly unkempt hair. Her clothes are clean, but drab and very creased
	Her eye contact is poor; she is slightly guarded in interaction, although appropriate, and is occasionally tearful
Speech	Her speech is monotonous, and reduced in rate and quantity
Mood	She describes feeling sad and worn out; objectively she appears sad and withdrawn
	She describes negative thoughts including hopelessness, guilt and worthlessness
Perceptions	No unusual experiences, such as hearing voices
Thoughts	No abnormal thoughts or delusions, but she is preoccupied with her own worthlessness
Cognitions	Her responses are slow, but she is fully orientated in time, place and person
Insight	She has some insight as she recognises she is different from her premorbid personality (a bit of a worrier but generally active, happy and sociable). However she believes she has brought this on herself due to her own inadequacies and does not believe treatment will help
Suicidal ideation	Sometimes she feels life isn't worth living and she has occasionally considered how she could end her life, but would not do so as she could not inflict such distress on her children

Table 3.1 Angela's mental state examination

Investigation	Indication
Investigations for affective disorders	
Full blood count	To exclude
	Anaemia (low Hb), Infection (high WCC), Delirium (secondary infection can mimic mania), High alcohol intake (macrocytosis, raised MCV)
Urea and electrolytes	Check renal function prior to prescribing any renally excreted medication
	Electrolyte imbalances possibly caused by medications, e.g. SSRIs and hyponatraemia
Liver function tests	Raised GGT to confirm suspicion of excessive alcohol use
	Baseline before prescribing medications that are metabolised by the liver
Thyroid function tests	Hypo - or hyperthyroidism can cause mood and energy changes
	Lithium causes abnormal thyroid function
Calcium and phosphate profile	Hypoparathyroidism presents with low mood
B12 and folate	If history indicates potential reason to be suspicious of a deficiency, e.g. malnutrition, family history
Urine drug screen	Substance misuse presents with low mood or manic symptoms
Syphilis (VDRL)	Increasing in prevalence recently, presents in many ways. Consider if history indicates potential risk factors
EEG/CT/MRI	If intracranial pathology such as epileptic focus or space occupying lesion is suspected
ECG	Patients with a cardiac history, as medications such as lithium and tricyclic antidepressants affect the QT interval

Table 3.2 Investigations for affective disorders. Hb, haemoglobin; MCV, mean cell volume; SSRI, selective serotonin reuptake inhibitor; VDRL, venereal disease research laboratory test; WCC, white cell count

Case 1 *continued*

She describes all three core symptoms of depression (**Figure 3.1**):

- Loss of energy (anergia)
- Loss of interest and enjoyment in usual things (anhedonia)
- A persistent depressed mood

Angela Bailey also exhibits four of the additional symptoms of depression:

- Poor concentration
- Disturbed sleep
- Poor appetite
- Guilt and self-blame

Her mental state examination (MSE) also indicates a diagnosis of depressive disorder (**Figure 3.1**). She is subjectively and objectively depressed with signs of self-neglect. Her speech and movements are slowed, indicating psychomotor retardation, but she has no psychotic features (delusions or hallucinations).

> **The delusions seen in depression tend to be 'mood congruent'.** This means they are understandable in the context of low mood and tend to focus on themes of loss, guilt and death. In extreme cases, patients believe they are dead or that their internal organs are rotting away (Cotard's syndrome).

Diagnosis

On the basis of her clinical history, physical examination and MSE, and the exclusion of endocrine, haematological or

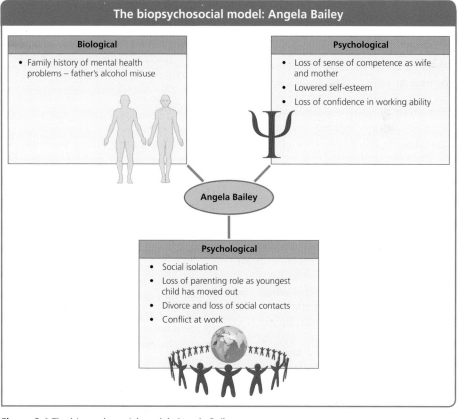

The biopsychosocial model: Angela Bailey

Biological
- Family history of mental health problems – father's alcohol misuse

Psychological
- Loss of sense of competence as wife and mother
- Lowered self-esteem
- Loss of confidence in working ability

Angela Bailey

Psychological
- Social isolation
- Loss of parenting role as youngest child has moved out
- Divorce and loss of social contacts
- Conflict at work

Figure 3.1 The biopsychosocial model: Angela Bailey.

Case 1 *continued*

metabolic problems through blood tests, Angela is diagnosed with a severe depressive episode. She has three core and four additional symptoms of depression that have been present for at least 2 months and are significantly impacting on her life, both socially and occupationally.

This is her first presentation with a mental health problem. Her family history and social circumstances are predisposing and precipitating factors, perpetuated by her difficulties at work because of her depression and her social withdrawal.

Her suicidal ideation demands immediate intervention to prevent further deterioration. Early evidence of self-neglect must be monitored to ensure she can meet her physical health and nutritional requirements.

Angela is briefly relieved that there is no serious physical illness but is quite negative that any treatment will be helpful. She says it is not worth the effort and that she should just pull herself together. The GP discusses the role of antidepressant medications and a psychology referral for cognitive behavioural therapy (CBT). After some persuasion, Angela agrees to both and accepts a further appointment the following week with the GP for a review.

Case 2 Overactivity

Presentation

Anita calls the student GP service. Her housemate John Feldman, a fellow medical student, has been behaving strangely and is not sleeping. He appears to have endless energy, talking continuously about having special powers and seeing a 'new order' in the world.

Initial interpretation

With this presentation, particularly in a student population, drugs and alcohol must be considered. Stress caused by university studies may be significant and can lead to substance use or a mood disorder.

The timescale of the onset of symptoms should be established to exclude infection and subsequent delirium (see Chapter 11). Excluding this and other organic disorders (such as frontal lobe lesions) requires a full neurological and physical examination.

Depression and numerous medical conditions can affect sleep. However, if sleep disturbance is combined with psychomotor agitation, a manic episode is a possible diagnosis. A past psychiatric history of any mood disturbance will inform the differential diagnosis.

History

Anita explains that John is normally quiet, reserved and hard working. For 3 weeks, he has been up all night playing loud music despite his forthcoming exams. He refuses to eat with his housemates, saying he is a 'superhuman machine' and does not need food. He has written bizarre passages all over his Facebook page.

At first John's 'new energy' and infectious mood were fun to be around, but he has become increasingly irritable and it is now impossible to have a conversation with him. Today's call was prompted by an incident the previous night when John was sexually inappropriate with one of the girls in their house and had to be restrained by two male housemates.

Anita does not think John has taken drugs and he has never mentioned any past mental health problems.

Case 2 *continued*

Mania: presentation

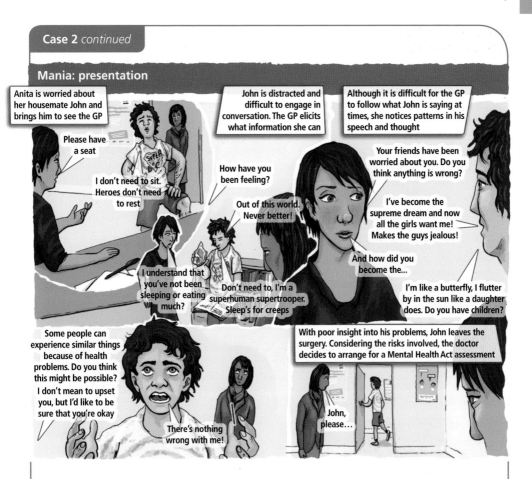

Anita is worried about her housemate John and brings him to see the GP

John is distracted and difficult to engage in conversation. The GP elicits what information she can

Although it is difficult for the GP to follow what John is saying at times, she notices patterns in his speech and thought

Please have a seat

I don't need to sit. Heroes don't need to rest

How have you been feeling?

Your friends have been worried about you. Do you think anything is wrong?

Out of this world. Never better!

I've become the supreme dream and now all the girls want me! Makes the guys jealous!

And how did you become the...

I understand that you've not been sleeping or eating much?

Don't need to, I'm a superhuman supertrooper. Sleep's for creeps

I'm like a butterfly, I flutter by in the sun like a daughter does. Do you have children?

Some people can experience similar things because of health problems. Do you think this might be possible?
I don't mean to upset you, but I'd like to be sure that you're okay

There's nothing wrong with me!

With poor insight into his problems, John leaves the surgery. Considering the risks involved, the doctor decides to arrange for a Mental Health Act assessment

John, please...

Asking yourself 'how does this patient make me feel?' is particularly useful in cases of mania and can help you to understand their mental state and reach a diagnosis. Patients who are elated or irritable are often 'infectious' and similar emotions can be felt when talking to them.

Interpretation of history

John is showing the characteristic features of an acute manic episode. For at least 1 week, he has had:

- Overactivity – a decreased need for sleep and increased energy
- Self-important ideas
- Accelerated thinking

- Elevated and irritable mood
- Impaired judgement and insight

A further examination of his mental state must elicit any further psychotic symptoms if schizophrenia and other psychotic disorders are to be considered as a diagnosis (see Tables 2.2–2.5).

Examination

John is persuaded to visit the GP with Anita later the same day. His body temperature is normal and has a slightly raised heart rate (110 bpm) but no other physical abnormalities are evident on a full physical examination. He talks to the doctor rapidly and openly about how he is feeling, and the GP conducts a full MSE (**Table 3.3**).

Case 2 *continued*

John's mental state examination	
Category	Description
Appearance and behaviour	Slim, dishevelled young man, wearing revealing shorts despite the cold weather and a tight, brightly-coloured, homemade t-shirt with 'Super Doc' written on it
	He is over-aroused, pacing the room, fiddling with various objects throughout the assessment
	He is over-familiar, flirting with the general practitioner
Speech	Increased in rate, volume and pitch and very difficult to interrupt. He displays tangentiality, circumstantiality and flight of ideas
Mood	Subjectively he feels 'out of this world'
	Objectively he is labile and irritable especially when asked direct questions
Perceptions	He describes perceptual disturbance, reporting that 'colours and sounds seem brighter and clearer'
Thoughts	He is preoccupied with his own 'super-human powers' (delusions of grandeur) so has no need for revision or food, and can see things in science and nature that others cannot
Cognitions	Not formally tested
Insight	He has no insight into his problems, laughing when asked if he thinks anything is wrong. He states that he needs no help as he is an invincible mastermind who can rise above base human needs

Table 3.3 John's mental state examination

> **Mania is difficult to distinguish from psychosis in an acute presentation.** Focus on recording a careful MSE that describes the presenting symptoms rather than immediately trying to differentiate the two.

Investigations

A full blood count, urea and electrolytes, C-reactive protein level as an inflammatory marker, thyroid and liver function tests, a urinary drug screen and blood alcohol level are all normal.

Diagnosis

The most likely diagnosis is of a manic episode with psychotic features, including secondary delusions of grandeur ('superhuman powers') and thought disorganisation (flight of ideas). A further past history from a relative may establish whether this is John's first presentation with a mood disorder. Previous episodes of low or elated mood may indicate bipolar disorder.

John quickly returns home after the consultation and the GP arranges for a mental health act assessment to be carried out as a matter of urgency. John has no insight into his problems, is not willing to engage in treatment and is a potential risk to others due to his sexual disinhibition. He is also a risk to himself through self-neglect and misadventure.

> **Manic episodes must be treated early. Patients quickly lose judgement and insight as they deteriorate, refusing to engage in treatment.** Admission to hospital under the provisions of mental health legislation is often required to manage the risks to themselves or others as a consequence of disinhibition and lack of judgement.

Depressive disorders

Classification

In the International Classification of Diseases 10th Revision (ICD-10; see Chapter 1), depression is classified into mild, moderate and severe according to the number and severity of symptoms (**Figure 3.2**). For a diagnosis of depression to be made, the symptoms must be present for at least 2 weeks.

Some patients experience only one episode of depression during their lifetime and make a complete recovery. For many, however, depression is a relapsing and remitting condition. A relapsing illness that is only ever characterised by depressive mood changes is referred to as a unipolar depressive illness. When episodes of mania also occur, it is called bipolar affective disorder.

Epidemiology

Depressive disorders are common, especially in women (**Table 3.4**): Depression affects up to one in six people at some point in their lifetime and approximately twice as many women as men are diagnosed with them. One in four women and one in 10 men require treatment during their lifetime.

Epidemiology of depressive disorders		
	Men	Women
Lifetime risk	1 in 10	1 in 4
Prevalence	30 per 1000	40–90 per 1000

Table 3.4 Epidemiology of depressive disorders in men and women

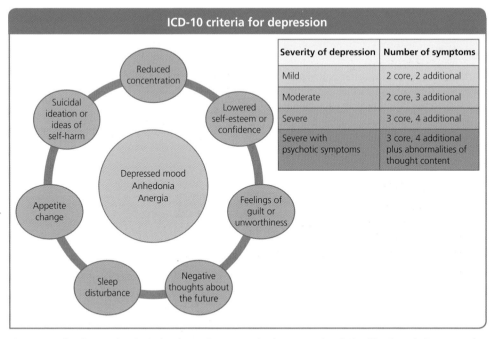

ICD-10 criteria for depression

Reduced concentration

Suicidal ideation or ideas of self-harm

Lowered self-esteem or confidence

Depressed mood
Anhedonia
Anergia

Appetite change

Feelings of guilt or unworthiness

Sleep disturbance

Negative thoughts about the future

Severity of depression	Number of symptoms
Mild	2 core, 2 additional
Moderate	2 core, 3 additional
Severe	3 core, 4 additional
Severe with psychotic symptoms	3 core, 4 additional plus abnormalities of thought content

Figure 3.2 The diagnostic criteria for depression set out in the International Classification of Diseases 10th Revision. The number of core symptoms (orange) and additional symptoms (purple) determines the severity of depression.

Depression results in more deaths by suicide than any other psychiatric disorder and is a cause of significant costs in terms of healthcare requirements and impairment of capacity for work and daily living.

Depression is:

- The third most common reason for GP consultations in the UK
- More common in divorcees, unemployed individuals and people with co-morbid physical health problems
- Increasing more quickly than would be expected if accounted for purely by better awareness and greater diagnosis

Depression is a serious but treatable condition that is underdiagnosed (up to 70% of cases being missed). Whichever area of medicine you decide to practise, always think to screen for depression, particularly in patients with other physical health conditions.

Aetiology

Genetic, endocrine, immunological and neurobiological factors all contribute to the complex aetiology of an individual's depressive illness. Social, psychological and cognitive factors must also be taken into account. The biopsychosocial model of illness (see page 52) is used to assess the relationship between the biological, psychological and social factors and inform the management. Biopsychosocial factors interact and are mediated through biological mechanisms including neurotransmitters and stress hormones (see Chapter 1) as well as psychological processes (**Figure 3.3**).

Affective disorders are more common in some families. The first-degree relatives of patients with a moderate to severe depressive disorder have a significantly greater lifetime risk of developing the disorder.

Twin studies suggest that this is genetically mediated as concordance rates for these disorders are the same in monozygotic twins reared together as in those reared apart. In addition, concordance rates for monozygotic twins are significantly higher than for dizygotic twins or siblings.

Similarly, the children of parents with depressive disorders who are adopted at an early age by patients without a history of serious depressive disorder have a higher prevalence of the disorder.

No single or multiple genes 'causing' depression have been identified. It is likely that multiple genes initially contribute to an increased risk of developing a mood disorder. This genetic predisposition then interacts with other environmental factors mediated by complex neurobiological, hormonal and physiological mechanisms.

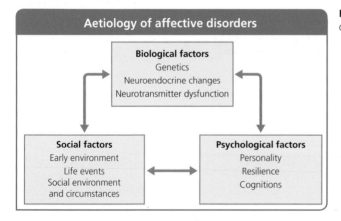

Figure 3.3 Aetiology of affective disorders.

Some people develop depression in the absence of any identifiable immediate stressor while others do not do so despite suffering multiple adverse life events. A genetic susceptibility to depression may be conferred by genes coding for neurotransmitter transporters, with different alleles leading to different susceptibilities.

Many physiological, hormonal and personality factors implicated in the aetiology of depression can also be linked with specific genetic coding. This further complicates the interplay between the different factors contributing to the development of depression. For example, environmental stresses such as childhood trauma, known to increase an individual's susceptibility to depression, result in changes in the responses of hypothalamic–pituitary–adrenal axis to stress (see page 15). This suggests that cortisol is involved in mediating biological changes that result in depression (**Figure 3.4**). These changes may then have more impact on genotypes with a predisposition to depression.

Some personality types, such as those characterised by high levels of anxiety and self-criticism, appear to confer a higher risk of developing mood disorders than others. Variations in personality may reflect the genetic factors that have contributed to the development of depression or to the specific physiological responses that predispose an individual to it.

Life events

Many episodes of depression occur in the immediate aftermath of significant life events, especially those involving loss. The incidence of depression rises sharply after stressful life events such as:

- Loss, including bereavement, separation or a change in relationships
- Challenges to self-esteem such as a loss of occupation
- Physical health problems or chronic disease, through added stress and/or by direct neurological effects (e.g. in endocrine disorders)
- Traumatic events such as assault

Existing social difficulties further increase an individual's susceptibility to depression in the face of negative life events. These include a lack of employment outside the home, poor social support and responsibility for looking after young children.

In addition, adverse life events in early childhood are associated with depression. These include:

- Parental separation in childhood
- Problems within the family, including a lack of appropriate care
- Physical or sexual abuse in childhood
- The death of a parent in childhood
- Parenting style, including both overprotective and non-caring parenting

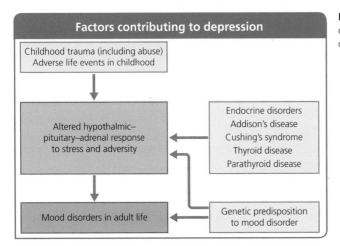

Figure 3.4 Interaction of factors contributing to the development of depression.

Pathophysiology

Studying the use of antidepressant drugs has led to an increased understanding of the changes in brain chemistry they cause. Abnormalities in neurotransmitter function have therefore been proposed as an underlying cause for mood disorders.

The monoamine hypothesis proposes that depression is caused by abnormalities in monoamine neurotransmitter systems at one or several sites in the brain (see Table 1.10). The monoamines serotonin (5-hydroxytryptamine or 5-HT), noradrenaline (norepinephrine) and dopamine are all known to play a role in our adaptive responses to stressful events. The use of antidepressant medications causes complex changes in, for example, the uptake of these neurotransmitters and the concentration of their receptors on the postsynaptic cells. A decrease in serotonin function is particularly implicated in causing depressive episodes.

> **Most antidepressant medications increase the amount of serotonin in the synaptic cleft and increase serotonergic activity.** This effect occurs immediately but the therapeutic benefit takes at least 2 weeks to establish. Therefore more subtle neurophysiological changes must also be involved.

More recent work has explored the role of the amino acid neurotransmitters glutamate and γ-aminobutyric acid in mood disorders and as treatment targets.

Cognitive theory

Negative thoughts are a characteristic of depressive disorders. Cognitive theory provides a psychological account of how depression may develop and become established, outlining the processing of information in ways that may both cause and prolong changes in mood.

This theory describes the 'vicious cycle' that can become established in which a patient feels sad and tired and so stops doing things. Negative thoughts such as 'there's no point' or 'I'm useless' are magnified and 'proven correct' by patients' inactivity (**Table 3.5**). In the absence of positive experiences to challenge these cognitive distortions, the inactivity generates further negativity.

These cognitive distortions are typical of depression and are the basis of treatment with cognitive behavioural therapy (CBT; see page 78). This challenges these automatic thoughts and the patient's resulting 'learned helplessness'. Although such distortions are a feature of established depressive illness, it is less clear whether they are implicated in causing depression in the first place rather than being a perpetuating factor after it has become established.

Clinical features

The clinical features of depression are outlined in **Table 3.6**.

Diagnosing depression may be difficult. Some patients present with mainly physical

Cognitive distortions in depression		
Cognitive distortion	Definition	Example
Arbitrary inference	Drawing a conclusion with no evidence for it	Believing someone dislikes you without any evidence
Selective abstraction	Focus on a detail while missing the broader context or features or a situation	Remembering the one awkward conversation you had at a party, but forgetting how pleased everyone was to see you
Overgeneralisation	Coming to a conclusion based on a single incident	Making one mistake at work and thinking that you will be bad at every task
Personalisation	Attributing external events to oneself in an unjustified way	A shop assistant is rude to you and you believe that you must have done something wrong without considering other explanations for their behaviour

Table 3.5 Cognitive distortions in depression

Eliciting clinical features during the mental state examination	
Symptoms	Example questions to elicit symptoms
Mood	
Depressed mood	'How have you been feeling lately?'
Cognitive symptoms	
Impaired concentration and attention, e.g. difficulty sustaining tasks, easily distracted, subjectively complain of memory problems	'Day to day, how are you getting on?' 'Are you finding it hard to concentrate at home or work?'
Low self-esteem	'How have you been feeling about yourself?' 'Do you think your mood has affected your confidence at all?'
Negative thoughts about the future and hopelessness	'You describe feeling very low at the minute, I wonder how you're feeling about the future?' 'Is there anything you are looking forward to?'
Suicidal ideation	'Sometimes, when people have been feeling low like this, they think about ending their life. Has that been happening to you?'
Guilt	'Are there thoughts that keep troubling you?' 'Are there any thoughts or memories you find yourself dwelling on or thinking about all the time?'
Psychotic symptoms	
Delusions	'Have you experienced anything you have found hard to explain lately?' 'Have you worried that your body wasn't working properly or that something terrible was happening to you?'
Hallucinations	'Have you felt as though people have been giving you a hard time lately or having a go at you?' 'Have you heard people criticising you or speaking about you when there was no one around?'
Biological symptoms	
Anhedonia	'Do you find that you are still interested in doing the things you used to?'
Anergia	'How are your energy levels?' 'Are you finding doing things difficult at all?'
Reduced emotional range or reactivity	'I wonder how the world feels to you at the minute. Do you ever feel slightly detached from everything going on around you?'
Diurnal variation in mood (worse in the morning)	'Have you found that your mood or energy levels change at all over the course of a day?'
Early morning wakening	'How are you sleeping?' 'Do you find any difficulty falling asleep or staying asleep?'
Psychomotor retardation	'Do you feel rather slowed down, or as if everything is difficult?'
Loss of appetite and/or weight loss	'How is your appetite?' 'Have you found you've lost any weight without trying?'
Loss of libido	'Sometimes when people are feeling low, they lose interest in everything, including sex. I wonder if you've been feeling like this?' 'Has it caused you any difficulties in your relationship?'
Non-specific physical complaints	'I wonder whether you've been feeling generally run down, with aches, pains or tummy troubles?'

Table 3.6 Symptom clusters and eliciting clinical features of depression during the mental state examination

symptoms such as aches and pains, and gastrointestinal or chest complaints (masked depression). Others may experience irritability rather than a classic low mood (agitated depression) or present with other patterns of symptoms recognised as a subtype of depression (**Table 3.7**).

An individual's cultural background may also affect their presentation and how they communicate their distress. Stigma and negative cognitions often prevent people from recognising or disclosing that there is something wrong.

Clinical patterns of depression	
Subtype of depression	Prominent clinical features
Agitated	Agitation. Commonly seen in elderly patients
Atypical	Reversal of typical biological symptoms: increased sleep and appetite
Retarded	Psychomotor retardation
Depressive stupor	Occurs in severe depression. Patient is 'stuporose' and may be mute, motionless and refuse to eat

Table 3.7 Clinical patterns of depression

> **Depression commonly co-presents with other health conditions such as heart disease, neurological conditions, diabetes or asthma.** It may be overlooked as the focus is often on the physical condition, leaving a treatable and distressing condition untreated. Co-morbid depression has been shown to impact negatively on mortality and morbidity.

In very severe depression, psychotic symptoms are prominent. Patients experience very distressing hallucinations and delusions. Hallucinations are usually auditory, taking the form of derogatory or accusatory voices that repeatedly remind the patient of their faults or imagined misdeeds from their past. Delusions tend to be persecutory or nihilistic, in which the patient believes that they are dead or rotting away inside.

> **'Clustering' the symptoms of depression into changes in mood, cognitive symptoms (depressive thoughts), biological symptoms (including changes in activity levels) and psychotic symptoms (Table 3.7)** helps you remember them and forms a framework to see their interrelation in an individual's case.

Diagnostic approach

A thorough assessment of depression should include:

1. The exclusion of an underlying physical cause by:
   - A full drug, alcohol and medication history
   - A full systems enquiry and physical examination
   - Blood tests (see **Table 3.2**) including a full blood count, urea and electrolytes and thyroid function tests
   - In cases where an organic cause is suspected, further investigations such as example neuroimaging

> **Blood tests and investigations should be guided by a thorough physical examination.** Based on the clinical presentation, always ask yourself why you are ordering each test. This is not only good clinical practice, but also cost-effective.

2. A full psychiatric and medical history:
   - A social and personal history
   - A history of the patient's childhood development to identify predisposing, precipitating and perpetuating factors

When assessing a patient with a mental health problem, always obtain collateral information from friends, family and other professionals. This should include a description of the patient's premorbid personality. This will give you a more thorough picture of the problems the person is experiencing and the impact on the patient and their life.

3. A screen for co-morbid psychiatric problems:
   - A full psychiatric history
   - A MSE (Table 3.6)
4. A grading of the severity of the mood episode:
   - According to the ICD-10 criteria
   - Noting the presence or absence of psychotic or somatic features (see Figure 3.1)
5. A risk and insight assessment:
   - Identify the most appropriate environment for the treatment, i.e. primary care, secondary care with a dedicated community mental health team or inpatient care

Always assess the risk of deliberate self-harm or suicide in all patients with a suspected depressive disorder. Specific questioning must focus on any ideas the patient might have about harming themselves. This risk must be reassessed at each review as it may appear at any point in the patient's illness.

Management

This is guided by:

- The severity of the depression and the potential risk to the patient or others
- The patient's circumstances and preferences
- The biopsychosocial formulation of the patient's problems
- The available local resources

Treatment can include pharmacological, psychological and social modalities.

Depression is graded by severity as mild, moderate or severe, and treatment options are recommended in line with this. Guidelines recommend a 'stepped' care model. Patients are treated according to the severity of the depression and moved up a 'step' if they are unresponsive to treatment or their symptoms worsen (Figure 3.5).

The least intrusive but most effective intervention should always be offered first. If a patient fails to improve with the interventions offered or declines them:

- Check the patient's concordance with current treatment
- Review the psychological and social causes
- Adjust the dosage of medication
- Consider alternative treatments such as combined therapy or pharmacological adjuncts from the next step up.

Psychological treatment

All patients suffering from a depressive disorder require some form of psychological intervention including, at minimum, education, support and reassurance. Basic advice about a healthy diet, exercise and sleeping should be offered to help the patient to re-establish normal routines.

Mild depression often resolves spontaneously with supportive counselling and regular review by the GP. Evidence suggests that antidepressant medication is little better than placebo in this group. Given the possible side effects of medication, psychological and social interventions are therefore the first choice in mild depression.

There are several types of psychological treatment with a very variable evidence base (see Chapter 2). Supportive counselling is enough for many patients with mild depression.

Stepped care model for depression

Step 1
Mild or suspected depression

Assess, support, provide psychoeducation, monitor and refer onwards as appropriate

Step 2
Mild to moderate depression

Consider interventions to address psychosocial problems
Psychological interventions (e.g CBT, self-help resources)
Antidepressant according to the patient's wishes and preferences

Step 3
No response or moderate to severe depression

Medication
High-intensity psychological interventions
Combined treatments and referral for specialist input as appropriate

Step 4
Severe and complex depression
Risk to life
Severe self-neglect

Medication and/or electroconvulsive therapy
High-intensity psychological interventions
Crisis service, combined treatments, multiprofessional and inpatient care

Figure 3.5 A stepped care model adapted from the National Institute for Health and Care Excellence guidelines for the management of depression. CBT, cognitive behavioural therapy.

CBT has become widely established as an effective psychological approach to treating patients with mild to moderate depression.

Social treatment

Social factors precipitate and perpetuate episodes of depression and, if not addressed, will limit many patients' recovery. They include:

- Finances
- Housing
- Relationships
- Caring responsibilities
- Employment and voluntary work
- Education and personal development
- Social activity

Pharmacological treatment

Antidepressant medications are widely prescribed in both general practice and secondary care. The evidence for efficacy of antidepressant medications is better for patients with moderate to severe depression.

Before prescribing antidepressants, identify and address any concerns the patient has about taking medication (**Table 3.8**) as these are particularly common in patients with mood disorders.

Concordance with medication is crucial for success so patients must understand the reasons for taking antidepressants. Some key facts must be emphasised to the patient:

- The full antidepressant effect develops gradually. Beneficial effects start after about 2 weeks, but it may take up to 6 weeks to achieve a full effect
- Medication must be taken as prescribed and at the same dose even when the symptoms are remitting
- Treatment must be continued for at least 6 months after the symptoms have remitted, and for longer in patients with recurrent depression
- Potential side effects vary for different classes of antidepressants (see page 82)
- Antidepressants may interact with other medications
- Discontinuation symptoms may occur if an antidepressant is stopped abruptly.

Patient concerns about antidepressant medication	
Concern	Response
'I don't want to get addicted to tablets. I'll be stuck on them forever'	'Antidepressants are not addictive and patients do not develop tolerance to them. Some provoke a withdrawal response if stopped abruptly, but this can be avoided by gradually decreasing the dose. Most patients discontinue antidepressants completely after adequate treatment'
'I've heard that they aren't safe. They have awful side-effects'	'Antidepressants vary in the side-effects they produce. Generally, initial side-effects settle quickly and are not dangerous'
'Will they turn me into a zombie?'	'Older antidepressants were very sedating. Modern antidepressants are not and you should not feel sedated or slowed down while taking them'
'I don't really need tablets. I just need to snap out of it'	'Many mild to moderate depressions resolve without antidepressants, although this may take months. For moderate to severe depression there is good evidence that medication relieves the symptoms of depression and shortens the episode'
'I don't want to take them because they will make me feel like a different person and interfere with the way I think and behave'	'Antidepressants treat the symptoms of depression and help to return people to their usual level of function and feeling. They do not change personality and their impact on thinking and feeling is positive, relieving the distressing symptoms of depression'
'The tablets will suppress the way I really feel and then I'll never be able to deal with it. It will all still be there when I stop taking them'	'Depressive disorders result from complex changes in the neurochemistry of the brain which causes you to think and feel differently. Antidepressants correct these and help you get back to your normal self, which allows you to get on with sorting out any other problems'
'I'm already taking other medications; these will interfere with them'	'It is usually possible to choose an antidepressant which is compatible with other medications to avoid interactions'
'Will I still be able to drive and work?'	'As with all medications, we advise caution when starting them but there are many antidepressants now which do not impair function In this way'

Table 3.8 Common patient concerns about taking antidepressant medication

This is particularly so for those drugs with a shorter half-life (such as paroxetine and venlafaxine)

Although a number of antidepressant medications are available, there is no clear 'winner' in terms of efficacy. All have some side effects and these differ between drugs (see page 82).

Some antidepressant medications work on one monoamine transmitter system (e.g. fluoxetine on serotonin), whereas others work on more than one (e.g. venlafaxine on serotonin and noradrenaline (see page 83). Prescribing is determined by the individual patient profile and depends upon a number of factors including:

- The side-effects and their likely impact on the patient. These may, however, be used beneficially, e.g. choosing a sedating antidepressant for a patient with severe insomnia

- Possible interactions with the patient's other medications
- Any past response to specific antidepressants
- Existing medical conditions and the likely impact of the medication on these
- The risk of suicide

Tricyclic antidepressants are contraindicated in patients with a high suicide risk as they are the most toxic antidepressant, causing potentially fatal arrhythmias in overdose.

Discontinuation reactions

Sudden discontinuation of an antidepressant can cause a discontinuation response that is subjectively very unpleasant. Symptoms include headaches, physical sensations often described as electric shocks, and symptoms such as anxiety, irritability, nausea and restlessness. Although these symptoms are not dangerous and subside in a few days, they are unpleasant. Therefore antidepressants should therefore be tapered off by gradually reducing the dose.

> Patients may stop their medication suddenly thinking they are well, or perhaps forget to take it when they go away. The sudden appearance of discontinuation symptoms is often interpreted by the patient as being a recurrence of their depressive illness.

The discontinuation response must be taken into account when a patient changes from one antidepressant medication to another. This may be necessary if the patient has not responded well to one antidepressant or has experienced intolerable side-effects. The preferred approach is to withdraw one antidepressant first and then, after a drug-free interval of a few days, begin the new antidepressant. This also avoids potentially dangerous interactions.

> Serotonin syndrome is a potentially dangerous interaction that occurs when more than one serotonin-blocking medication is used at the same time. It presents with restlessness, sweating, seizures and confusion and is potentially fatal (see page 81).

Some patients do not respond effectively to the first antidepressant medication they are prescribed despite full concordance with the medication regime for a protracted period. Patients are considered to be resistant to treatment if they have had two full therapeutic trials of antidepressants from different classes for a minimum of 6–8 weeks but remain symptomatic.

Many strategies can then be adopted. The dose of medication can be increased above standard dosing levels or other medications, for example lithium, can be added. Alternatives to medication, such as electroconvulsive therapy (ECT), can also be considered. Specialist psychiatric treatment is the norm in this situation.

Electroconvulsive therapy

This is a highly effective treatment for severe depression, particularly psychotic depression, and will produce benefit more swiftly than antidepressants. It carries the risks associated with a general anaesthetic (see page 94).

It is indicated when:

■ There is no response to antidepressant medications despite adequate trials of more than one medication
■ A rapid response is required due to a high risk of suicide, severe self-neglect or severe psychomotor retardation

Prognosis

Unipolar and bipolar depressive disorder are chronic conditions characterised by relapse and recurrence (**Table 3.9**).

Relapse prevention

Prevention of relapse requires psychoeducation informing the patient about:

■ the nature of their condition
■ treatment choices
■ how to identify triggers that cause them to relapse, such as work stress
■ how to recognise early warning signs, such as changes in sleep patterns at the start of an illness

Every patient should be actively involved in formulating a care plan that they feel works for them.

Prevention strategies should be personalised to the individual and their specific experience of a disorder. Strategies include ensuring concordance with medication, cognitive therapy focusing on staying well and identifying depressed forms of thinking, lifestyle changes (e.g. addressing relationship or occupational stressors and triggers to illness), identifying early warning signs and agreeing an action plan with the health professionals involved in their care and the relevant family or friends.

Course and prognosis of affective disorders		
	Unipolar depression	Bipolar disorder
Recurrence rates	80% with major depression have further episodes (recurrent severe depression) 50% with moderate depressive episode will have another episode	90% of patients experiencing a manic episode will have further episodes of severe mood disturbance
Length of episode	Average 6 months, reduced to 2–3 with treatment 25% have episodes that last >1 year 10–20% develop unremitting chronic illness	Average length of treated or untreated manic episode is 6 months
Recurrence frequency over 25 years	Average 4 further episodes	Average 10 major episodes of mood disturbance
Pattern of recurrence	Interval between episodes gets progressively shorter	Interval between episodes gets progressively shorter
Remission	Over 80% achieve periods of symptom resolution, to the point where good social and occupational functioning is achieved	Approximately 25% achieve periods of symptom resolution, to the point where good social and occupational functioning is achieved
Standardised mortality rates	Twice that of general population	Twice that of general population
Suicide rates	10% with severe depressive disorder commit suicide	15% with bipolar affective disorder commit suicide (long-term treatment with mood-stabilising agents reduces this to general population levels)
Prognostic factors	Most significant predictor of disorder course is the history of previous episodes Higher risk of future episodes affected by: ■ History of several previous episodes ■ Incomplete remission of symptoms between episodes ■ Early age of onset ■ Co-morbid substance misuse ■ Co-morbid personality disorder	

Table 3.9 Course and prognosis of affective disorders

Bipolar affective disorder

Classification

In the ICD-10, bipolar affective disorder is described as a major affective disorder characterised by severe mood swings and changes in activity level (both elevated and depressed mood) with complete recovery between episodes and subsequent recurrence of the symptoms.

A diagnosis of bipolar disorder requires the patient to have experienced at least two episodes of mood disturbance, one of which must be mania, hypomania or a mixed affective state (**Table 3.11**).

In 'mixed affective states', manic and depressive symptoms appear together. Patients are overactive and restless with depressive thoughts and mood. Some patients have 'alternating mood states' in which their mood fluctuates rapidly between mania and depression.

Recurrent episodes of abnormal mood that always involve symptoms of depression but never symptoms of mania are diagnosed as recurrent depressive disorder.

The central features of mania include:

- A significant elevation of mood – elation and marked feelings of well-being or irritability
- Psychomotor agitation – increased activity
- Grandiosity – ideas of self-importance

Unlike with depression, it is not necessary to have a specific number of symptoms to make a diagnosis of a manic episode. Manic episodes are defined by the severity of the symptoms, their duration and the impact on an individual's functioning.

An extreme mood of elation severely affecting a person's functioning is called 'mania'. When it is less severe without gross disruption of an individual's work or social interactions, it is called 'hypomania' (**Table 3.10**).

Epidemiology

Bipolar affective disorder is less common than recurrent depression (**Table 3.11**). Prevalence estimates range from 0.4% to 1%, with little variation internationally. The lifetime risk is approximately 1 in 100 and equal in men and women.

The average age of onset is the early 20s, although there is a second 'peak' of onset in later life. First episodes of mania occurring much after the age of 50 years should be thoroughly investigated for an organic cause.

Aetiology

The causes of bipolar disorder are thought to be similar to depressive disorders although data on bipolar disorder are more limited.

Many patients with bipolar disorder have a positive family history of it. Patients with a first-degree relative with the condition have a 15% risk of developing it (**Table 3.11**). This increase in heritability relates to bipolar disorder alone: the first-degree relatives of a patient with depression are at greater risk of developing depression but not at greater risk of developing bipolar disorder. Conversely, the first-degree relatives of a patient with bipolar disorder have an increased risk of developing both depression and bipolar disorder compared with the general population.

In monozygotic twins, the concordance rate for bipolar affective disorder (79%) is higher than that for depressive disorders, suggesting a stronger genetic component than for other psychiatric disorders.

A number of organic factors can provoke a manic episode, including:

- Medication, e.g. corticosteroids
- Endocrine disorders, e.g. Cushing's syndrome and hyperparathyroidism
- Dopamine-agonist medications, e.g. bromocriptine. As dopamine-receptor-antagonist drugs (e.g. haloperidol) are also helpful in treating mania, this suggests a role for dopamine in the genesis of manic symptoms
- Antidepressant medications in patients with a family history of bipolar disorder or a predisposition to developing this illness

ICD-10 categorisation of severity of manic episodes	
Name	Psychopathological features
Hypomania	Slightly elevated or irritable mood lasting several days
	Some interference, but not severe disruption of work or social functioning
Mania without psychotic symptoms	Greatly elevated or irritable mood
	Marked over-activity, significant social impairment
Mania with psychotic symptoms	Incoherent thinking
	Delusions which may be bizarre
	Hallucinations
Manic stupor	Immobility replaces over-activity
	Reduced or absent speech

Table 3.10 ICD-10 categorisation of severity of manic episodes

Epidemiology of affective disorders		
	Bipolar disorder	Recurrent depression
Lifetime risk (LR)	1%	5%
LR if 1st degree relative bipolar	15%	15%
LR if 1st degree relative unipolar	1%	9%
Average age of onset	21 years	27 years
Sex ratio (M:F)	1:1	1:2

Table 3.11 Epidemiology of affective disorders

Neuroendocrine abnormalities have been demonstrated in some manic patients, with high levels of circulating cortisol and a diminished response to dexamethasone. As with depressive disorders, this may reflect underlying genetic variations contributing to the complex interplay between genetic, biological and environmental factors in the aetiology of mania.

> **Abruptly discontinuing medication for bipolar disorder against medical advice can precipitate a sudden relapse of mania.** Patients often want to discontinue their medication when they feel they are back to normal and dislike the feeling that medication is controlling their moods.

Personality

Cyclothymic personality disorder is characterised by regular mood fluctuations that are more marked than for most people but do not amount to discrete episodes of mania or depression. Bipolar disorder may be more common in people with with this personality type, perhaps reflecting a common genetic predisposition to both conditions.

Social factors

The links between significant adverse life events and episodes of disease are less evident than for depression. Notably, mania is often precipitated by stressful events that would be expected to produce a depressive mood change, such as a bereavement. However, many manic episodes occur without any obvious precipitating event.

Clinical features

Table 3.12 describes the clinical features of mania.

Diagnostic approach

Symptoms of mania must be present for no less than 1 week to qualify for a diagnosis of mania. The diagnostic approach is outlined in **Figure 3.6**.

> **Always consider risk very broadly in patients presenting with mania.** Significant risks arise as a consequence of disinhibition and impairment of judgement, resulting in a diminished regard for personal needs and safety.

Management

The management of manic episodes depends on the severity and impact of the disinhibition, and altered mood and behaviour on social functioning. These, as well as the associated risk of harm to the patient or others, must be addressed in the management plan. The combination of elation, loss of judgement and grandiose ideas means that many patients require compulsory admission as they fail to recognise they are unwell or at risk. Prompt community treatment may be a feasible alternative where the identified risks are low.

As with all psychiatric disorders, a plan addressing the individual's full biological, psychological and social needs should be formulated.

General principles in the management of a manic episode are as follows:

- Referral to psychiatric services should take place immediately
- Mania should be treated promptly to minimise the social and personal consequences for the patient
- Medication is invariably required. Mood stabilisers and antipsychotics are the mainstay of pharmacological therapy. The strength, combination and duration of drug treatment should be determined by the clinical history, the previous response to drug treatment, and an observation of mental state, sleep patterns and activity levels. Early discontinuation should be avoided to prevent relapse.
- Monitor for the development of severe depressive symptoms and suicidal ideation as the clinical picture can rapidly change from mania to depression. Persistent depressive symptoms may require cautious treatment with an antidepressant to avoid further relapses of mania.

Eliciting clinical features of mania during the MSE	
Symptom/clinical feature	Example questions to elicit symptoms
Mood	
Elevated mood: irritability or elation	'How have you been feeling lately?'
	'Have you felt in a particularly good mood, or so full of energy that you feel irritable and frustrated?'
	'Have your friends or family commented on your mood, energy or what it's like to be around you?'
Cognitive symptoms	
Inflated self esteem/grandiosity	'How have you been feeling about yourself?'
	'Have you felt more confident or sure in yourself?'
	'Have you been feeling that you've got special abilities that mark you out as different or superior to others?'
Poor attention and concentration	'How is your concentration?'
	'Have you found that you're so full of thoughts and ideas that it can be difficult to concentrate on one thing?'
Increased speech (content and rate)	'Have people commented that it is difficult to talk to you or that you've been dominating conversations?'
Accelerated thinking	'Do you find that you've had lots of thoughts and ideas that are rushing through your head that you need to 'get out' or share with people?'
Loss of normal social and sexual inhibitions and impaired judgment	'Have you been finding that you've been doing new or exciting things that you wouldn't normally do?'
Participation in gratifying activities without considering consequences, e.g. gambling, excessive spending, sexual indiscretions	'How have you been spending your time lately?'
	'Have you been doing lots of shopping or going out more than you would usually?'
	'What about gambling or seeing lots of women/men?'
	'Have you found that your sex drive has increased at all?'
Biological symptoms	
Over activity/psychomotor agitation	'What are your energy levels like?'
	'Have you been finding it difficult to sit still?'
Reduced need for sleep	'How are you sleeping?'
	'Are you finding you don't need to or can't sleep?'
Psychotic symptoms	
Disorder of the form of thought	'Do you find that people have been finding it difficult to follow you and all these ideas and thoughts you have?'
	'Have people been frustrating you at all, by not following your ideas and thoughts?'
Secondary delusions (mood congruent)	'Do you feel that anything special has happened to you lately?'
	'Do you feel that you're special and different to others in any ways?'
	'Have you got any special abilities or powers?'
Perceptual disturbance	'How does the world seem and feel to you at the minute?'
	'Have you found that sounds seem louder or clearer, or colours brighter and more vivid?'

Table 3.12 Symptom clusters and eliciting clinical features of mania during the mental state examination (MSE)

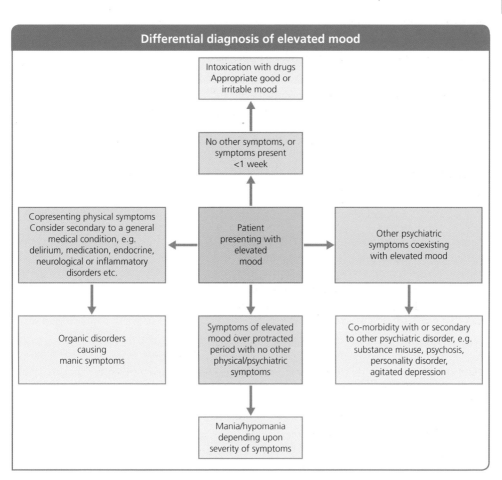

Figure 3.6 The differential diagnosis of an elevated mood

Collateral information from friends and relatives may be vital in clarifying:

- The impact of the symptoms on the patient's immediate physical health, nutritional needs and risk of misadventure
- The impact of the illness on their day-to-day life, e.g. their work and finances
- Potential precipitating factors, e.g. recent illnesses, operations and drug treatments
- The available social resources, e.g. family members who may be able to monitor and support the patient
- The needs of any dependants (e.g. children) who may be affected by the patient's illness and require support

When the patient has recovered from the manic episode, a clear plan should be made to identify the trigger factors or prodromal features that indicate the start of an episode of illness. A shared care plan of how to respond to these can then be developed to help the patient, relatives and even employers, where appropriate, to note early changes in the patient's mood or behaviour that may herald the start of another episode.

As bipolar affective disorder is a relapsing condition, continued treatment after an episode has settled and prophylaxis with mood-stabilising agents can diminish the frequency and severity of future episodes (see page 92).

Table 3.13 summarises the range of treatments used in manic and depressive episodes in patients with bipolar disorder and in the longer term treatment of recurrent disorder.

Treatment for bipolar disorder			
Treatment option	Manic episode	Bipolar depression	Bipolar affective disorder
Antipsychotic medications	Newer atypical antipsychotics better tolerated, e.g. olanzapine, quetiapine, risperidone	Quetiapine useful but not first-line. Low-risk of precipitating manic episode	Long-term treatment limited to those with recurrent psychotic symptoms or second/ third-line
Antidepressant medications	Not used in manic phase	Effective, but 5–10% risk of precipitating manic episode so prescribed with mood stabiliser/anti manic medication	Not used to prevent relapse
Benzodiazepines	For behavioural disturbance associated with mania (better tolerated than high-dose antipsychotics), e.g. lorazepam	Not indicated	Not used to prevent relapse
Lithium	Less effective and slower onset in acute mania relative to antipsychotics. Difficult to use safely in very disturbed patients. Can be used in combination with antipsychotics May be initiated in combination during milder manic episode if intent to use long-term in prophylaxis of relapse	Less effective in bipolar depression than mania but useful in milder illness when its use in long term treatment planned. Dose can be increased for patients already established on lithium at beginning of new illness	Reduces risk of relapse. More effective at preventing manic than depressive episodes. Risks of side-effects to be weighed up against risk of relapse. Requires plasma level drug monitoring blood tests
Antiepileptic medications	Slightly less effective than antipsychotics but fewer side effects. Can be given at higher loading doses than lithium, e.g. valproate and carbamazepine	No good evidence for valproate or carbamazepine. Some evidence for efficacy of lamotrigine	Valproate reduces risk of relapse but unclear if as effective as lithium. Lamotrigine effective in preventing depressive relapses. Carbamazepine less effective than lithium
ECT	Poor formal evidence base but known efficacy in acute mania. Indicated only if antipsychotics not tolerated or ineffective	Indicated in severe or treatment resistant episodes	No routine role in maintenance
Psychological therapies	Generally not able to engage during acute mania	CBT/IPT helpful	Family therapy can prevent relapse. Role of CBT unclear. Education about signs of manic relapse very helpful

Table 3.13 Treatment for acute mania, acute bipolar depression and long-term (continuation) treatment of bipolar affective disorder. CBT, cognitive behavioural therapy; ECT, electroconvulsive therapy; IPT, interpersonal therapy

Prognosis

The course and prognosis of bipolar disorder is shown in **Table 3.9**. Episodes of depression and mania can be followed by a relapse into a mood change in either direction. Some individuals are at risk of rapidly cycling illness. Many go on to develop a chronic recurrent illness characterised by periods of relapse.

A worse prognosis is associated with:

- An early onset
- A lower socioeconomic status
- Poor social support

- Ongoing psychosocial stressors
- Longer periods of depression
- Psychotic features
- Frequent relapses
- Substance misuse

Persistent mood disorders

Some people experience persistent mood disorders that fluctuate in severity throughout their lifetime but are rarely severe enough to meet criteria for hypomania or mild depression. Opinions differ but a known genetic link to mood disorders has led to these being grouped as personality types that confer an increased risk of developing mood disorders (Table 3.14).

Clinical features

Cyclothymia or cyclothymic personality disorder is defined as a persistent mood instability in which the individual experiences many periods of mild elation and mild depression. It starts early in adult life and lasts through most of the life course. Many people never come to the attention of mental health services and view themselves simply as being prone to mood swings.

Dysthymia is defined as a chronic low mood that does not meet the criteria for a diagnosis of a depressive disorder. Individuals with dysthymia tend to be of low energy and feel tired, inadequate and low all the time, although they have small intervals where they feel comparatively better. The balance between periods of 'normality' and low mood is very variable.

Features of dysthymia and cyclothymia		
	Dysthymia	Cyclothymia
Lifetime risk	0.9%	0.4–4.0%
Male:female ratio	More common in women	Equal
Treatment	Hospitalisation not required	Hospitalisation not required
	Psychotherapy and lithium have some evidence of efficacy	CBT, individual psychotherapy or if severe antidepressants may have efficacy

Table 3.14 Features of dysthymia and cyclothymia. CBT, cognitive behavioural therapy

Answers to starter questions

1. Not all patients with depression should be given medication. Depression is treated according to severity and many mild depressive episodes respond well to psychological and social treatments alone. Antidepressants are usually indicated for moderate and severe depressive illnesses.

2. Some patients' depression is so severe that they are acutely at risk of harming themselves or others. Antidepressants take some time to begin to work (2–3 weeks) so electroconvulsive therapy (ECT) is sometimes used because it is effective more quickly. Some patients do not respond to adequate doses of different antidepressants, but respond to ECT. Psychotic depression responds more quickly to ECT.

3. Not all patients with a depressive illness have further episodes. Some have an episode following a significant stressor in their life, from which they make a good recovery and which does not recur. However, in the most severe depressions 80% of patients experience further episodes, while 50% of people experiencing a moderate depression have a recurrence.

4. In patients with a predisposition to mania, antidepressants can trigger development of a manic mood state. This means that treatment of patients who have both manic and depressive episodes is difficult; they usually require a mood-stabilising agent in addition to antidepressants and antipsychotics for acute episodes of depression and mania. Other medications (e.g. steroids) and recreational drugs (e.g. amphetamines) also precipitate manic mood states.

5. Many people will have only one episode of depression, from which they make a full recovery. For others it is treatable rather than curable; 80% of people experiencing depressive illness recover good social and occupational functioning. The average length of time a depressive episode lasts is 6 months if untreated or 2–3 months with treatment. However, it is an illness which recurs for many patients, with an average of four episodes during a lifetime.

6. Many patients enjoy the early symptoms of a hypomanic mood change and describe themselves as feeling 'on top of the world', full of energy and positivity and enjoying life to the full. However, for some the initial mood change will present as irritability rather than elation, with outbursts of anger. For most that progress to a more severe manic mood change the over-activity, inability to focus on any one activity, lack of sleep and disinhibition leading to risk-taking behaviours soon overwhelm the more positive aspects of a more minor elevation of mood.

7. Antidepressants are not addictive because they do not result in the development of tolerance (in which higher doses are required to achieve the same beneficial effects). However, if they are discontinued abruptly many provoke a withdrawal syndrome which lasts for a few days, including unpleasant physical symptoms, so they should be withdrawn gradually.

Chapter 4
Schizophrenia and psychotic illness

Introduction. 123
Case 3 Auditory hallucinations . . . 124
Case 4 Self-neglect. 127

Schizophrenia. 128
Other psychotic disorders 138

Starter questions

Answers to the following questions are on pages 140–141.

1. Are people with schizophrenia dangerous?
2. Do people with schizophrenia need to stay on medication for the rest of their life?
3. Does cannabis cause schizophrenia?
4. Can you empathise with someone with psychotic symptoms when it is hard to imagine what they feel like?
5. Do people with psychosis ever realise how strange their psychotic experiences appear to others?
6. Do patients with psychosis remember their symptoms when they are better?

Introduction

Schizophrenia is the most serious of a group of disorders characterised by psychotic symptoms. These include 'positive' symptoms – delusions, hallucinations and distortions of thinking – that appear within a wide spectrum of presentations. Patients with psychotic illnesses lose contact with reality, with distressing, often harrowing, symptoms that dominate everyday life and prevent normal functioning.

Although some acute psychotic disorders, including those induced by illicit drugs, can rapidly remit, many have a chronic, relapsing course. As they tend to present for the first time in young people, they can have a profound effect on all aspects of the patient's life.

Many patients also experience disabling 'negative' symptoms: including lack of motivation, apathy, social withdrawal and a decrease in their ability to respond normally to everyday events. These have a major impact on their ability to function socially.

Case 3 Auditory hallucinations

Presentation

Catherine Gibson is 26 years old and has been brought to the emergency department by her sister Julia. In the last 4 weeks, Catherine has been behaving oddly and has recently stopped going to work. Today, at her sister's house, she became very upset. She accused her brother-in-law, Mark, of spying on her and poisoning her food as it smelled of lavender. She refused to see her own general practitioner (GP) but agreed to come to hospital to check that the poison in her food had not harmed her. She is, however, refusing to speak to the doctor, saying she has been told that she 'cannot trust him and should say nothing'.

Initial interpretation

This sudden change in behaviour suggests an acute psychiatric disorder. Catherine appears to be expressing delusional ideas about Mark and her comment about being told she cannot trust the doctor suggests she may be experiencing auditory hallucinations. This could be caused by a number of physical conditions, medications or illicit drugs, or may be an evolving psychotic illness.

History

Julia says her sister was her usual self until 4 weeks ago and has never behaved like this before. Catherine is an insurance clerk and has a steady group of friends but recently stopped going out with them. She has not been to work for 10 days; her manager suggested she should have some time off but Catherine will not say why.

Catherine agrees to talk to a female doctor, Dr Martin, insisting they should speak in a closed room away from the main

Psychosis: presentation

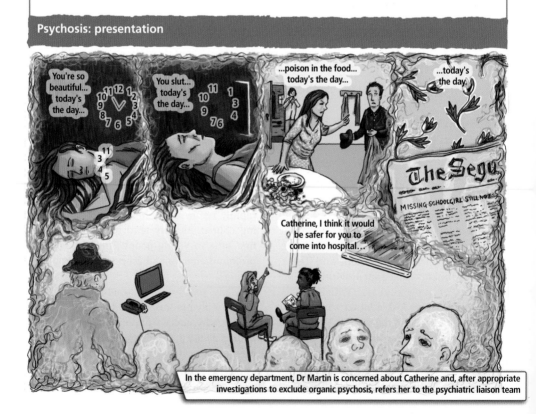

In the emergency department, Dr Martin is concerned about Catherine and, after appropriate investigations to exclude organic psychosis, refers her to the psychiatric liaison team

Case 3 *continued*

ward so Mark cannot hear them. Whispering, she tells Dr Martin that Mark has poisoned her and is angry because she has refused his sexual approaches. He wants to kill her to prevent her telling her sister. Mark talks to her at night, whispering to her in the dark and commenting on how beautiful she is.

At first Mark commented on everything she was doing, but more recently he has started to say unpleasant things, accusing her of sleeping with other men and saying she is worthless and deserves to die. Catherine has become increasingly afraid of him. She does not know how he is able to see everything she is doing, but she has stopped going out as she knows he will follow her and kill her.

She did not expect him to be at his house today. She knew at once he would try to harm her as he had moved the furniture around and left a newspaper open at a page detailing the recent disappearance of a local schoolgirl. As soon as she entered the house, Catherine heard him repeat 'Today's the day' in a sinister tone of voice.

Catherine is physically fit and is not taking any medication. She becomes upset when Dr Martin asks if she uses illicit drugs and denies this angrily. She says Mark would like that because then he would be able to make her do what he wants.

Interpretation of history

Catherine is describing both 'running commentary' and second-person (Table 2.10) auditory hallucinations, hearing her brother-in-law's voice speaking to her when she is alone at home. She is describing the delusional belief that he wishes to kill her and believes that he attempted to poison her today.

In the absence of any evidence of substance abuse or acute physical illness, the most likely diagnosis at this point is a psychotic illness. Underlying physical illness such as neurological, autoimmune and endocrine disorders must, however, be excluded before a diagnosis can be made.

Further history

Catherine has never behaved like this before and is usually healthy. She is quiet and shy but has a good circle of friends. She drinks socially only at weekends, does not smoke and has never used illicit drugs.

She has no significant medical history and takes no prescribed medication. A full physical systems enquiry reveals no physical symptoms.

Julia says this behaviour is completely out of character. Catherine was a straightforward child and has always got on well with the family, including Mark. Julia is particularly worried that this may be a serious mental illness as her maternal uncle became unwell in his 20s and never recovered. She does not know much detail but says her uncle had lengthy admissions to psychiatric care.

Examination

A full physical examination does not reveal any abnormal findings. A full mental state examination is recorded in **Table 4.1**.

Interpretation of findings

Catherine is demonstrating the signs and symptoms of a psychotic disorder. She denies using illicit drugs and is not taking any medication. There is no evidence that this is the consequence of a physical disorder. She has a family history of severe mental illness, although the diagnosis is unknown.

Investigations

Dr Martin arranges an initial assessment by the liaison psychiatry team. She also recommends taking blood for a full blood

Case 3 *continued*

Catherine's mental state examination

Category	Description
Appearance and behaviour	Catherine is appropriately dressed, clean and tidy. She is wearing no make-up and keeps her coat buttoned up during the interview. She is restless and wary. She repeatedly asks for reassurance that no-one is listening and looks out of the window frequently
Speech	Catherine whispers, pulling Dr Martin close so that she can hear, speaking quickly and urgently
Mood	Catherine appears suspicious and fearful. She says she must keep checking out of the window as she knows Mark is on his way
	She describes feeling restless and unable to settle. For the last 3 weeks she has been unable to sleep in her bedroom as she knows Mark will come and speak to her there. She keeps watch from her window and has been unable to do any of her usual activities. She denies being low in mood, but feels exhausted.
Perceptions	Catherine describes hearing Mark talking directly to her, particularly at night time. It is always his voice and she can now hear him wherever she is. Today he has said 'today's the day' repeatedly and she knows he means to kill her
	She may also be experiencing olfactory hallucinations, smelling lavender when she was eating
Thoughts	Catherine believes Mark wishes to kill her because she rejected his sexual advances. She says that he leaves signs for her, moving things around, letting her know he has been in her flat, though she does not know how he gets in and has never seen him there
Cognitions	Catherine is not demonstrating any cognitive abnormalities
Insight	Catherine is demonstrating little insight. She believes she is being poisoned by her brother-in-law and agreed to come to hospital only to ensure that she received appropriate treatment for that
Suicidal ideation	Catherine is not expressing any suicidal ideation. She is terrified that Mark wishes to kill her and does not want that to happen

Table 4.1 Catherine's mental state examination (MSE)

count, thyroid and liver function tests, urea and electrolytes and random blood glucose to check for any physical abnormalities not revealed by the history and examination.

Diagnosis

The most likely diagnosis is an acute psychotic disorder with no evidence of psychotic illness caused by underlying organic illness. There are no precipitating events or evident stressors. Dr Martin is concerned that Catherine may be in the early stages of a schizophrenic illness, although she has not yet had symptoms for the required 4 week period for schizophrenia to be diagnosed. Catherine is agitated and fearful for her life and agrees to see the liaison psychiatry team.

The liaison psychiatry doctor recommends admission to the local psychiatric hospital for investigations. These are to include the blood tests recommended in the emergency department, a CT scan of Catherine's head to exclude intracranial pathology and a close observation of her daily activity to ensure her safety and provide further analysis of her mental state.

Case 4 Self-neglect

Presentation

Matthew Barker's mother has requested that his GP visits them at home. Matthew is 18 years old and finished school 6 months ago. He achieved much lower grades than expected in his A levels so could not take up his university place to study engineering. At first, his parents thought he was low in mood because of this, but over the last 3 months they have become increasingly concerned about him. He no longer leaves the house, has no contact with friends and lies on his bed all day listening to music.

Initial interpretation

Matthew's change in behaviour could be a consequence of a number of psychiatric disorders such as depression, anxiety, a psychotic illness or substance abuse. Physical disorders, for example endocrine disorders and chronic infections, must also be considered.

Further history

Matthew is lying in his bed, looking at the ceiling with his headphones on. He is willing to speak with the doctor but does not initiate conversation. He drifts off in the middle of sentences and seems unable to hold the thread of the conversation. His eye contact is poor, and his speech is sparse and monotonous.

His hair is long and unwashed, and he is wearing old, stained jeans and a scruffy T-shirt. His room is a mess, with piles of screwed-up papers in the corners. He says the paper is there because he is always trying to answer the questions but it never works out; he cannot explain this further.

Matthew says his mood is okay and that he doesn't really want to do anything as he has everything he needs here. He cannot understand why his mother is worried about him. He admits he regularly used cannabis with friends when he was 14–18

years old but has now stopped as he cannot be bothered to go out and get it.

Examination

Matthew declines a physical examination. His mental state examination is recorded in **Table 4.2**.

Interpretation of findings

There has been a marked deterioration in Matthew's educational, personal and social functioning over the last few months. The use of cannabis at a young age is a risk factor for the development of schizophrenia in susceptible individuals. Matthew's symptoms have been present consistently for some months. Although he has no acute florid psychotic symptoms he is showing negative symptoms and a significant change in his personal behaviour. This suggests he does have at least two symptoms required for a diagnosis of schizophrenia.

Investigations

The doctor wants to take a blood sample for a full blood count, thyroid and liver function tests, urea and electrolytes, random blood glucose and Epstein–Barr virus to exclude glandular fever but Matthew will not consent to this at present.

Diagnosis

Matthew does not have particularly florid symptoms but the deterioration in his functioning and social withdrawal are very marked. The GP calls the local Early Intervention in Psychosis team to arrange an urgent assessment. He thinks Matthew is likely to be suffering from schizophrenia, which will require medication and psychosocial support.

Case 4 *continued*

Matthew's mental state examination	
Category	Description
Appearance and behaviour	Matthew is unkempt, untidy and smells unwashed. He is co-operative but unreactive, lying still on his bed throughout
Speech	Matthew speaks slowly, says very little and does not initiate conversation. His voice is monotonous and he frequently loses his train of thought and drifts off. He is vague in conversation and uses stock phrases repeatedly, e.g. 'the music has all of the truth in it'
Mood	Matthew's mood is flat and unreactive. He denies feeling low and says he doesn't feel anything, not even bored. He has no depressive symptoms, says he eats well because his mum brings him meals regularly and sleeps a lot. He has no overt concerns and no suicidal ideation
Perceptions	He denies having hallucinations, though he agrees that the music he is listening too has 'all of the truth in it' and particular messages for him
Thoughts	Matthew says he is trying to work everything out but 'it's all very complicated'. He is sure that there must be some special purpose for him and no-one will tell him what it is. He believes he has to wait to find this out and all will become clear.
	He cannot say why he keeps losing the train of his thoughts saying 'they just aren't there anymore'
Cognitions	Matthew is not demonstrating any cognitive abnormalities
Insight	Matthew is demonstrating little insight. He believes he is fine, just waiting and does not really understand why his mother has called the doctor
Suicidal ideation	Matthew has no suicidal ideation

Table 4.2 Matthew's mental state examination (MSE)

Schizophrenia

Schizophrenia is the most serious form of psychotic illness. The core feature of psychotic illness is the individual's loss of contact with reality. This is demonstrated by the development of fixed, false beliefs (delusions) that have a major impact upon the person's behaviour. Abnormal perceptions (hallucinations) are characteristic and take many forms. Although the course of schizophrenia varies enormously, it is for many patients a chronic, relapsing condition that starts at a young age.

Acute and chronic syndromes

The presentation of schizophrenia can be divided into two distinct syndromes or phases: acute and chronic.

The acute syndrome is characterised by 'positive' symptoms that represent a loss of contact with reality. These include hallucinations, delusions and marked disturbances in behaviour, often in response to these abnormal beliefs and perceptions.

The chronic syndrome develops over a much longer time period and is characterised by an accumulation of 'negative' symptoms. These include lack of motivation, underactivity, reduced speech, reduced emotion, social withdrawal and thought disorder.

A further phase, the 'at-risk mental state', is increasingly being recognised as a period during which lower grade symptoms such as social withdrawal and apathy predominate without formal psychotic symptoms. This often appears in teenagers and can be hard to distinguish from normal adolescent behavioural changes, depression, social anxiety and substance misuse. Many, but not all, individuals presenting with this will develop a full psychotic illness.

between the ages of 15 and 30 years. Women tend to develop symptoms several years later than this, with a higher incidence in women after the age of 30 (**Figure 4.1**). Schizophrenia and psychotic disorders are very rare in children under the age of 10 but can appear for the first time in adults over the age of 50.

> **Treating an evolving psychosis as early as possible improves its prognosis.** A long duration of untreated psychosis is associated with increasing damage to social functioning, cognitive ability and overall recovery.

Classification

The ICD-10 groups schizophrenia and psychoses together. This category includes schizophrenia and its immediately related disorders, delusional disorders and psychotic disorders with an accompanying affective (mood) component (**Table 4.3**).

> **Psychosis presenting for the first time in an elderly person mandates careful assessment to distinguish it from an organic psychosis,** particularly one related to medication or caused by the underlying cognitive changes in dementia.

Epidemiology

Schizophrenia has a lifetime prevalence of 1% with an annual incidence of 10–20 cases per 100,000 population. There is little variation in the incidence and prevalence of schizophrenia internationally. However, the prevalence is higher in areas of socioeconomic deprivation.

> **Schizophrenia is more common in deprived urban areas and lower socioeconomic classes.** It is present in 10% of the homeless population. This may be a consequence of the downward 'social drift' caused by the disorder and its impact on the individual's life rather than homelessness being an aetiological factor.

Schizophrenia typically begins in early adulthood. Men tend to develop schizophrenia

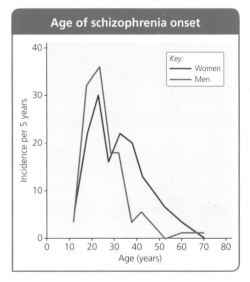

Figure 4.1 Gender differences and age of onset in schizophrenia.

Schizophrenia and related disorders: ICD categorisation	
ICD Category	**Description**
Schizophrenia	All forms of schizophrenia (paranoid, catatonic, simple etc) in which the characteristic distortions of thinking and perception occur
Persistent delusional disorders	Characterised by the presence of delusions, which are persistent and often lifelong, usually without the presence of accompanying hallucinations
Acute and transient psychotic disorders	Acute onset, sometimes arising as a response to stress , usually remitting completely within 2–3 months
Schizoaffective disorders	Episodic illnesses in which affective and psychotic symptoms are equally prominent within the same episode of illness

Table 4.3 Schizophrenia and related disorders: ICD categorisation

Aetiology

The aetiology of schizophrenia is multifactorial and wide-ranging (**Table 4.4**).

Prevention

There is a complex interrelationship between the many causative factors of schizophrenia so specific prevention is difficult. Medical management, however, aims to prevent relapses by focusing on many of the risk factors listed in **Table 4.4**.

Pathogenesis

Although some psychological theories have been suggested to explain the development

Aetiological factors for schizophrenia	
Factor	Risk
Predisposing factors	
Increased lifetime risk of first degree relatives of patients with schizophrenia	1–10% for first degree relatives 50% for children of two parents with schizophrenia
Concordance between twins for schizophrenia	Monozygotic twins concordance 40–50% Dizygotic twins concordance 15%
Environmental factors	Slightly increased risk in people born in winter months
Maternal factors during pregnancy	Slightly increased risk in those born to mothers with a virus (e.g. flu) during pregnancy or abnormalities of pregnancy (pre-eclampsia, bleeding, diabetes)
Obstetric difficulties	Emergency caesarean section and asphyxia during delivery
Fetal development	Low birth weight Congenital abnormalities
Migration	Increased risk in first and second-generation immigrant populations, especially Afro-Caribbean
Personality	Personality disorders, particularly those with schizoid traits
Early adverse life experience	Physical abuse Neglect Sexual abuse
Substance misuse	Cannabis, amphetamines, cocaine, hallucinogenic drugs produce symptoms akin to schizophrenia Cannabis with high concentrations of THC (tetrahydrocannabinol) used extensively as a teenager increases the risk six-fold
Precipitating factors	
Stress and life events	Acute adverse life events (bereavement, separation, change of home, loss of employment, etc.)
Substance misuse	Returning to cannabis or hallucinogenic drugs can provoke a relapse of symptoms in predisposed individuals
Perpetuating factors	
Adverse social circumstances	Poor housing, financial difficulties, lack of social activity and poor personal relationships all contribute
Non-concordance with medication	Taking medication inconsistently is highly correlate with continued symptoms
High expressed emotion	Relatives may be very critical of the behaviour of individuals with schizophrenia Highly 'expressed emotion' is associated with relapse
Substance misuse	Continued use of drugs and alcohol inhibit recovery

Table 4.4 Aetiological factors for schizophrenia

of schizophrenia, much more compelling evidence implicates neurodevelopmental and neurotransmitter changes.

Neurotransmitter theories

Antipsychotic medications act predominantly on receptors on the dopaminergic neurones. This has given rise to the dopaminergic theory of schizophrenia, which suggests that it arises from overactivity of the dopaminergic neurones (see Table 1.10 and; **Table 4.5**).

The changes in dopaminergic function that occur in schizophrenia do not, however, fully explain the disease. Antipsychotic medications do not reduce the symptoms in all patients. In addition, they are effective in many other conditions, including delirium and dementia. Other receptor activity has also been implicated in schizophrenia as newer effective antipsychotic medications act on serotonergic and histaminergic receptors as well.

> **There is always a therapeutic delay before antipsychotic medication takes effect** even though dopaminergic activity is blocked immediately. In most individuals, side effects appear long before the medications have had their full effect.

Neurodevelopmental theories

Neuroimaging techniques show structural abnormalities in the brains of patients with schizophrenia, such as enlarged ventricles which are associated with negative symptoms. There is a general reduction in brain size due to cell loss, especially in the:

- Frontal and temporal lobes
- Hippocampus
- Amygdala
- Parahippocampal gyrus

Newer imaging techniques such as positron emission tomography and functional MRI allow the functional levels in the brain to be assessed by measuring the regional blood flow. These techniques have demonstrated that schizophrenia is associated with diminished activity in the frontal lobes.

People who develop schizophrenia are also more likely to have had developmental problems during childhood and a lower average premorbid intelligence quotient.

Clinical features

Acute-phase symptoms

In the acute phase, the symptoms are characteristically florid. The central features are delusions and hallucinations, which may take varied and bizarre forms (see Chapter 2).

Some patients appear to have entirely normal behaviour, only describing their psychotic experiences when directly asked. For many, however, there are marked disturbances in behaviour. Patients may be:

The dopamine theory of schizophrenia			
Neural pathway	Physiological function	Dopamine theory	Evidence
Mesolimbic tract	Motivated and goal-directed behaviours, promotion and reinforcement of learning. Implicated in the neurobiology of addiction	Positive symptoms of schizophrenia could result from excessive dopaminergic activity in this tract	All effective antipsychotic medication blocks dopamine receptors
			Potency of dopamine receptor blockade is positively correlated with efficacy against positive symptoms
			Drugs such as amphetamines which cause release of dopamine mimic positive psychotic symptoms
Nigrostriatal tract	Initiation and control of movement	Negative symptoms could result from dopamine under-activity in this area	Antipsychotic medications (further reducing dopaminergic activity) make little impact upon negative symptoms

Table 4.5 Evidence for the dopamine theory of schizophrenia

- Restless, agitated and noisy
- Awkward in their social behaviour
- Withdrawn and preoccupied
- Perplexed and anxious

Their speech may be difficult to follow, reflecting their disturbed ability to think. It may also be vague and difficult to grasp, or entirely preoccupied with the patient's current concerns and ideas.

Hallucinations can occur in any sensory modality but are most commonly auditory. Particularly diagnostic of schizophrenia are hallucinations of:

- Hearing people talking about the patient as if they were not there, usually making derogatory or critical comments
- Voices describing everything the patient is doing (running commentary)
- Hearing their own thoughts spoken out loud (thought echo)

Command hallucinations, in which a voice speaks directly to the patient, may present particular risks if they instruct the patient to do something that may be harmful to themselves or to others.

Some patients locate the voice as coming from a particular part of their own body or from a speaker or microphone hidden in the room. They then develop delusional explanations to support this. Auditory hallucinations may be transitory and associated with particular circumstances, or persistent and accompanying everything the patient does.

Never ask patients about 'their voices'. To the patient, the auditory hallucination has all the qualities of any real voice and cannot be distinguished from one, making it all the more disturbing. Instead ask the patient to describe what they are hearing, what is being said and who is speaking to get a clear picture of their experience.

Delusions can relate to any aspect of the patient's life. They are often persecutory and understandable as a response to the

auditory hallucinations the patient is experiencing (see Tables 2.10 and 2.12). Delusions of control (Table 2.12) including interference with the patient's thoughts (withdrawal, broadcasting or insertion), movements and feelings are particularly characteristic of schizophrenia. These delusions can terrify the patient, leading them to extreme action to evade their perceived persecutors.

Some patients experience delusions that could be true. For example, they may become convinced their partner is having an affair or stealing money from them but offer bizarre evidence for this belief. A collateral history from a close relative may be necessary to clarify this.

Insight is characteristically impaired in the acute phase of schizophrenia. The hallucinations and delusions are real and compelling to the patient, and consequently affect their behaviour. This lack of insight also impacts upon the patient's willingness to accept medical advice or treatment. Some patients can only be treated after admission to hospital against their will.

Assessing the patient's insight is a key part of the risk assessment. A lack of insight may cause them to expose themselves or others to risk if they act in response to their auditory hallucinations or delusions.

Chronic-phase symptoms

Although some patients make a good recovery from the acute phase of the illness, some enter a more chronic phase characterised by 'negative symptoms'. Although these may be less immediately obvious, they are extremely disabling and difficult to treat (**Table 4.6**).

In addition, some positive symptoms of hallucinations and delusions often persist. The delusions may become more complex but be held separately from the rest of the patient's life and associated with less emotional response than in the acute phase. This allows

Negative symptoms of schizophrenia	
Symptom	**Description**
Lack of motivation (volition)	Inactivity, loss of initiative and interest in usual activities with protracted inactivity if left to their own devices
Loss of social skills and self-care	Neglect of personal hygiene and appearance
	Poor nutrition with marked changes in weight
	Withdrawal from social activity
	Inappropriate social behaviour, e.g. approaching strangers in the street or sexual disinhibition
	Lack of care of home and surroundings
	Preoccupation with a narrow specific range of activity
Blunted affect	Lack of appropriate responses to emotional events which may extend to an incongruous affect (e.g. laughing when hearing of someone's death)
Poverty of thought and speech and thought disorder	See Table 2.11
	May be profound and make conversation hard to understand
Movement disorders	Although many abnormal movements are caused by medication, some patients will also show stereotypies (repetitive purposeless movements) and mannerisms (repeated odd but goal-directed movements)

Table 4.6 Negative symptoms of schizophrenia

the patient to function more effectively than they did during the acute phase. Although patients may still not accept that they are ill, they may come to recognise their auditory hallucinations as different from everyday experience, allowing them to get on with their life.

> **Many patients develop a partial insight into the acute phases of their illness,** recognising that they were unwell but still believing that this was as a real consequence of the persecution they were experiencing at the time.

Diagnostic approach

In the ICD classification, symptoms of schizophrenia must be continuously present for at least 1 month (**Table 4.7**). Many psychotic episodes remit before a month has elapsed and therefore do not warrant a diagnosis of schizophrenia. These would be diagnosed as an acute psychotic disorder (see page 139).

As with most psychiatric diagnosis, a careful history and an examination involving the mental state examination are key. Particular attention must be given to:

1. **A full psychiatric history,** including the social and personal history and childhood development. This is to identify predisposing, precipitating and perpetuating factors. Make a detailed exploration of any hallucinations and delusions, specifically checking for the symptoms outlined in **Table 4.7**.

> **Ask the patient to tell you more about their hallucinations just as you would for anyone who told you people were saying horrible things about them.** Ask what the voices are saying, when they hear them and who they think is speaking. Your interest will reassure the patient that you are taking them seriously and encourage them to tell you more.

2. **A collateral history** from a close informant if the patient is too unwell to give a good account
3. **A consideration of other psychiatric disorders** which include psychotic symptoms during your psychiatric assessment, e.g. bipolar disorder, dementia, delirium and severe depression

ICD-10 criteria for schizophrenia	
Diagnosis must include either:	
One (or more) of the following symptoms*	Two (or more) of the following symptoms*
Thought echo, insertion or withdrawal	Persistent hallucinations of any type accompanied by fleeting delusions without clear emotional content, or persistent over-valued ideas
Delusions of control, influence or passivity or delusional perceptions	Breaks in the train of thought, incoherent or irrelevant speech and/or neologisms
Hallucinatory voices giving a running commentary on behaviour, discussing the patient in the third person or other hallucinatory voices arising elsewhere	Catatonic behaviour (excitement, waxy flexibility or posturing, stupor or negativism)
Delusions of a bizarre nature (e.g. with religious or superhuman content)	Negative symptoms (apathy, paucity of speech, blunting of affect, social withdrawal and loss of function). These must not be attributable to medication or other psychiatric disorder
	Significant persistent change in personal behaviour with social withdrawal and an aimlessness and self-absorbed attitude.

* All symptoms must be clearly present for most of the time for at least 1 month

Table 4.7 ICD-10 criteria for schizophrenia

4. **The exclusion of any underlying causative physical disorder.** The most likely organic cause of psychosis, particularly in young patients presenting for the first time, is substance misuse. Amphetamines, ecstasy, ketamine, phencyclidine, cocaine, cannabis and inhalants can all precipitate a psychosis, as can alcohol withdrawal and intoxication. Several prescribed medications, including morphine and steroids, have the same effect. Less common physical disorders presenting with psychosis include neurological disorders (brain tumours and degenerative disorders), strokes, autoimmune disorders, HIV/AIDS and hereditary disorders

5. **A full medical history, physical examination and investigations** (see page 134). Any abnormal results must be investigated further

Investigations

A number of investigations will help to rule out an organic cause for the psychosis and to establish the patient's current state of health prior to commencing medication (**Table 4.8**).

Management

Most patients presenting with a psychosis for the first time ('first-episode psychosis' – FEP) require assessment and treatment by specialist psychiatric services. In the UK, this is via the Early Intervention in Psychosis Team, referral to outpatient psychiatric services or admission to psychiatric hospital depending upon severity and attendant risks. The sooner a psychotic illness can be treated the better, as the prognosis in terms of long-term functioning worsens the longer the initial psychosis goes untreated. This can be particularly problematic when the early signs of illness are subtle and develop slowly. Such presentations must be treated with a high degree of suspicion and referred for expert attention.

The first interview with a patient with a psychotic illness can be very difficult, especially if the patient does not think they are ill. Do not challenge their beliefs or experiences no matter how bizarre. Remember they are completely real and distressing to the patient – you should respond empathically and uncritically.

The importance of treating a psychosis as swiftly as possible has led many countries to develop dedicated psychosis services such as the UK's, Early Intervention in Psychosis Services, which provides a rapid-response assessment of patients who appear to have early symptoms suggestive of psychotic illness.

Investigations for a patient presenting with psychotic symptoms		
Investigation	Details	Reasons for investigations
Blood tests	FBC, U&E, LFT, TFT, CRP, fasting blood glucose, glycosylated haemoglobin (HbA1C)	Assessing for anaemia, infection, thyroid abnormalities, evidence of alcohol misuse, diabetes, abnormalities of renal/liver function
	If indicated from history HIV testing, syphilis serology and other autoimmune markers	Also necessary for baseline blood values prior to commencing medication
Urine testing	MSU with/without drug screening	Evidence of drug misuse, infection screen
Pregnancy testing	Prior to starting any medication for fertile females wherever indicated	Teratogenicity of medications will need to be considered if patient is pregnant
Lipid levels	Prior to starting treatment with antipsychotic medication	Atypical antipsychotic medications raise lipid levels: assay required for baseline level
Neuroimaging	CT scan of head if pathology suspected	Checking for intracranial pathology which may be contributing to presentation

Table 4.8 Investigations for psychotic patients. CRP, C-reactive protein; FBC, full blood count; LFT, liver function tests; MSU, midstream urine; TFT, thyroid function tests; U&E, urea and elctrolytes

Patients with psychotic symptoms come to the attention of medical services via numerous routes. These include GP services, accident and emergency departments and non-medical services such as the police.

Many patients attend because their relatives or neighbours are concerned about them, despite the patients not knowing they are ill themselves.

Management should include psychological support, education about the illness and activities suitable to the patient's abilities and interests.

Risk assessment

Some patients may present a significant acute risk to their own safety or to the safety of others as a consequence of their behavioural disturbance (**Table 4.9**). Although only a minority of patients with schizophrenia are violent, the immediate risk assessment must also consider where and how the patient should be assessed. It may be unsafe for them to be seen alone in their own home so assessment may have to take place in a place of safety such as a police station.

Antipsychotic medication

If it is safe, it is preferable to have a brief period of assessment without medication during which investigations can be undertaken and the patient's symptoms explored further. Some drug-induced psychoses settle quickly when the ingested drug is discontinued and recover with supportive treatment alone.

Risks to consider in schizophrenic patients		
Risks to self	Risks to others	Risks from others
Attempted suicide (10–15%). More common in young male patients at an early stage of illness and in those with depressive symptoms	**Violence**. More likely with past history of violence and substance misuse, during acute phase of psychosis. Increased in patients with personality disorder and access to weapons	**Vulnerable to abuse** from others during psychosis including violent crime, sexual assault and financial corruption
Self-neglect. Immediate loss of interest in self-care and nutrition, employment, management of finances, care for ongoing medical conditions, etc.	**Inadvertent risk due to immediate chaotic behaviour**, e.g. disinhibition, lack of awareness of danger, driving whilst unwell	**Stigma and bullying**
Self-awareness. Risk-taking behaviour in response to hallucinations/delusions		

Table 4.9 Risks to consider in schizophrenic patients

Although a biopsychosocial approach to treatment should be adopted, the core effective treatment for an established diagnosis of psychosis is antipsychotic medication. The overall approach to the use of antipsychotic medication is summarised in **Figure 4.2**.

In general, antipsychotic medications should only be initiated by a psychiatrist (other clinicians issue repeat prescriptions for maintenance therapy once symptoms are under control). As described in more detail in Chapter 2, these drugs are dopamine antagonists and fall into two groups, typical and atypical antipsychotics. Their side effects arise from the effect of dopamine blockade on dopaminergic pathways in the brain (**Figure 4.3**). The two groups have differing side-effects (see Chapter 2), and their advantages and disadvantages should be discussed in detail with the patient and their immediate carer or close relative before starting therapy. Baseline investigations are also required before therapy starts.

Atypical antipsychotics are usually the first-line treatment for newly diagnosed schizophrenia. Treatment is initiated with a single antipsychotic at the lowest dose that effectively controls the symptoms. The dose is titrated upwards if necessary. This approach is preferable to starting with a high dose that may induce intolerable side-effects before any beneficial effects have occurred.

Typical antipsychotic medications are still widely used despite the extrapyramidal and hormonal side effects (e.g. hypoprolactinaemia) caused by their widespread blockade of dopamine receptors. Unlike most of the atypical antipsychotics, they are available in long-acting injectable format (depot injections), which are useful for patients who are unable to adhere to daily medication regimens.

Atypical antipsychotics are the first choice for new patients with a psychotic illness. However, patients who are stable on long-term therapy with typical antipsychotics do not need to be transferred to these newer medications. Atypical medications are less troublesome for patients in terms of the side effects produced by dopamine blockade. However, it has become increasingly apparent that they cause a range of metabolic disturbances, including changes in glucose and lipid metabolism and weight gain.

Antipsychotic medication is likely to be taken for protracted periods over months or years. Understanding the effects and side effects is central to improving patients' commitment to the their treatment.

Some patients' symptoms do not remit with medication. If the first medication does not produce symptom remission after being

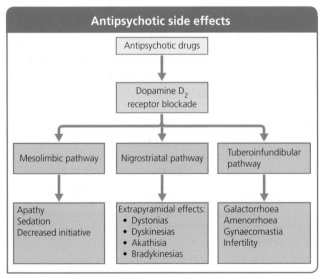

Antipsychotic side effects

Antipsychotic drugs

↓

Dopamine D$_2$ receptor blockade

↓

| Mesolimbic pathway | Nigrostriatal pathway | Tuberoinfundibular pathway |

| Apathy Sedation Decreased initiative | Extrapyramidal effects: • Dystonias • Dyskinesias • Akathisia • Bradykinesias | Galactorrhoea Amenorrhoea Gynaecomastia Infertility |

Figure 4.2 Side effects of antipsychotic drugs.

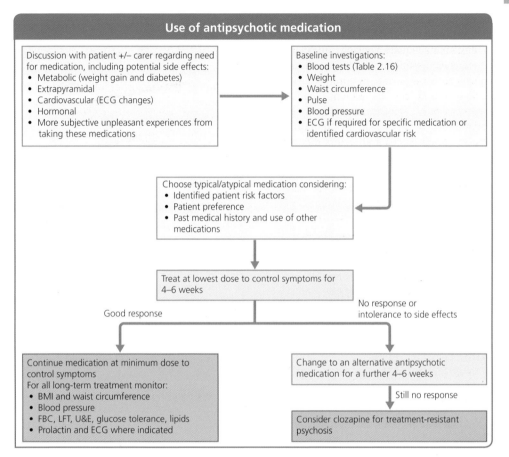

Figure 4.3 Use of antipsychotic medication.

used at full dose for 6 weeks an alternative should be prescribed for a further 6 weeks. Patients who do not respond to two or more antipsychotics for a full 6 weeks are considered to be 'treatment resistant'. Patients with treatment-resistant schizophrenia (TRS) are prescribed clozapine. This is beneficial when most other medications have proved ineffective but requires weekly to monthly white cell monitoring for potentially fatal agranulocytosis (see Chapter 2, page 88). All antipsychotics are more effective at treating the positive symptoms than the negative symptoms of schizophrenia.

Psychological treatment

Cognitive behavioural treatment is often used in schizophrenia and may help some patients to manage their symptoms and challenge their own unusual beliefs and experiences. Some patients are able to manage their own experiences highly effectively using this approach, with significant benefit to their social and personal functioning. Family therapy and couple therapy including the patient's nearest relatives and partner can also be used.

Social treatments

Patients with schizophrenia and psychotic illness now spend much less time in hospital environments than has historically been the case. However, the majority of patients experiencing their first episode still require an initial period of hospitalisation. Subsequent treatment focuses on maximising function in the community, including social skills and communications skills training, improving access to work, training and education, and developing personal skills.

Ensuring adequate housing and financing, and engaging patients in appropriate social activity are all important in minimising stresses and supporting the patient's continued recovery after a significant psychotic illness. Prevention of relapses includes attention to the misuse of substances and factors that trigger relapses for the individual patient. Care should be coordinated via a multidisciplinary team who can consider all aspects of the patient's psychological, medical and social care.

> Many patients function more highly if discharged from hospital to a hostel or other supported living environment rather than to the family home. This is likely to be due to both the availability of social support/structure, and the decreased 'expressed emotion' or critical emotionally over-involved attitudes which may be expressed to a family member with a disorder.

Prognosis

Contrary to public perceptions, a significant proportion of patients make a full recovery from a significant schizophrenic episode and never have another one (**Table 4.10**). A number of factors are, however, associated with a poor prognosis (**Table 4.11**).

The patient's physical health must be monitored during treatment (**Figure 4.1**), and any concurrent physical illness must be treated appropriately. Patients with severe and enduring mental health problems such as schizophrenia are likely to die an average of 15–20 years earlier than the general population. Many of these deaths are related to raised cardiovascular risk, which can be decreased by management of weight, blood pressure, diet and lifestyle factors.

Prognosis in schizophrenia	
Outcome	Percentage (%)
Full recovery from acute episode	20–30
Recurrent episodes of illness	20–30
Recurrent episodes of illness with diminishing recovery between episodes	20–30
Severe continuous illness and disability from the outset	10
Suicide	10–15

Table 4.10 Prognosis in schizophrenia

Prognostic factors in schizophrenia	
Good prognosis	Poor prognosis
Female	Male
Later acute onset	Slowly developing illness at a young age
Concordance with medication	
Good social support	Long duration of untreated psychosis (DUP)
Employment and social engagement	Prominent negative symptoms
Marital status: better for those in stable relationships	Continued misuse of drugs or alcohol
	Family history of schizophrenia
	Previous psychiatric history or premorbid personality disorder

Table 4.11 Prognostic factors in schizophrenia

Other psychotic disorders

Persistent delusional disorders

This group of psychotic illnesses is considered separately from schizophrenia because the most prominent, and often the only, symptom is delusions. Persistent delusional disorders are less common than schizophrenia and tend to develop gradually from the fifth decade onwards.

Clinical features

Delusions may be single or multiple but often become intricate and complex. Their content is variable but they are often persecutory, grandiose or focused on litigation against some perceived wrongdoing. For a diagnosis of delusional disorder to be made, delusions must be present for more than 3 months in the absence of other symptoms or an underlying physical cause.

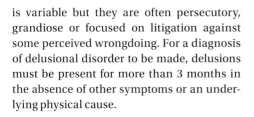

Pathological jealousy (Othello syndrome) is a delusional disorder in which the patient believes their partner is being sexually unfaithful to them. They produce irrational reasoning for this belief and spurious evidence for the perceived betrayal. It is more common in men and they may become violent towards their partner.

Despite the complexity of their delusional system, many patients are able to continue with their everyday life remarkably well. Hallucinations are not part of this disorder, and the patient's affect, speech and behaviour are usually normal outside discussion of the delusional content. Some delusions are understandable in the context of the patient's life experience but will develop to become implausible and incredible to others.

Management

The assessment must include a full psychiatric assessment to consider other diagnoses including schizophrenia, depressive psychosis and bipolar disorder. Assessment must also rule out causative organic factors, such as endocrine disorders, medications, drugs and alcohol.

A risk assessment in terms of the consequences of the patient's beliefs should be made. Many patients are not willing to undertake treatment as they lack insight into their condition. A few require treatment in hospital if they are presenting a risk to themselves or others.

Medication

Antipsychotic medication may diminish the intensity of the patient's delusional beliefs and decrease any emotional distress they are causing. For many patients, the delusions will persist despite treatment but can be managed by the patient. In this way, they can carry on with their ordinary daily activities.

Acute and transient psychotic disorders

These disorders have much in common with schizophrenia but are generally of very acute onset and remission and may arise in response to acutely stressful life events.

Clinical features

The psychotic symptoms appear rapidly (within 2 weeks or less, and sometimes within as little as 48 hours) in a previously completely well person. The presentation includes hallucinations and delusions accompanied by a markedly changeable emotional state ranging from elation to irritability and anxiety. In some patients, these symptoms arise soon after an acute stress such as a bereavement, job loss, marital breakdown or severe physical threat such as combat.

Patients usually make a full recovery. For many, this takes only a few days or weeks and it is certainly complete within 2–3 months.

Management

An acute disturbance may be severe enough to require acute admission to hospital. Treatment with antipsychotic medication will provide symptomatic relief and remission of the symptoms. It should be possible to cautiously withdraw the medication when the patient is symptom-free.

Patients who do not recover fully should be offered continued psychiatric outpatient treatment as this may be the first presentation of a more severe schizophrenic illness.

Schizoaffective disorders

These are disorders in which both psychotic and affective (mood) changes are equally apparent throughout the disorder. They must be differentiated from a depressive episode developing in a patient with previously diagnosed schizophrenia.

Clinical features

A schizoaffective disorder should only be diagnosed when symptoms of schizophrenia and mood change are present simultaneously.

> Patients who have recently recovered from a severe psychotic episode commonly become clinically depressed without new psychotic symptoms. This should not be diagnosed as a schizoaffective disorder.

In schizoaffective disorder, patients present with delusions and hallucinations accompanied by either a depressive or a manic mood state.

Patients with the depressive type demonstrate characteristic symptoms of depression alongside typical schizophrenic symptoms. Patients with manic schizoaffective disorder are likely to present with more florid manic symptoms including overactivity, elation, excitement and disinhibited behaviour.

> A depressive schizoaffective disorder is sometimes difficult to distinguish from a depressive psychosis. A careful mental state examination should focus on eliciting the core characteristic symptoms of schizophrenia, which go beyond the mood-congruent hallucinations expected with a depressive psychosis. These include delusions of control or interference and hallucinations.

Management

After a thorough psychiatric assessment and mental state examination, treatment should be instituted to manage the symptoms of both the schizophrenia and the attendant mood disorder. Hospital treatment should be considered for patients whose behavioural disturbance or risk of harm to themselves or others is significant.

Many patients recover well from the acute episode of illness but experience recurrent episodes of illness requiring ongoing treatment.

Answers to starter questions

1. It is commonly thought that patients with schizophrenia are dangerous. The vast majority are not and account for less than 5% of violent crime. They can, however, be a risk to themselves (lifetime risk of suicide 10%) and to others as a consequence of their erratic behaviour. Patients with schizophrenia are more likely to be frightened and confused than violent, and are often at risk from crime and victimisation as a consequence of their illness.

2. Some patients only have one episode of illness and their medication can be gradually withdrawn following full recovery. Patients who experience relapses need to remain on the lowest achievable dose of medication for the foreseeable future to control their symptoms and reduce the risk of relapses.

3. Many illicit drugs produce psychotic symptoms, but the majority of people who use cannabis do not develop schizophrenia. However, cannabis with high concentrations of THC (tetrahydrocannabinol) used extensively as a teenager increases the risk of developing schizophrenia six-fold.

4. Unlike depression, which is an exaggeration of a mood state that we can relate to, schizophrenia includes symptoms such as delusions and hallucinations that are not part of our ordinary experience. Although what the patient says is often completely impossible, try to put yourself in their place and imagine how you would feel if the things they are describing were actually happening.

Answers *continued*

5. Insight into the abnormal nature of their experience varies between patients. Some understand that their symptoms are difficult for others to believe in or understand, but many do not. After successful treatment, some patients recover full insight and realise that their beliefs and experiences were part of an illness, while others will always think their experiences were real but have now stopped happening.

6. Some patients with very acute florid psychosis have limited recall of their symptoms when they recover. Other patients remember their symptoms clearly and are able to give a full account of the things that they believed were happening when they were unwell.

Chapter 5
Anxiety disorders

Introduction. 143
Case 5 Persistent pervasive
      symptoms of anxiety 144
Generalised anxiety disorder 147
Panic disorder 150
Phobias. 151
Obsessive compulsive disorder . . . 154
Acute stress reaction and post-
    traumatic stress disorder. 157

Starter questions

Answers to the following questions are on page 160.

1. Why are women more prone to anxiety disorders than men?
2. Is there a difference between panic disorder and agoraphobia?
3. How do people with obsessive compulsive disorder develop their compulsive behaviours?

Introduction

Everyone experiences symptoms of anxiety during their lifetime. It is a normal physical and psychological response to stress, mediated through adrenaline (epinephrine) and noradrenaline (norepinephrine).

Anxiety disorders are extreme or pervasive versions of this response, and include a spectrum of different conditions (**Figure 5.1**).

In the UK, approximately 15–20% of the population experience an anxiety disorder at some stage in their life. These can, however, be difficult to diagnose accurately as they are often co-morbid with each other or with other mental illnesses. They also frequently present as physical illnesses such as heart or gastrointestinal conditions.

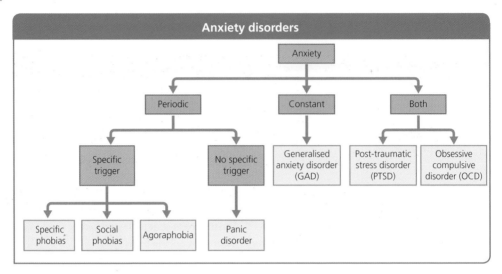

Figure 5.1 Anxiety disorders.

Case 5 Persistent pervasive symptoms of anxiety

Presentation

Annabel Pascoe is a 64-year-old woman who has reluctantly visited her general practitioner (GP) with a relative who is worried about her isolation and constant worrying. Annabel is obviously very anxious, sitting on the edge of her chair and digging her nails into her hands.

Initial interpretation

Many people are anxious about visiting their GP; however, Annabel's level of anxiety coupled with her relative's concerns should raise suspicion that she has an anxiety disorder. Symptoms of anxiety can also be caused by many other conditions, including as hyperthyroidism, heart conditions and depression.

Further history

Annabel has been feeling anxious for several months. She thinks it started soon after being burgled, which made her feel insecure in her own home. Over the last 6

months, she has been unable to sleep well due to her anxiety. She feels worried about little everyday things such as what to wear and when the mail will come. These worries often cause additional physical symptoms such as sweating, nausea and palpitations. On one occasion, she even called an ambulance as she thought she was having a heart attack.

Annabel has lost some weight because she has felt too sick to eat. Sometimes she feels low because of how much she worries, but she does not always feel like this and never thinks that life is not worth living.

She says she has had no previous medical problems and is not taking any medications. She does not drink alcohol or take any recreational drugs. She went through the menopause 8 years ago and does not have any troubling symptoms from it.

Examination

A full physical examination looking for signs of hyperthyroidism, cardiac disease and lung conditions such as asthma

Case 5 *continued*

Generalised anxiety disorder: presentation

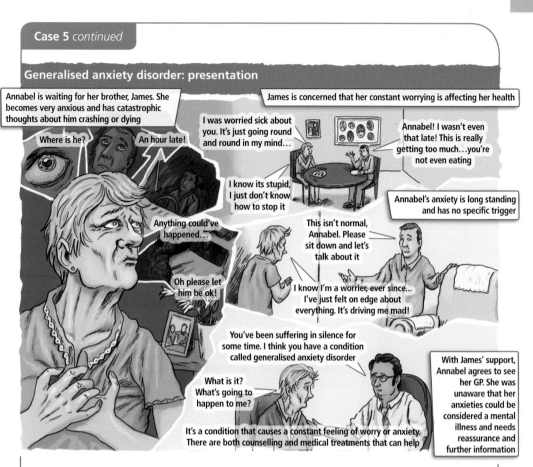

or chronic obstructive pulmonary disease reveals no abnormalities. Her blood pressure is also normal. The GP conducts a simple memory test (the mini mental state examination) to rule out dementia as a cause for her anxiety.

Interpretation of findings

The history of long-term anxiety about small problems is indicative of a generalised anxiety disorder (GAD). Annabel's symptoms of nausea, sweating, palpitations and difficulty sleeping are typical of this condition. People with GAD have occasional panic attacks, which is probably what occurred when Annabel thought she was having a heart attack.

There are no symptoms to suggest depression as the cause of her anxiety – she does not have pervasive low mood or suicidal thoughts. Drug or alcohol abuse commonly cause symptoms of anxiety and should always be excluded. As there were no hormonal problems associated with Annabel's menopause, they are unlikely to be the cause. However, other hormone problems such as hyperthyroidism should be ruled out.

A normal physical examination suggests that there is no physical cause for her symptoms, but this must be backed up by appropriate investigations.

Investigations

The GP orders blood tests:

- Glucose to exclude diabetes
- Urea and electrolytes to exclude kidney failure and electrolyte imbalances
- Thyroid function tests to exclude

Case 5 *continued*

hyperthyroidism
- A full blood count to exclude anaemia
- Bone profile to help exclude conditions such as hyperparathyroidism
- Liver function tests to exclude liver problems
- An ECG to exclude cardiac conditions

All the test results are normal.

Phaeochromocytoma is a rare tumour that causes anxiety as it releases adrenaline. This causes high blood pressure, palpitations and headaches. If it is suspected, a 24-hour urine test for catecholamines should be ordered.

Diagnosis

As Annabel's physical examination and investigations are all normal, the diagnosis is GAD (**Figure 5.2**). Annabel's GP talks to her about this condition and the possible treatment options. Psychological treatment, in particular cognitive behavioural therapy (CBT), is the best option for long-term recovery. Antidepressant medication can also be used. Annabel opts for CBT and is referred to a psychological therapist.

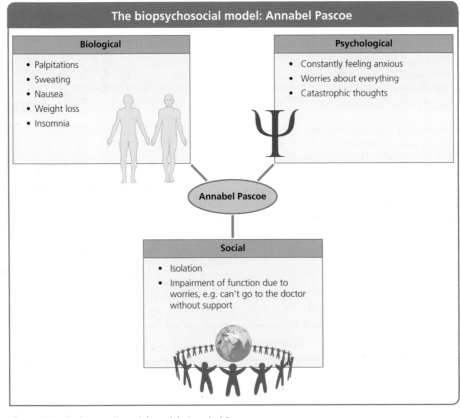

Figure 5.2 The biopsychosocial model: Annabel Pascoe.

Generalised anxiety disorder

Constant pervasive anxiety is extremely disabling and greatly reduces a person's quality of life. Although it is a relatively common condition, many people are not diagnosed for several months. This is partly due to their anxiety and reluctance to engage with medical services, but it is also because GAD is a poorly understood condition that many doctors find hard to diagnose.

Epidemiology

The lifetime prevalence of GAD is around 5%. It is twice as common in women as it is in men. The average age of onset is 21 years, but it can also occur later in life after a stressful event.

> **Anxiety disorders are more common in women.** This is partly due to the protective effects of testosterone against certain stress hormones, but mostly it is due to a cultural expectation that women will feel more anxiety and an acceptance that they will seek help.

Aetiology

The heritability of GAD is approximately 30%: environmental factors have more impact than genetic ones. No single causative gene has been identified, and it is thought that a number of genetic variations come together to create a vulnerability to a variety of anxiety disorders, including GAD. Multiple environmental factors cause GAD (**Table 5.1**).

Pathogenesis

This is not fully understood but it appears to involve multiple neurotransmitters and affects many different parts of the brain (**Figure 5.3**).

Clinical features

GAD is typified by constant free-floating anxiety. This means that individuals feel anxious and worry about normal, everyday occurrences such as having a shower or making a meal. The symptoms of anxiety are wide ranging (**Table 5.2**) as adrenaline has an

Aetiology of GAD	
Factors	Risk increased through
Childhood	Insecure attachment
	Poor parenting: overprotective/lacking warmth
	Abuse or neglect
Life events perceived as threatening/dangerous	Chronic anxiety post-event
Personality/temperament	Neurotic traits
	Selective or over attention given to potential threats
	Over estimation of threats in the environment
Substance misuse	Direct anxiety provoking effects of stimulants
	Rebound anxiety effects as the drug/alcohol is metabolised
	Altered thinking: more prone to assess situations as threatening
Isolation/poor support	Unemployment: less distractions, more insecurity
	Single status: feelings of insecurity

Table 5.1 Aetiology of generalised anxiety disorder (GAD)

effect on almost every organ in the body. The presentation can therefore be markedly different depending on the symptoms the person is experiencing.

Diagnostic approach

GAD is a chronic illness so symptoms should be present for at least 6 months for it to be diagnosed. Four or more of the symptoms shown in **Table 5.2** should occur with no particular trigger causing them.

GAD is often co-morbid with other mental illnesses such as depression. By establishing which came first and which is the most severe, it is usually possible to determine which is the primary illness. Although occasional panic attacks are common in GAD, consideration should be given to a dual diagnosis of panic disorder and GAD if they occur frequently.

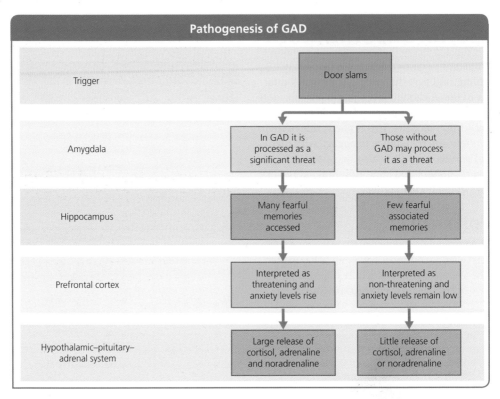

Figure 5.3 Pathogenesis of generalised anxiety disorder (GAD).

Investigations

GAD is a diagnosis of exclusion so it is vital to rule out any physical conditions (**Table 5.3**) or medications that could be mimicking the symptoms.

Antihypertensives, bronchodilators, thyroxine and many neurological and psychiatric drugs cause symptoms of anxiety, either while the patient is taking them or when they are suddenly withdrawn. Substance misuse should also be considered, given that many recreational drugs cause anxiety. A full physical examination, ECG and appropriate blood tests are required to rule these out.

> Caffeine consumption should always be considered as it is known to exacerbate or even cause symptoms of anxiety.

Management

The mainstay of management is psychological intervention for mild symptoms, self-help and psychoeducation are used, such as CBT booklets or mindfulness apps.

Many patients with GAD require more formal psychological therapy. CBT helps by teaching patients not to interpret small events as threats and to improve their emotional regulation. Other psychological therapies for GAD include motivational interviewing, problem-solving therapy, interpersonal therapy and intolerance of uncertainty therapy.

Social interventions improve quality of life through help with anxiety-provoking tasks, teaching life skills (e.g. work experience) and the use of support groups.

Selective serotonin reuptake inhibitors (SSRIs) are used if psychological treatment is ineffective or refused. If antidepressant medications do not work, pregabalin is sometimes effective. Benzodiazepines are no longer recommended for GAD except for crisis situations where the person poses a significant risk to themselves, or for short-term use while psychological or other medical treatment is being started.

Benzodiazepines were widely prescribed in the 1960s and 1970s, often to housewives suffering from anxiety. This led them to be known as 'Mother's little helper'. Dependency and difficult withdrawal led to recommendation for short-term use only.

Prognosis

As GAD is a chronic disorder, approximately 60% of patients have residual symptoms 6 years after being treated. GAD also often leads to other conditions such as depression or phobias (**Table 5.4**).

Symptoms of anxiety	
System	**Symptom**
Cardiovascular	Palpitations
	Tachycardia
	Chest pain/tightness
Respiratory	Sensation of being unable to breathe
	Tachypnoea (rapid breathing)
Gastrointestinal	Dry mouth
	Choking sensation/feel unable to swallow
	Nausea/vomiting
	Heart burn
	Abdominal pain
	Diarrhoea or sensation of urgency
Neurological	Feeling faint
	Altered sensation in hands and feet
	Generalised pain
	Sweating/hot flush
	Tremor
Psychological	Hyper-alert
	Feeling of being out of control
	Feeling unreal
	Restless
	Poor concentration
	Poor sleep

Table 5.2 Symptoms of anxiety

Conditions that mimic anxiety	
System	**Condition**
Cardiovascular	Myocardial infarction/angina
	Arrhythmias
	Valve disease
	Congestive cardiac failure
Respiratory	Asthma
	Chronic obstructive pulmonary disease
	Pulmonary embolism
Haemological	Anaemia
Neurological	Brain tumour
	Epilepsy
Endocrine	Hyperthyroidism
	Hypoparathyroidism
	Diabetes
	Phaeochromocytoma

Table 5.3 Conditions with symptoms that mimic anxiety

Comorbidities of GAD	
Condition	**Rate of comorbidity (%)**
Depression	17
Alcohol/substance misuse	30
Social phobia	22
Agoraphobia	9
Panic disorder	3

Table 5.4 Comorbidities of generalised anxiety disorder (GAD)

Panic disorder

A panic attack is an abrupt intense feeling of anxiety that lasts for around 10–20 minutes and is accompanied by psychological and physical symptoms. Approximately 25% of the population will experience one or more during their lifetime. The difference between someone who has panic attacks and someone with a panic disorder is the lack of trigger events in the latter condition and its impact on quality of life.

Epidemiology

Panic disorder has a lifetime prevalence of 5%. There are two peaks in the age of onset, one at around 24 years, and the second at 50 years. Women are two to three times more likely to develop a disorder than men. Both genders have an increased risk if they have previously been married, i.e. if they are separated, divorced or widowed.

Panic disorder frequently occurs in the context of other psychiatric conditions, with a co-morbidity of 30% with both alcohol misuse and agoraphobia.

Aetiology

The heritability of panic disorder is 30%, suggesting that environmental factors are more significant than genetic factors. The contributory factors are similar to those for the development of GAD (see **Table 5.1**). In addition, hypersensitivity to slight increases in carbon dioxide or sodium lactate in the brainstem could trigger development of panic disorder as the brain responds to what is falsely perceived to be suffocation.

Clinical features

The clinical symptoms of panic disorder are diverse (these are the symptoms of anxiety seen in **Table 5.2**) and are often confused with medical disorders such as ischaemic heart disease.

> It is an unfortunate irony that having panic disorder increases a person's risk of developing ischaemic heart disease. Therefore warning symptoms such as chest pain should never be dismissed without investigation.

For this reason, panic disorder should be considered for any patient with four or more symptoms of anxiety if other conditions that present in a similar way have been excluded. For a diagnosis of panic disorder, the panic attacks should not be triggered by a stressful or upsetting event and should occur unpredictably. This affects the person's quality of life as they worry about when the next attack will occur.

Diagnostic approach

A diagnosis of panic disorder should only be made when other causes have been ruled out. A careful history must look for signs of other mental illness such as depression or schizophrenia.

Physical illness should be excluded by a full history and examination. The history should include questions about the use of drugs and alcohol, including prescribed medications. Smoking, coffee and alcohol all trigger or exacerbate symptoms of anxiety.

Investigations

There are no specific investigations for panic disorder. However, physical illness should be fully excluded, so blood tests and an ECG are often performed.

> Although antidepressants are used to treat panic disorder, they also occasionally cause it or exacerbate the symptoms.

Management

Panic disorder is often successfully treated with self-help or CBT. As CBT produces a recovery rate of 80%, other therapies are rarely offered. If CBT is declined or fails, antidepressants are considered. Benzodiazepines are no longer recommended for panic disorder as tolerance and dependency quickly develop.

Other conditions co-occurring with the panic disorder should also be treated. In particular, substance misuse should be treated as a priority because many recreational drugs, including alcohol, nicotine and caffeine, sometimes trigger or worsen panic disorder and lessen the effectiveness of CBT.

Phobias

A phobia is a marked fear of a specific situation or object that results in attempts to avoid or limit exposure to it. Phobias are fairly common, with 10–20% of the UK population experiencing some form of phobia during their lifetime.

Many people with a specific phobia do not seek professional help because as long as the phobic object or situation is avoidable, there is minimal impact on their quality of life. In contrast, social phobia and agoraphobia often have a significant negative effect on quality of life.

most common ones are shown in **Table 5.5**. Many people suffer from more than one type of phobia.

Epidemiology

The lifetime prevalence of specific phobias is 12.5%. Women are two to three times more likely to be diagnosed than men for all phobia types except blood and injury phobias; there is no difference for these. Phobias commonly occur for the first time during adolescence but also develop during adulthood. It is rare for a phobia to develop in old age.

Specific phobias

Types

There are hundreds of specific phobias that cover almost any object or situation. The

Aetiology

Many genes contribute to making someone more vulnerable to developing a phobia. Heritability is around 20–40%, therefore,

Types of phobia		
Phobia type	Example	Lifetime prevalence (%)
Animals	Arachnophobia (spiders)	3–7
Environment (water, storms etc.)	Aquaphobia (water)	2–4
Heights	Acrophobia	3–5
Flying	Aviophobia	2
Enclosed places	Claustrophobia	3
Injury/blood/needles	Haemophobia (blood)	3–5
Professions (doctors, dentists etc.)	Dentophobia (dentists)	5
Situations (being in a tunnel, on an escalator etc.)	Escalaphobia (escalators)	1–3

Table 5.5 Types of phobia

environmental factors have a greater impact. A negative experience of an object or situation, particularly during childhood, increases the risk of developing a phobia. The more often this negative experience is repeated, the more likely the phobia is to develop. Some phobias probably have an evolutionary basis as an aid to survival; these include fears of spiders, snakes, heights and blood.

> 'Little Albert' was a 1-year-old boy who was conditioned to fear white fur by a researcher repeatedly presenting a white rabbit along with an unpleasantly loud noise. Albert developed a phobic response to white fur, which also unfortunately included Santa Claus's white beard. The research, published in 1920, and which would be considered unethical today, did not include treatment for the phobia.

Prevention

There is no universal strategy to prevent phobias, but parents are often given advice on how to prevent their own phobias developing in their children. When children visit dentists, or doctors' surgeries for injections, positive associations are made through the use of small rewards such as stickers. This reduces any potentially negative associations.

Clinical features

The patient experiences symptoms of anxiety (Table 5.2) when confronted with, or thinking about, the trigger situation or object. The patient therefore tries to avoid the trigger. With claustrophobia, for example, shopping, lifts and public transport are avoided.

The patient usually shows attentional bias towards the trigger. For example, those with a phobia of spiders often see spiders before others do and sometimes misinterpret objects such as tomato stalks as spiders.

Blood phobia is different from other phobias in that it has not been shown to have an attentional bias. In addition, patients often faint when exposed to the trigger, which is rare with other specific phobias.

> One possible reason for the association between fainting and seeing blood is that it had the evolutionary advantage of reducing blood flow to the extremities and maximising blood flow to vital organs. It also has the advantage of 'playing dead', which perhaps prevented further harm

Management

Specific phobias respond well to CBT and to self-help that uses CBT strategies.

The CBT usually focuses on desensitising the patient to the trigger through gradually increasing their exposure to it. A version of desensitisation called 'flooding' is occasionally used. In this, the patient undergoes prolonged exposure to the trigger until they no longer have an anxiety response. Online self-help programmes expose the patient to the trigger through the use of pictures and video.

Medications are rarely used for phobias, but antidepressants are used if CBT fails or is refused.

Social phobia

Social phobia is also called social anxiety disorder and is a form of extreme shyness. Most people experience some form of social anxiety in new or difficult social situations. However, those with social phobia find that everyday social interactions become a source of anxiety that is more extreme and intense than the discomfort of shyness. This ultimately leads people with social phobia to avoid these situations.

Epidemiology

The prevalence of social phobia in the UK is around 10%. It affects women two to three times more often than men. It usually starts in early adolescence and reduces in incidence after the age of 65 years.

Aetiology

Environmental factors have a stronger influence than genetics on its development: the more negative social experiences the person has, the more vulnerable they are to developing a social phobia. Childhood stammering is also known to increase the risk. This is due to the increased anxiety related to trying to communicate effectively in social situations and the negative response these children sometimes receive.

Clinical features

People with social phobia experience symptoms of anxiety (see **Table 5.2**) in situations where they feel the centre of attention or believe they may act in an embarrassing way. Anxiety symptoms that others could discern, such as blushing, needing to defecate or urinate and vomiting, are particularly feared. Safety behaviours such as drinking alcohol, avoiding eye contact and never asking questions may be used to minimise the anxiety. Individuals try to avoid social situations, leading to their isolation.

Approximately 19% of people with social phobia develop depression. Patients are also at risk of misusing drugs and alcohol, and from developing other anxiety disorders such as GAD or agoraphobia.

> Assessing a person with social anxiety disorder or agoraphobia requires some flexibility in where and how they are initially assessed because those with severe symptoms often feel unable to leave their homes. It is sometimes best to see them in the home or make contact using more indirect means, such as telephoning or emailing.

Management

Mild social phobia is improved by self-help in the form of a graded exposure to anxiety-provoking situations, relaxation techniques and practising positive thinking. CBT and social skills training are useful for those with more severe social phobia.

If these do not work or are declined, antidepressants, usually SSRIs, can be tried. Beta-blockers such as atenolol are occasionally used for tremor and palpitations. This is particularly advantageous for performance-related anxiety, for example in musicians.

Agoraphobia

Agoraphobia is a fear of being unable to escape or control the environment the person is in. Although it literally means 'open space' phobia, it is more easily understood as being a fear of feeling unsafe, because the person often feels anxious in crowds and enclosed spaces as well as open areas.

Epidemiology

There are two peaks in the onset of agoraphobia, one in the early 20s and the second in the 30s. As with most anxiety disorders, it is more common in women. The lifetime prevalence of agoraphobia is 2%.

Aetiology

There is a possible evolutionary basis to agoraphobia: there would be a survival advantage in fearing large open spaces where it would be difficult to escape from predators. This suggests that some people might have a genetic predisposition towards developing agoraphobia.

People with agoraphobia often learn to fear certain places after having a negative experience there, usually in the form of a panic attack. The person then becomes concerned that the situation will trigger the same response, and this becomes a self-fulfilling prophecy – the person is so anxious about going into the trigger situation that a panic attack is very likely.

Another contributory factor is a fault in the vestibular system, which helps people balance. Some patients have been shown to rely more on their visual and proprioceptive systems to balance. This results in feelings of being 'unsafe' when there are too few stimuli, such as in wide open spaces, or when there is too much stimulation, for example in crowds.

Clinical features

For a diagnosis of agoraphobia, symptoms of anxiety need to be experienced in two or more of the following situations:

- Public places
- Crowds

- Travel away from home
- Travelling alone

Patients often feel anticipatory anxiety when preparing or thinking about going into a situation that triggers anxiety (**Figure 5.4**). Concurrent social anxiety also often occurs as the person fears having a panic attack in front of strangers.

People with agoraphobia develop strategies to help them cope with their fears, such as only leaving home accompanied by a trusted friend, doing their shopping over the internet or only travelling to certain destinations. Those with more severe symptoms may become housebound. This can lead to self-neglect and can be life threatening if they refuse to leave their home even in a medical emergency.

Management

As with all types of phobia, CBT is the most effective treatment and should be offered first. For those with mild agoraphobia, self-help and support groups reduce the symptoms to a manageable level.

If the symptoms are so severe that CBT is not possible or it is not the patient's preference, antidepressants such as SSRIs are used. Hypnotic medications such as benzodiazepines are not routinely recommended for agoraphobia as they cause dependence and rebound anxiety when the dose is reduced. They are occasionally used when the patient is in crisis or needs to leave their home for medical reasons.

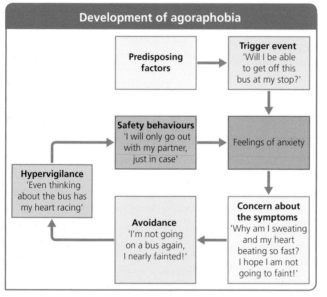

Figure 5.4 The development of agoraphobia.

Obsessive compulsive disorder

Obsessive compulsive disorder (OCD) is often mistakenly used to describe people who are fastidious or meticulous in their actions, particularly in regard to cleaning. However, the anxious thoughts in true OCD lead to widely differing behaviours. Although some people with OCD have certain rituals that they are very fastidious about, others have what many would consider to be extremely slovenly lives.

Many people without OCD experience anxious thoughts about whether they have locked a door or turned off the lights, and this sometimes results in rechecking behaviours. For those with OCD, however, the anxious thought is far more intense and the behaviour markedly abnormal.

Epidemiology

OCD has a lifetime prevalence of 2%, with most people developing OCD before their twenties. Unlike most other anxiety disorders, there is no significant difference in incidence between the sexes.

Aetiology

Unlike other anxiety disorders, OCD that develops during before 12 years of age has an heritance of around 65%. There are differences in the striatum of the brain (an area involved in movement and decision making) and reduced levels of serotonin in those with OCD. Environmental factors that contribute to these changes include:

- An overprotective parenting style
- Learnt OCD behaviours from the parents
- Stressful life events
- Streptococcal infection

> **Streptococcal infection in children who have a genetic vulnerability to OCD can result in the rapid development of symptoms.** This is thought to be because the antibodies that are produced to fight the infection also harm certain receptors in the brain.

Clinical features

The symptoms of OCD are extremely wide ranging (**Table 5.6**). The obsessive thoughts are usually fears that something will happen or that the person has done or will do something negative or harmful. These thoughts are repetitive and result in symptoms of anxiety. This then results in the development of behaviours that become compulsive to try to decrease the anxiety.

A cycle of anxiety-provoking thoughts therefore develops that results in compulsive behaviours (**Figure 5.5**). This has a significant impact on the person's quality of life as they often spend long periods of their day engaged in these behaviours.

> **The thoughts and behaviours of OCD can merge with religious practices,** such as praying compulsively to avoid harm or disaster. It is important to untangle the person's usual practices and beliefs from the symptoms of their disorder. This may involve talking to relatives or religious leaders.

Diagnostic approach

A careful history should be taken to rule out other mental illnesses. Psychosis in particular can present in a similar manner to OCD. The thoughts in OCD are extremely intense, but unlike delusional beliefs, there is room for doubt. The Yale–Brown Obsessive Compulsive Scale aids diagnosis and assesses the severity.

Management

OCD is treated with psychological therapy or medication. A specific form of CBT called exposure and response prevention is used. In this, the person's obsessive thoughts are triggered but they do not carry out the compulsive behaviour (**Figure 5.6**). This aims to break the cycle by teaching the person that there is no association between their compulsions and the thoughts they are having.

SSRIs are as effective as CBT in treating OCD in patients over 18 years. For those with severe OCD, a combination of an SSRI and CBT is used. Antipsychotics or other antidepressants are occasionally used if these treatments are ineffective. Social interventions such as support groups and measures to improve the person's quality of life are also beneficial.

Prognosis

Although there is usually a significant improvement in the symptoms with medication and/or psychological therapy, 70% of people with OCD continue to have some low-level residual symptoms and 5% develop chronic OCD. OCD frequently occurs with other mental illnesses, particularly depression.

Types of OCD

Behaviour type	Examples	Commonly associated fear(s)
Checking	Taps	Flooding
	Doors	Burglary
	Windows	Burglary
	Lights	Fire
	People (e.g. by texting)	Loved one harmed or dead
	Where they have been	Causing harm
Cleaning and contamination	Avoiding public facilities	Germs or dirt that could cause harm to themselves or loved ones
	Avoiding crowds	
	Washing after shaking hands	
	Avoiding dark or red colours	
	Cleaning objects before touching	
Hoarding	Unable to throw away unneeded items	Losing memories particularly pleasurable ones
	Keeps letters/newspapers and junk mail	Wastefulness or losing important information
	Collecting unusual items (e.g. takeaway menus from restaurants) to an extreme degree	Losing memories or wastefulness
Repetitive thinking	Repeating a 'magical' number or word	They will harm themselves or others
	Specific phrases	
Avoidance	Objects that could cause harm, e.g. knives/scissors	They will harm themselves or others
	Potentially 'dangerous' situations, e.g. train platforms	
	Certain numbers/letters/places	Harm or disaster will occur
Orderliness	Symmetry required in various ways, e.g. how towels hang	Disaster or harm will occur
	Objects having a correct place	
	Doing things a certain number of times	

Table 5.6 Types of obsessive compulsive disorder (OCD)

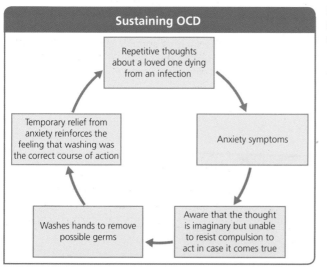

Sustaining OCD

Repetitive thoughts about a loved one dying from an infection

Anxiety symptoms

Aware that the thought is imaginary but unable to resist compulsion to act in case it comes true

Washes hands to remove possible germs

Temporary relief from anxiety reinforces the feeling that washing was the correct course of action

Figure 5.5 Example of a cycle sustaining obsessive compulsive disorder (OCD).

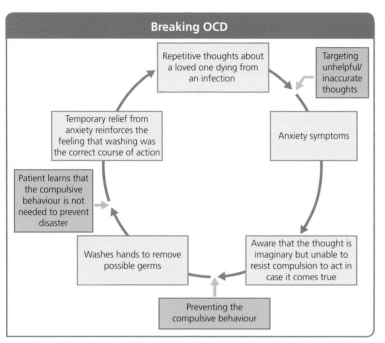

Figure 5.6 Breaking the cycle of obsessive compulsive disorder (OCD) using cognitive behavioural therapy.

Acute stress reaction and post-traumatic stress disorder

Both acute stress reactions and post-traumatic stress reactions occur after an exceptional stressor. They occur at any age, although they often present slightly differently in young children.

Many people mistakenly believe that post-traumatic stress disorder (PTSD) or acute stress reactions only occur when a person has been through or witnessed something horrific. However, any event that the person interpreted as being life threatening, even if it was not, can leave that person vulnerable to these disorders. Stressors such as divorce and job loss are not associated with PTSD and acute stress reactions.

Acute stress reaction

By definition, this starts acutely, usually within an hour, after exposure to a stressor. When the stressor is removed, the symptoms start to resolve within 8 hours. To be classified as acute stress reaction, there should be no residual symptoms after a few days.

'Nervous breakdown' is a lay term and does not exist as a diagnosis. It most closely resembles an acute stress reaction.

Clinical features

The symptoms and duration of the reaction are closely linked to adrenaline and noradrenaline levels that cause symptoms of anxiety (see **Table 5.2**). Other symptoms include:

- Narrowing of attention
- Despair or hopelessness
- Withdrawal
- Aggression
- Restlessness

The most severe form of acute stress reaction can cause a dissociative stupor, in which the person is unresponsive but not unconscious.

Management

The management of an acute stress reaction is mainly supportive. The person should if possible be removed from the source of the stressor and cared for in a place of safety. This might involve admission to either a medical or a psychiatric ward. Benzodiazepines are sometimes used to reduce the severity of the symptoms in the short term (reduced then stopped after a few days). The risk of suicide and/or harm to others is monitored closely depending on the symptoms displayed.

Some acute stress reactions lead to PTSD, particularly in individuals exposed to rape or disasters that included fatalities. In these cases, it is beneficial to consider trauma-focused CBT or psychoeducation on the body and brain's reaction to traumatic events to help prevent PTSD developing or reduce its severity.

> Although 'debriefing' after a traumatic event is common there is no evidence that this reduces the incidence of acute stress reaction or reduces its severity.

Post-traumatic stress disorder

In 75% of people, some symptoms of PTSD appear as soon as the stressor occurs, but only a minority seek help at this time. Guidelines stipulate that the symptoms have to have been present within 6 months of the stressor to warrant a diagnosis of PTSD. However, the person may have been suffering for several months or years before seeking help.

> PTSD was originally called 'shell shock' after soldiers returning from World War I exhibited symptoms of chronic anxiety having being exposed to shell fire. Up to 40% of those who fought in the Battle of the Somme developed shell shock.

Epidemiology

PTSD has a 7% lifetime prevalence, with women having a higher risk than men of developing it. Those exposed to sexual abuse, war or natural disaster are particularly vulnerable to developing PTSD. Approximately 25–30% of individuals exposed to extreme stress develop PTDS.

Clinical features

One of the hallmark symptoms of PTSD is reliving the event, frequently with a similar level of detail and emotion as for the actual event (**Figure 5.7**). This reliving occurs in the form of intense memories, flashbacks or nightmares. The patient attempts to avoid situations that are reminders of the event. For example, someone who was in a car crash might avoid driving.

If the person is unable to avoid the situation, they experience symptoms of anxiety (see **Table 5.2**). Other symptoms include:

- Poor concentration
- Irritability and increased aggression

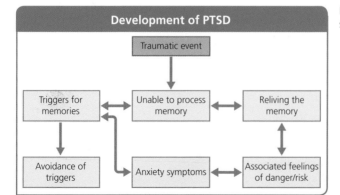

Figure 5.7 How post-traumatic stress disorder (PTSD) develops.

- Poor sleep
- Hypervigilance and an increased startle reflex
- Poor memory, particularly for the period around the event

> The reliving that occurs in PTSD is thought to be due to the brain repeatedly attempting to process the memory but being unable to do so due to its intensity.

Diagnostic approach

Those who have experienced a major disaster or are refugees from a conflict zone should be screened around 1 month after the event for symptoms of PTSD.

For those presenting with symptoms of PTSD, a full psychosocial history should be taken to rule out other mental illnesses such as depression or psychosis. Co-morbid substance misuse such as alcohol dependence is also seen as patients try to self-medicate to deal with their symptoms. Physical illnesses that can mimic anxiety (see **Table 5.3**) should also be excluded.

Management

PTSD is treated with trauma-focused CBT or eye movement desensitisation and reprocessing therapy:

- Trauma-focused CBT is similar to standard CBT but focuses more on the memories of the traumatic event. It targets the associated unhelpful thoughts and behaviours that have arisen from it.
- Eye movement desensitisation and reprocessing reduces the symptoms by helping the brain to correctly process the traumatic memory. It does this by alternating a stimulus, usually visual, from left to right while focusing on the traumatic memory. This alternating stimulation is believed to help process memories more effectively.

Antidepressant medications are also effective. They are used as an alternative if psychological therapy is declined or is ineffective. The SSRI paroxetine has the most evidence to support its use but other antidepressants such as mirtazapine are also used. Co-morbid conditions should also occur be treated.

Social support is also beneficial, especially in the early stages after the trauma. This support focuses on reducing the sequelae of the trauma, such as isolation and ruminating on negative thoughts.

> The computer game Tetris has been found to help the brain to process trauma if it is played immediately after the traumatic event. It is thought that it distracts the brain from repeatedly replaying the event, thus reducing the intensity of the memory.

Prognosis

PTSD can be treated even years after the traumatic event. However, it is less likely that treatment will be effective if the condition remains undiagnosed for several months. In 80% of patients, PTSD is complicated by other co-morbid mental health conditions. Due to both of these factors, 33% of patients develop chronic symptoms and another 33% have residual symptoms or relapse.

Early treatment with protection against re-exposure to the trauma and good social support increases the probability that PTSD will be successfully treated.

Answers to starter questions

1. There are many possible explanations as to why women develop anxiety disorders more frequently than men. Women are more likely to communicate their feelings and it is culturally more acceptable for women to feel anxiety. This makes it easier for them to seek help for the symptoms they are experiencing. It could also be due to men being more likely to 'self-medicate' with substances such as alcohol in an effort to mask anxiety symptoms.

2. Agoraphobia used to be considered as a form of panic disorder due to the large range of situations that could trigger anxiety. It is now felt that the two are separate although often comorbid with each other. Agoraphobia has multiple triggers, including any situation where the person feels unsafe. Patients feel unsafe when experiencing symptoms of anxiety and this fear of anxiety then triggers symptoms. Panic disorder has no trigger but patients have frequent sudden feelings of panic. This develops into a trigger in itself, similar to agoraphobia.

3. People with obsessive compulsive disorder (OCD) have repetitive thoughts that cause anxiety symptoms. In order to control these thoughts and their associated unpleasant effects, the person develops behaviours they feel might prevent the thought from becoming reality. Some resemble 'normal' behaviours, such as rechecking the oven to ensure it has been turned off. For someone with OCD this behaviour only provides temporary relief before the thoughts return and they have to repeat the behaviour. In this way the behaviours become compulsive.

Chapter 6
Suicide and self-harm

Introduction 161
Case 6 A serious overdose 162
Case 7 Repeated self-harm 164

Self-harm 166
Suicide 172

Starter questions

Answers to the following questions are on page 176.

1. Is there a difference between self-harm and attempted suicide?
2. Why are people who self-harm more likely to commit suicide?

Introduction

Attempted suicide and self-harm are two of the most upsetting and worrying situations a clinician encounters. Health professionals who encounter people who self-harm or attempt suicide can feel helpless and worried about how to approach the situation. This is exacerbated by having no definitive diagnostic criteria or clear treatment approaches.

In psychiatry, attempted suicide and self-harm are routinely examined for in almost every clinical encounter, and the risk of future attempts must be quantified as far as possible. Clinicians in other specialties often feel uneasy with this 'crystal ball' approach. Although it lacks specific physical investigations to underpin the prediction of risk, it is similar to weighing up the risk of sending someone home after a myocardial infarction or deciding what level of anticoagulation a patient requires for their atrial fibrillation.

It is relatively common to encounter a self-harming or suicidal patient. Approximately 20% of all teenagers in the UK, for example, have had thoughts of suicide, if only fleetingly, and 15% admit to engaging in self-harming behaviours. Unfortunately, significant cultural stigma still surrounds self-harm and suicide, which means that many individuals do not present to health professionals until they are in crisis.

Case 6 A serious overdose

Presentation

George Walker, a 57-year-old man, has been brought to the emergency department by ambulance after his neighbour Christina found him semi-conscious with empty medication packages and alcohol bottles next to him. He is assessed by Dr Trent.

Initial interpretation

Empty medication boxes are a strong indication that George has taken an overdose, although this could be a coincidental finding. A full history and examination are required to rule out other causes of an altered mental state. These include stroke, trauma, myocardial infarction, infection, dehydration, diabetic crisis and other hormonal abnormalities , such as severe hyperparathyroidism or hypothyroidism.

Further history

Dr Trent asks Christina about George. She tells him that George recently had a difficult divorce from his wife. Since then, he has been increasingly isolated, quitting his job as a store clerk and spending all his time at home.

Christina has been visiting him fairly regularly and has been worried about the state of his home and his clothes. She has noticed he has not been eating well and 'can't be bothered' with anything. George has told her he feels he has no future but he has never mentioned contemplating suicide. She decided to visit that day as she had received a text from him saying, 'I'm so sorry.' When he did not answer the door, Christina rang the police. She does not think George has any health problems or takes any prescribed medication.

George talks about having nothing to live for and seems upset that he is in hospital. He asks Dr Trent not to bother with him and becomes tearful when Dr Trent talks about treatment. He says he wanted to die and has done so for a number of months. Over the last few weeks, he has been collecting paracetamol and sleeping tablets from various chemists. He took them with alcohol late last night and had not expected to wake up this morning.

> In 1998 the amount of paracetamol that could be bought at a pharmacy in the UK was limited to a maximum of 32. This has reduced the death rate from paracetamol overdose by 43%.

Examination

George has a Glasgow Coma Scale Score of 13 out of 15 indicating minor brain injury, but his examination is otherwise essentially normal. His abdomen is slightly tender but there is no sign of infection or neurological deficit that would suggest a stroke. Dr Trent examines the medication packages that the ambulance has brought; they are a mixture of paracetamol and a sedative antihistamine. From the boxes, he estimates George has taken 60 paracetamol and 15 antihistamines.

Interpretation of findings

George has taken a substantial amount of medication with the intention of dying. His examination does not suggest any other cause for his altered mental state. He has been neglecting himself and possibly drinking alcohol to excess, so liver failure, infection and heart conditions have not yet been fully excluded.

Case 6 *continued*

Investigations

Routine tests including blood pressure, temperature and a urine dip stick (looking for urinary infection or glucose) are all normal. Dr Trent orders a range of blood tests (**Table 6.1**). The results show high blood paracetamol levels that must be treated to prevent liver failure. An ECG is performed; this shows no sign that George's admission was associated with any heart condition.

Diagnosis

George has taken a serious overdose of paracetamol. His blood tests and ECG show no evidence of another cause for his altered mental state.

As the overdose took place approximately 12 hours previously, Dr Trent does not give activated charcoal, which is only useful in the first few hours after an overdose. He uses **Figure 6.1** to determine whether treatment with acetylcysteine is required. The area above the treatment line (which is lower for those with liver damage) indicates a need to administer acetylcysteine. As George's level of paracetamol is above the treatment line, Dr Trent admits George and starts an acetylcysteine drip of to prevent liver toxicity.

Dr Trent decides that a specialist psychiatric nurse or doctor should carry out a psychosocial assessment to assess the risk of further suicide attempts and for any mental illness. He therefore lets the local mental health team know about George's admission to hospital.

> **Activated charcoal works by reducing the absorption of many drugs from the gut.** It reduces the harm caused by overdosing by binding to the drug but only works when given within 2 hours after taking the overdose.

George's blood test results		
Blood tests ordered	Results	Interpretation
Urea and electrolytes	Urea 8 mmol/L (normal 3–7 mmol/L) Creatinine 1.56 mg/dL (normal 0.6–1.3 mg/dL)	Probably slightly dehydrated
Liver function tests	GGT 110 U/L (normal 0–51 U/L)	Been drinking alcohol but overdose taken less than 24 hours ago so no other LFT results affected
Inflammatory markers (CRP or ESR)	CRP 4 mg/L (normal <6 mg/L)	No infection
Full blood count	Haemoglobin 15 g/L (normal 120–170 g/L) White blood cells (normal 3.5–10 x10^9/L)	Not anaemic Normal white cell count rules out infection
Blood gas	pH 7.42 (normal 7.34–7.45)	Rules out hypoxia and CO poisoning. Acidosis is only seen in very serious paracetamol overdose
Glucose	5.1 mmol/L (normal 4.4–7.8 mmol/L)	Rules out diabetic crisis
Clotting	Prothrombin time 11 s (normal 10–15 s)	Deranged if overdose taken over 72 hours ago or was staggered
Paracetamol	110 mg/L (normal <40 mg/L at 12 hours)	Requires treatment for overdose
Salicylate	10 mg/dL (normal <30 mg/dL)	Did not take aspirin as part of overdose

Table 6.1 George's blood test results. CRP, C-reactive protein; ESR, erythrocyte sedimentation rate; GGT, gamma-glutamyl transferase

Case 6 *continued*

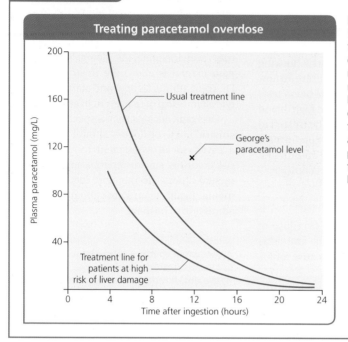

Figure 6.1 Determining the need for acetylcysteine treatment post-paracetamol overdose: treatment is needed if the patient's result is to the right of the line. Patients at high risk of liver damage include those on medication, alcohol dependents and patients with hepatitis: their threshold for treatment is lower.

Case 7 Repeated self-harm

Presentation

Jessica Milne, a 16-year-old girl, has been taken to see Dr Denby, the general practitioner (GP), by her mother. This has been prompted by Jessica's school expressing concerns about cuts and scars on her arms. Her mother states that she had noticed some scars a few months ago when Jessica was being bullied. She thought it had stopped after the school had moved her away from the pupils who were bullying her.

Initial interpretation

Self-harm is triggered by many different causes including mental illnesses such as depression, borderline personality disorder or psychosis. It also occurs in the context of stressful situations, with abuse and in those with low self-esteem. It is important to establish whether the cuts represent self-harm or attempted suicide as this can affect the treatment given.

Further history

Dr Denby invites Jessica to talk without her mother present. When her mother has left the room, Jessica says she has been low for a number of months because of the ongoing bullying she is experiencing. The bullying started approximately a year ago after she told a friend she thought she might be a lesbian. Since then she has been frequently teased about this both at school and on social media sites.

Jessica started cutting using a razor about 4 months ago. At first she just cut her arms but now she cuts her stomach and

Case 7 *continued*

legs as well. Jessica feels that cutting helps release the pain she is feeling. This somehow makes her feel slightly better and able to cope with what she is feeling. She has had thoughts of suicide but has never cut with that purpose.

> **Homosexual and bisexual people are twice as likely to self-harm compared with heterosexual people.** This is felt to be due to the stigma, isolation and victimisation they often experience.

Dr Denby asks Jessica more about her mood to establish whether she has symptoms of depression or another mental illness. Jessica states she has been low in mood for about 5 months and has become more withdrawn in recent months. Her mood does not vary much during the day

and she does not remember the last time she felt happy or excited. Her sleep is quite poor as she often lies awake thinking about what is being said online. This means she usually feels very tired during the day.

Jessica denies seeing or hearing things that other people do not (hallucinations) or having any unusual worries or thoughts (which could indicate delusional beliefs). She has a close relationship with her mother and has some friends, although she is currently seeing less of them. She denies having any problems making or keeping friends.

Examination

On a review of Jessica's wounds, Dr Denby finds multiple old scars and other wounds at various stages of healing. There is no evidence of infection that would require treatment. There are no bruises or other marks to suggest physical abuse.

Self-harm: presentation

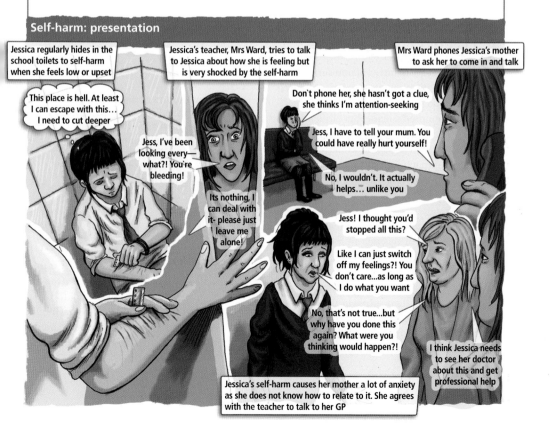

Case 7 *continued*

Interpretation of findings

Jessica describes a history of self-harming as a way of coping with the bullying she is experiencing. The symptoms of low mood, poor energy levels and sleep, along with thoughts of suicide and increased withdrawal, suggest that Jessica could be suffering from depression. The history provides no evidence of a borderline personality disorder, such as unstable relationships or emotional instability. Psychosis is also unlikely as she has no hallucinations or delusions.

Investigations

As Jessica has signs of depression, Dr Denby orders blood tests to determine thyroid function, glucose level and a full blood count to rule out medical conditions that mimic depressive symptoms.

Diagnosis

Self-harm by itself is not usually classified as a mental illness but this does not mean the person does not need help. In Jessica's case, there are symptoms of depression so Dr Denby refers her to the local Child and Adolescent Mental Health team for further assessment.

He talks to Jessica and her mother about managing self-harm and using self-help websites. He also talks about the triggers for self-harm and how these could be addressed, for example discussions with the school, reporting online bullies and possibly a support group for Jessica to explore her sexuality.

Self-harm

Self-harm refers to all forms of non-fatal injury conducted for psychological relief. Research studies often do not differentiate between self-harm and attempted suicide, but clinically it is essential to distinguish the two: a person who uses self-harming as a coping strategy requires a different approach to treatment from someone who is self-harming with an intent to die.

What is considered a self-harming behaviour also depends on the person's cultural background. Ritual cutting to create scars is considered a rite of passage in some African tribes but is usually considered to be a form of self-harm in Europe, for example. Some definitions of self-harm also include situations where the person has put themselves in danger, such as walking down the middle of a busy road or showing sexual promiscuity, where their aim is to reduce their emotional pain or punish themselves.

Self-harm used to be termed 'deliberate self-harm' to indicate that it was done purposely rather than accidentally. However, some self-harming occurs while in a dissociative state, so the term was challenged as it was felt to be stigmatising and inaccurate.

Types

Cutting and scratching are the most common types of self-harm, accounting for around 50% of all self-harming episodes (**Figure 6.2**). It is, however, very difficult to determine accurately which methods are commonly used as most instances do not require medical attention and many people who self-harm use more than one method.

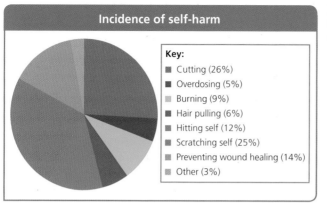

Incidence of self-harm

Key:
- Cutting (26%)
- Overdosing (5%)
- Burning (9%)
- Hair pulling (6%)
- Hitting self (12%)
- Scratching self (25%)
- Preventing wound healing (14%)
- Other (3%)

Figure 6.2 The incidence of different types of self-harm in the community.

Overdosing or self-poisoning is difficult to differentiate from attempted suicide and in studies is often grouped with attempted suicide. This is because the individual's motivation is often a combination of self-harm and attempted suicide.

Epidemiology

Approximately 4–5% of all people in the UK have self-harmed. Self-harm is far more prevalent in young people, being seen in 15% of all under 18s. It is estimated that there are over 140,000 presentations to hospital after self-harm in England each year. Most are episodes of overdose, although these represent only a small proportion of instances of self-harm.

The most common age to self-harm in females is between 15 and 19 years, and in males is 20–24. Females are more likely to self-harm than males, particularly through cutting or overdosing. People who self-harm are 100 times more likely to attempt suicide than those who do not. Almost all forms of mental illness increase the risk of self-harming behaviours, but borderline personality disorder has the highest incidence (**Table 6.2**).

Self-harm in the UK began to increase in the 1960s. The reasons for this included the increased recognition of mental illness and self-harm, the decriminalisation of suicide attempts and possibly a cultural shift that allowed more freedom of expression.

Incidence of self-harm in mental illness

Mental illness	Incidence of self-harm (%)
Borderline personality disorder	70–75
Psychosis	50
Depression	40
Alcohol dependence	25–33
Anxiety disorders	20–30
Autism spectrum disorder	20–30
Eating disorders	15–50

Table 6.2 Incidence of self-harm in mental illnesses

Aetiology

There is no one main cause or trigger for a self-harming episode – multiple factors combine to increase the risk. Although it seems counter-intuitive, a genetic vulnerability to self-harm has been identified, with a heritability of around 45%. It is likely that this is due to genetic influences on impulsivity and mood rather than being a direct link between genetics and self-harming behaviours.

The rare genetic disorder Lesch–Nyhan syndrome causes severe self-harming behaviours along with other symptoms including neurological dysfunction and intellectual impairment. Other factors that increase the risk of self-harming behaviours are shown in **Table 6.3**.

Personality traits linked to self-harming behaviours include:

- Pessimism
- Perfectionism
- Impulsivity
- Neuroticism

Factors increasing risk of self-harm		
Areas	Factor	Impact
Family	Family member self-harming	Modelling behaviour
	Parents separated/divorce, foster care, or being a single parent	Reduced support, feelings of uncertainty and increased stress
	Severe mental illness or substance misuse in the parent(s)	Reduced support, caring role which entails stress and uncertainty
	Marital discord/domestic violence	Fear, stress and reduced support
Relationships	Breakdown of a sexual relationship	Anxiety, negativity and low self-esteem
	Bullying/victimisation	Anxiety, negativity, low self-esteem, isolation
	Friend(s) self-harming	Modelling behaviour
Individual	Mental or physical illness	Anxiety, low mood, low self-esteem, isolation
	Intellectual disability	Anxiety, impulsivity, frustration, isolation
	Alcohol/substance misuse	Reduced impulse control, labile emotions
	Homosexual, bisexual or transgender identity	Stigma, bullying, feelings of isolation
	Past or present abuse	Anxiety, low mood, low self-esteem, self-loathing, isolation

Table 6.3 Factors that increase the risk of self-harm

Subcultures such as 'Goths' and 'Emos' show an increased risk of self-harming behaviours. This could reflect the type of person who is attracted to these group but could, in part, also be due to the acceptance (or sometimes even encouragement) of self-harm within these subcultures.

Prevention

Most people self-harm privately and do not seek help. It is therefore very difficult to develop a strategy to effectively prevent self-harm. Education and raising awareness have helped in understanding the triggers and reducing the associated stigma. However, the number of individuals self-harming has not decreased.

There is no prevention strategy that specifically targets self-harm, but strategies that improve a young person's welfare can have an impact. These include family support for vulnerable families and anti-bullying campaigns.

Pathogenesis

Self-harm is used as a coping strategy for two main reasons relating to two different thought processes (**Figure 6.3**). First, the person feels it reduces stress and feels 'relieving'. Second, it induces sensations, making the person feel 'alive'. Individuals who experience a sense of relief often feel this is due to the physical pain 'overriding' the emotional pain they are feeling. Other reasons to self-harm include self-punishment, to feel in control and to express frustration.

The trigger event for an episode of self-harm is anything from a friend not making contact to being sexually abused. Drinking alcohol acts as a trigger, probably by increasing impulsivity and inducing or increasing feelings of dysphoria.

Clinical features

As it includes a large range of behaviours, it is impossible to generalise about the symptoms and signs of self-harm. Most people have no outward indicators. Those who injure their

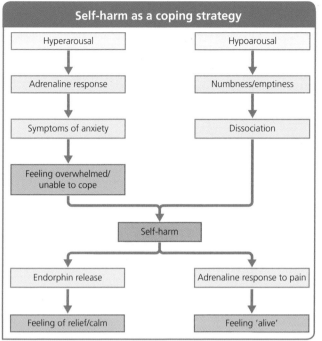

Figure 6.3 Self-harm as a coping strategy.

skin often try to cover the wounds and scars; this may seem unusual behaviour, especially during the summer.

When examining for self-harm, look for unusual injuries on the body, particularly the arms, abdomen and legs (**Figure 6.4**). There are often old scars and marks from previous self-harm. The size and depth of the cuts give an indication of whether the patient was self-harming or attempting suicide (**Figure 6.5**).

Diagnostic approach

A detailed history of the background risk factors and current triggers is crucial when self-harm is suspected. It is also important to assess for mental illness and suicidal thoughts.

Investigations

If possible, undertake a full physical examination to assess the severity of the self-harm. If overdosing or self-poisoning is suspected, blood tests are required to assess for organ damage, particularly the liver and kidneys.

Management

The immediate management of self-harm is to treat the injury or overdose with appropriate measures, for example suturing any cuts or intravenous acetylcysteine for paracetamol overdose. In the longer term, strategies should be given to improve the person's emotional regulation and ability to cope. These:

- Address underlying difficulties, such as mental illness
- Provide support for families
- Intervene to stop bullying

Substance misuse and alcohol dependence can be addressed via mental health services or voluntary organisations. There is no effective medication for self-harming behaviours.

Therapies such as cognitive behavioural therapy and dialectical behavioural therapy help to address difficulties with emotional regulation and impulsivity. They also provide coping strategies, e.g. relaxation and seeking appropriate sources of support. Family

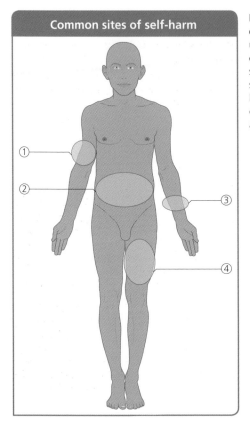

Common sites of self-harm

Figure 6.4 Common sites of self-harm. ① Cutting often extends up the whole arm. In the summer the upper arm may be cut in preference so that T-shirts can be worn. ② Cutting to the abdomen and sometimes the chest occurs particularly in those who self harm regularly. ③ Cutting is very common on the lower arm. If left-handed the patient will generally cut on the right arm and vice versa. ④ Cuts to the thighs are common as they are easily hidden from view.

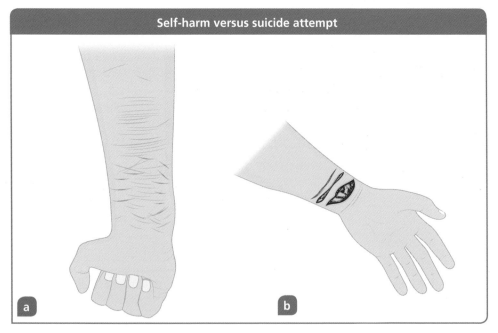

Self-harm versus suicide attempt

a

b

Figure 6.5 Distinguishing between self-harm and a suicide attempt. (a) Multiple superficial cuts up the arm often indicate self-harming behaviour. (b) Deep lacerations through the fat layer, particularly on the anterior wrist should be considered as a possible suicide attempt.

therapy and parenting classes are useful, particularly for children and teenagers, if the family background is complex. Distraction techniques are often used to prevent an episode of self-harm when a trigger event has occurred. These include exercise, watching television and listening to music. Self-help guides and websites are used either alone or with the above interventions.

The focus of these interventions is to reduce or stop the self-harming behaviours but this is not always possible, at least in the short term. In this situation, education about self-harm and how to minimise it should be given. This includes discussions about alternatives to self-harm, where on the body to cut (e.g. over fatty areas and away from arteries and ligaments) and how to keep the wound as sterile as possible to reduce infection (**Figure 6.6**).

Safer alternative methods of self-harming

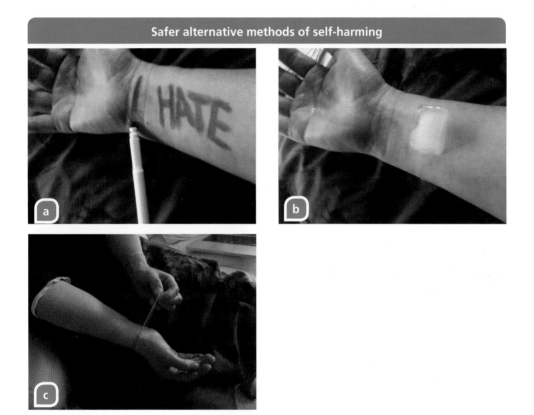

Figure 6.6 Safer alternative methods of self-harming. (a) Red pen marks mimic the marks and blood created by cutting, and can be used to write down some of the feelings the person is experiencing. (b) Ice burns create a similar feeling of pain to cutting while being harmless. (c) Elastic bands simulate the marks and pain of cutting.

Suicide

Suicide is one of the main causes of death of people under 34 years in the UK. Attempted suicide is distinct from self-harm as the actions are carried out with intent of dying rather than hurting oneself. This means that an injury or action that causes little harm can still be classified as a suicide attempt if the person did it believing they would die as a result.

Suicide attempts usually occur in a context of despair and distress. However, they also occurs with religious extremism, cult beliefs or extreme social pressure.

> People still often use the term **'committing suicide'** because until 1961 (1993 for Ireland) suicide was a criminal offence in the UK. Those attempting suicide were prosecuted and often imprisoned. A more appropriate term is 'die by suicide'.

Types

The prevalence of suicide and the method used varies considerably worldwide (**Figure 6.7**).

In the USA, most suicides involve firearms. In the UK, where there is limited access to this method, the most common method is hanging. Inhaling gases from either a domestic supply or car exhaust was previously the most popular method in the UK. However, this is now less used because changes in domestic supplies of gas and the use of catalytic convertors in car exhaust systems have made them safer.

Globally, pesticides are one of the leading methods of dying by suicide. In farming communities in Britain, this also is a common method, as is the use of firearms.

Epidemiology

In the UK, over 6700 suicides were recorded in 2013, which equates to one person dying through suicide every 2 hours. In addition, statistics record that approximately 100,000 people attempt suicide in the UK each year. The actual figure could be much higher, given that many individuals do not present to health-care providers.

Thirty per cent of those who attempt suicide will reattempt within 5 years. They are 48 times more likely than average to die by suicide.

Aetiology

Usually multiple aetiological factors combine to increase a person's suicide risk (**Table 6.4**). A genetic link has been found in twin

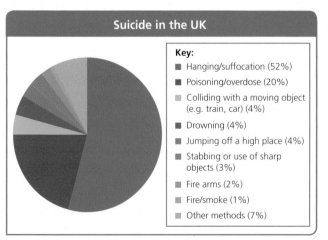

Suicide in the UK

Key:
- Hanging/suffocation (52%)
- Poisoning/overdose (20%)
- Colliding with a moving object (e.g. train, car) (4%)
- Drowning (4%)
- Jumping off a high place (4%)
- Stabbing or use of sharp objects (3%)
- Fire arms (2%)
- Fire/smoke (1%)
- Other methods (7%)

Figure 6.7 Methods of suicide in the UK and their incidence as a percentage of presenting patients.

Factors increasing and reducing suicide risk			
Raise risk			Reduce risk
Personality/psychological	Environmental	Cultural	
Impulsive	Abuse (past or present)	Stigma	Family support
Aggressive	Socially isolated	Media portrayal of suicide	Resilience to stress
Neurotic	Lack of support	Reduced access to help	Good problem-solving skills
Pessimistic	Loss of a significant relationship	Poor access to treatment for mental illness/ substance abuse	Strong support structures
Hopelessness			Restricted access to means of suicide
External locus of control (believe they have no control)	Dramatic reduction in income or job role	Religious/ cultural acceptance or encouragement	
Poor problem-solving	Physical illness		
Poor coping strategies	Family dysfunction or history of suicide		
	Poor childhood experiences		

Table 6.4 Factors that increase and reduce risk of suicide

and adoption studies. It is thought that some people have a genetic dysregulation in their serotonin system that makes them more likely to become depressed and impulsive, increasing their risk of suicide.

One of the main risk factors is mental illness. Approximately 90% of those who die by suicide have a mental illness (often diagnosed retrospectively through psychological autopsy) at the time of death. Around 5% of all people with schizophrenia die by suicide. Depression also significantly increases the risk of suicide, especially if there is co-morbid substance misuse such as alcoholism.

Prevention

Universal prevention strategies focus on reducing access to lethal methods, for examples fencing and nets on bridges and railway lines and reduced access to pesticides and other poisons. For example in Britain, only 16 paracetamol tablets can be bought in one purchase (32 in pharmacies), which has reduced the number of fatalities from overdose. Notices advertising helplines are put up in places where suicide attempts are common.

The main form of prevention is early detection and treatment of those found to be at risk. Educating teachers, social workers and health workers on the signs of mental illness and how to identify vulnerabilities such as adverse life events helps to detect those at increased risk. Risk monitoring is an essential part of ongoing assessment for people who have been diagnosed with a mental illness. If necessary, mental health legislation is invoked to prevent suicide in someone with a known or suspected mental illness.

Clinical features

There are no defining features to identify someone who is suicidal. Even in the context of mental illness, some people never contemplate suicide. However, there are risk factors (**Table 6.5**) present more often in people who are suicidal, and protective factors seen in those who are not. As some people who are suicidal keep their plans private even if questioned sensitively, the presence of multiple risk factors and few or no protective factors should raise suspicion.

> Some professionals worry that they will make a suicide attempt more likely by asking about thoughts of suicide. However, there is no increased risk of suicide just from asking about it.

Diagnostic approach

Many questionnaires have been developed to assess the risk of suicide. These range from the simple four-question assessment of the

Assessing risk of suicide		
Example questions	Example high-risk answer	Example low-risk answer
'Have you ever had thoughts about ending your life?'	'Yes, frequently'	'Very rarely'
'Have you ever attempted suicide?'	'Yes, about 1 month ago, but it didn't work so I didn't tell anyone'	'No, I could never do that to my family'
'Have the thoughts of suicide ever lead you to make a plan of how to end your life?'	'Yes, I have a plan to hang myself, I have already bought the rope and know when I want to do it'	'No, the thoughts never get to that level'
'Have you been organising things for after you have died, e.g. writing a will?'	'I have written a will and paid a few bills, the rest doesn't matter anymore'	'No, nothing like that'
'Have you written a suicide note or said your goodbyes to anyone?'	'I have written a note to my children which I have asked to be given to them when I'm dead'	'No, it would upset them too much and I don't want to hurt them'
'What would stop you from attempting suicide?'	'I don't think anything could now. My life is nothing now'	'My family is the main thing I think about that stops me, I could never do it to them'
'Can you see a way out of how you are feeling if you got help?'	'No, I think it is too late for help now, I'd rather just die'	'I really want to get better, I don't want to die, it's just difficult sometimes'

Table 6.5 Assessing the risk of suicide. High-risk answers indicate a significant risk the person will attempt suicide, while a low-risk answer indicates little or no risk that the person will attempt suicide

Manchester Self-Harm Rule to the lengthy approach of the Suicide Assessment Scale. Unfortunately, no matter how much detail they include, questionnaires do not accurately predict future suicide attempts. At present, no diagnostic measure other than taking a detailed history is recommended when assessing suicidality.

In a history related to thoughts of suicide, it is important to measure the predicted risk of an attempt occurring. This is usually divided into three categories: low, moderate and high risk (**Table 6.5**). Questions about thoughts of suicide and previous suicide attempts should be coupled with a comprehensive psychosocial history exploring the individual's risk factors.

Investigations

A physical examination is often conducted due to the presence of other symptoms such as low mood, which is sometimes caused by physical illness , e.g. hypothyrodism or brain tumours. In the elderly, dementia should also be considered.

If no evidence of physical illness is found, further investigations are rarely required in those with thoughts of suicide.

Management

The management of people with thoughts of suicide aims to:

1. Keep the person safe
2. Treat any underlying cause for their thoughts of suicide.

In the context of a suicide attempt, physical treatment should take priority, although the risk of a repeat attempt should be considered as soon as possible. Some patients attempt suicide but refuse admission to hospital, in which case detention under the mental health act may have to be considered (see page 283).

Community care

People who are having thoughts of suicide are often willing to accept help, with the result that the intensity of suicidal thoughts diminishes. The community mental health team, or occasionally the patient's GP, see these patients regularly for ongoing assessments of risk while interventions are being implemented.

Crisis care

Other individuals have stronger thoughts and more risk factors that make the risk too high for community care. Crisis or rapid response teams have therefore been set up in most areas of the UK to provide intensive support while longer term management is being set up and implemented. These teams are made up of mental health professionals who visit the patient daily if required. In most areas, they run a 24-hour service.

The individual's risk is occasionally deemed too high for them to remain at home. When this occurs, admission to a mental health unit is usually recommended in the short term, (usually a few days) even though this is not ideal for the patient. If they do not wish to be admitted to hospital and they have a suspected mental illness, they are assessed under mental health legislation for involuntary detention.

> Although the primary aim of any short-term management is to keep the patient safe, this has to be weighed against removing the patient's sense of autonomy, independence and sense of responsibility. This could jeopardise the individual's longer term recovery, especially if a borderline personality disorder is present.

Long-term care

Longer term strategies aim to address the modifiable risk factors that were identified in the history. These are usually split into psychological, social and biological interventions.

Psychological interventions include talking therapy for any mental illness that has been identified, for example cognitive behavioural therapy for depression. Problem-solving skills and improving emotional control are often taught either through self-help or by a member of the mental health team.

Dialectical behavioural therapy is targeted at those with borderline personality disorder who have often made multiple suicidal attempts. It aims to improve tolerance to distress using techniques such as mindfulness.

It also improves individuals' skill sets to change their behaviour away from repeated suicide attempts.

> **Selective serotonin reuptake inhibitors slightly increase the risk of suicidal thoughts** because they increase impulsivity and motivation before they act on low mood. Consequently, the patient feels low for a few weeks, but with more motivation to do something about it, increasing their thoughts of suicide.

Social interventions aim to improve modifiable environmental factors. They include assessing what support a person requires at home, giving financial or career advice and accessing help for physical illness and related difficulties. Mental health teams often include an occupational therapist and a social worker to provide expertise in these areas. Family work is conducted to improve family functioning and family support. Improving access to support also includes encouraging the person to join local groups or voluntary services.

Biological interventions target underlying mental or physical illness that is contributing to the thoughts of suicide. There is no recommended medication for suicidal thoughts without an underlying condition. Occasionally, usually in a hospital setting, benzodiazepines are used as a short-term solution for those who are extremely agitated or distressed by their thoughts. However, this is becoming increasingly rare as people are identified earlier and offered targeted help in a timely fashion.

In those with mental illness, only lithium has been shown to reduce suicide attempts. Other drugs, such as antidepressants, reduce the risk but only through treating the underlying mental illness. Selective serotonin reuptake inhibitors occasionally increase the risk of suicidal thoughts in the short term in those under 25 years of age.

Answers to starter questions

1. In many research studies no distinction is made between self-harm and attempted suicide, but there are clinical differences. Self-harm is not done for the purpose of ending the person's life, but as a means of finding relief from emotional distress. In attempted suicide, a person may be engaging in the same, or even less lethal, actions than someone who self-harms, but with the purpose of ending their life. Often, particularly in those who self-harm through overdose, both thoughts of self-harm and suicide are present. For this reason self-harm and suicide are often seen as being on the same spectrum.

2. People who self-harm have a similar risk factor profile to those who attempt suicide. Self-harm is a dysfunctional way of coping with distress, often used as a form of self-punishment or relief from pain. This is similar to suicide attempts where the person no longer sees the physical damage or pain as something that would prevent the attempt. Those who self-harm often feel there is no other means of helping themselves, which again is similar to those attempting suicide who feel there is no other way out of the situation. Self-harm as a coping strategy often requires escalating levels of harm as the person becomes desensitised to pain or damage caused, resulting in more lethal means of self-harm being utilised.

Chapter 7
Personality disorders

Introduction.................. 177
Case 8 Emotional instability and
         relationship difficulties ... 178

Personality disorders........... 180

Starter questions

Answers to the following questions are on page 184.

1. Why would some personality disorders be found in company executives?
2. Why is there such a negative stigma attached to personality disorders?
3. Can you teach patients with antisocial personality disorder to be empathic?

Introduction

Personality is defined as the characteristics we have that influence our thoughts, emotions and behaviours in different situations. It develops during childhood and is fully formed by early adulthood.

Most personality types learn from their life experiences and as a result develop coping strategies. With a personality disorder, however, the emotions, thoughts and behaviours are abnormal so individuals have significant difficulty learning from experience. People with personality disorders exhibit abnormal behaviours and problems in social interactions in many situations. A personality disorder is a chronic condition, although people can go into remission, i.e. they have a decrease or disappearance of signs and symptoms. The condition often reduces in severity with age.

Until the advent of dialectical behavioural therapy, there was no effective treatment for personality disorders and they were often considered 'incurable'. Because of the chronic nature of the disorder and the poor response to treatment, people with personality disorders were often stigmatised by medical professionals. This sometimes led to them having difficulty accessing the help they required.

Case 8 Emotional instability and relationship difficulties

Presentation

Rachel Sherwood, who is 23 years old, attends a psychiatric outpatient clinic complaining she has a low mood and feels 'empty' inside. This has led to frequent self-harming and on, a few occasions, suicide attempts

Initial interpretation

Rachel's presentation suggests she is suffering from depression or a borderline personality disorder. It is important to determine whether the symptoms are chronic, which could indicate a personality disorder, or more acute in onset, possibly in relation to a life event (which could indicate depression).

Further history

Rachel says she has felt this way for a number of years, only feeling happy when she is in a relationship. However, she has not had much luck with relationships as they always break down, usually after only a few weeks. It is often after a break-up that she harms herself or attempts suicide.

Rachel talks about her emotions as being on a roller coaster, one moment high and happy, the next low or angry. She finds it difficult to predict her emotions and does not know what triggers a change in them. She occasionally drinks alcohol to help her manage her moods but denies taking any recreational drugs.

Borderline personality disorder: a patient's experience

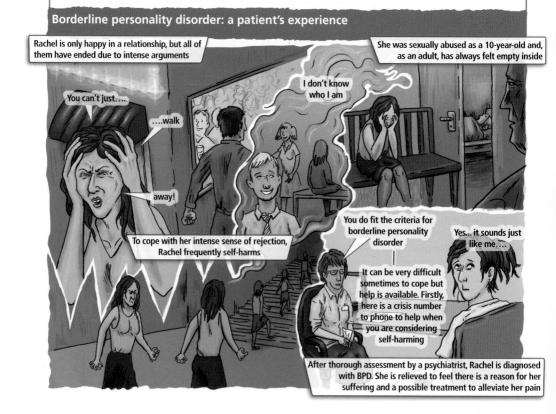

Case 8 *continued*

When Rachel was 10 years old, her stepfather sexually abused her. At the time she tried to tell her mother, who did not believe her. The abuse continued for a number of years until her mother and stepfather separated.

Examination

Rachel has numerous scars and healing injuries on her arms, thighs and stomach. She says these were caused by her cutting with a razor blade. There is no evidence that the cuts are infected.

Interpretation of findings

Rachel's unstable mood is evidence of a personality disorder rather than depression. Her difficulty with relationships also supports this diagnosis. Many people who develop a personality disorder have been abused during childhood. As is common in borderline personality disorder, Rachel's self-harming and suicide attempts are her way of coping when faced with rejection.

It is important to rule out drug and alcohol abuse when considering this diagnosis as it imitates the symptoms. Drug abuse and personality disorder are also often co-morbid conditions, which should be considered in the treatment plan.

Investigations

As a borderline personality disorder is suspected, the psychiatrist meets with Rachel more than once to reassess her symptoms and to confirm they are chronic. This will confirm the

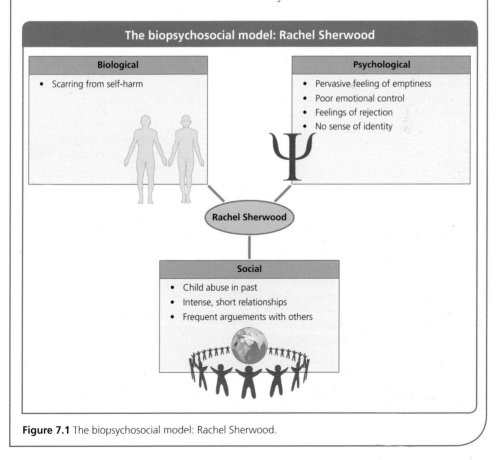

Figure 7.1 The biopsychosocial model: Rachel Sherwood.

Case 8 *continued*

diagnosis of personality disorder rather than an emerging depression or other mental illness.

A risk assessment is also performed as Rachel regularly self-harms and has previously attempted suicide. The first priority in managing Rachel's symptoms is to keep her safe from serious injury by identifying and managing the triggers for her risky behaviours.

Diagnosis

Given her history and the chronicity of her symptoms, it is determined that Rachel has a borderline personality disorder (**Figure 7.1**). The psychiatrist assessing Rachel is aware that this diagnosis carries a negative stigma and therefore carefully talks though with her what it means, emphasising that it can be treated effectively. The doctor discusses ways to cope that do not involve self-harm or attempts at suicide, and gives Rachel a crisis call card to use if she feels suicidal at any time.

Personality disorders

The International Classification of Diseases 10th Revision (ICD-10) and Diagnostic and Statistical Manual of Mental Disorders, 4th edition (DSM-IV) classify the many subtypes of personality disorder, which is useful when choosing a treatment package. Recently, however, it has become clear that the severity is usually more important than the actual subtype in terms of prognosis and treatment, and this is reflected in ICD-11, the latest revision of the ICD.

Types

Personality disorder is traditionally divided into three main types: A, B and C (**Figure 7.1**). It also has four 'dimensions', indicating its severity:

1. Traits of one or many personality disorders without reaching the full criteria for any
2. Meets the criteria for one or more personality disorders in the same cluster
3. Meets the criteria for more than one personality disorder in more than one cluster
4. As for dimension 3 but causes severe disruption to the individual and society

A person with severe antisocial personality disorder is sometimes termed a 'psychopath' as the lack of empathy and disregard for other people's rights often leads them to commit serious crimes, such as murder.

Epidemiology

In the general population in the UK, 1 in 20 people have a personality disorder. In the prison population, however, this rises to 50–70%.

The most common types of personality disorder are borderline (also called emotionally unstable), schizotypal and antisocial (**Figure 7.2**). Men develop personality disorders more frequently than women, except for borderline, dependent and histrionic personality disorders, which are more often diagnosed in women.

Aetiology

The heritability of personality disorders in general is around 20–60%. For some types, such as obsessive compulsive and

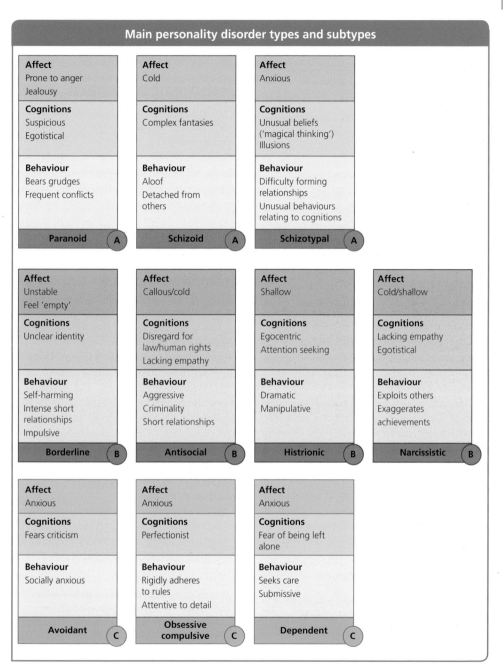

Figure 7.2 Main personality disorder types and subtypes. (A) Paranoid/odd types. (B) Emotional/dramatic types. (C) Anxious/fearful types.

schizotypal disorder, the heritability is higher, at around 50–70%. It is the combination of genetic factors creating a personality that is then vulnerable to negative experiences.

Experiences during childhood appear to play a larger role than genetics in the development of personality disorders. Abuse in childhood is linked to an increased risk, but only 20% of those who have been abused later develop a personality disorder. Borderline personality disorder has the strongest association with physical or sexual abuse in childhood.

Conduct disorder and ADHD are linked to an increased risk of developing antisocial personality disorder in adulthood.

Clinical features

The symptoms of a personality disorder are apparent in many different situations, affecting the person's social and occupational functioning. Many people with milder symptoms manage to function well except when in crisis.

The symptoms are relatively stable as personality disorders do not follow a relapsing and remitting course like some other mental illnesses, such as bipolar or recurrent depression. However, people with personality disorder often enter into a crisis precipitated by relatively minor causes, e.g. an argument with a friend. During a crisis episode, there is an exacerbation in symptoms and a subsequent reduction in functioning.

> A study examining high-earning executives found that not all personality disorders have a negative impact on the workplace. Histrionic, narcissistic and obsessive compulsive disorders have been found to be more common in high-earning executives than psychiatric inpatients.

A personality disorder affects a person's emotional control, thought processes and impulse control. Symptoms start to manifest in adolescence and are usually apparent by early adulthood. As the person passes through adulthood, the symptoms diminish in severity.

Although all personality disorders have common features, they present in significantly different ways (**Table 7.1**).

Diagnostic approach

A patient with a suspected personality disorder should be carefully assessed on more than one occasion. This ensures their symptoms are not being caused by another mental illness, such as schizophrenia or depression. If the person is in crisis when they present, the diagnosis should ideally not be made until the crisis has passed as they may function well at other times.

The diagnosis is rarely made in children because their personalities are still forming and are therefore unstable. Young people in their teens who experience symptoms of personality disorder are often described as having an emerging personality disorder unless the symptoms are very severe.

Assessment should take a biopsychosocial approach and involve a history incorporating childhood experiences. Risk assessment is very important because many patients with personality disorders engage in behaviours that cause risk to either themselves or others. Personality disorders are often co-morbid with other disorders (**Table 7.2**), which should be carefully assessed and treated alongside the personality disorder.

Antisocial personality disorder requires a specialist forensic psychiatry assessment and a structured diagnostic interview, such as the Psychopathy Checklist–Revised (**Table 7.3**).

> Personality disorder is one of the most controversial mental illnesses due to the significant negative stigma attached and the perception that no treatments help.

Management

This depends on the severity of the condition. Most patients receive social education to improve their interpersonal relationship skills.

Psychoeducation helps patients understand their condition and identify triggers for crises. As personality disorders are chronic, psychological input tends to involve longer term therapies such as dynamic psychotherapy or interpersonal therapy. Dialectical behavioural therapy is used with borderline personality disorder. This is a modified form of cognitive behavioural therapy and mindfulness, which involves individual and group therapy. For antisocial personality disorder, residential therapies are more effective than outpatient care.

There is no recommended drug treatment for personality disorders. Drugs such as sedatives are occasionally used in the short term (usually no more than a few days) if the

Common presentations of personality disorders	
Personality disorder	Example presentation
Paranoid	Presents after a conflict where the other party suggests a need for psychiatric treatment. Is extremely difficult to develop a therapeutic relationship with, as they are very mistrustful of your motivations
Schizoid	Referred as possibly having mild autism spectrum disorder. Has very few friends and appears cold and aloof during the assessment
Schizotypal	Referred for possible psychosis, appears very anxious and describes some unusual thoughts and illusions
Borderline	Presents after attempting suicide, describes a history of self-harming behaviour often triggered by minor events
Antisocial	Police request an assessment after they are arrested for a serious assault. Appear to have no remorse for their actions and are charming and grandiose during the assessment
Narcissistic	Asked to attend after coming into conflict with their employer. Grandiose and arrogant at assessment
Histrionic	Referred themselves having had a breakdown at work after being criticised. Very emotional during assessment and use dramatic language
Avoidant	Referred with possible anxiety disorder. They want to have friends, but fear what is required to do so, in particular being rejected
Dependent	You are asked to visit the home of a patient who is living with their parents and rarely leaves their room. Their parents care for them and never leave them alone as they become so distressed
Obsessive compulsive (anankastic)	Referred for possible OCD, they desire perfection in their environment and struggle at work as colleagues do not live up to their expectations

Table 7.1 Common presentations of personality disorders

Conditions comorbid with personality disorders	
Personality disorder	Associated conditions
Schizotypal	Psychotic disorders, anxiety disorders, drug/alcohol abuse
Schizoid	Depression, anxiety disorders
Paranoid	Pathological jealousy, delusional disorder, depression, anxiety disorders
Borderline	Depression, anxiety disorders, bipolar disorder, eating disorders, drug and alcohol abuse
Antisocial personality disorder	Depression, anxiety disorders, drug and alcohol abuse, ADHD
Histrionic/narcissistic	Depression, anxiety disorders, drug and alcohol abuse
Avoidant/dependent	Anxiety disorders, depression, drug and alcohol abuse
Obsessive compulsive (Anankastic)	Obsessive compulsive disorder and other anxiety disorders, depression, drug and alcohol abuse

Table 7.2 Conditions comorbid commonly associated with personality disorders

Psychopathy checklist	
Aspects assessed	Examining for
Interpersonal	Compulsive lying
	Grandiosity
	Manipulative
Affect	Shallow emotions
	Lacking empathy/feelings of guilt
Lifestyle	Irresponsible
	Lack of long-term goals
	Impulsive
Antisocial behaviour	Criminal behaviour
	Childhood criminality
	Poor behavioural control
Sexual behaviour	Multiple sexual partners
	Short-term relationships

Table 7.3 Overview of the psychopathy checklist

patient is in crisis or suffering from severe insomnia. Long-term treatment is avoided to prevent abuse or dependency. Mood stabilisers or antipsychotics are occasionally used in severe personality disorder but have limited effect. Any co-morbid mental illness must be treated appropriately, for example with antidepressants if the patient develops depression.

Each patient requires an individualised treatment plan specific to their difficulties, including how to manage crisis episodes.

During crisis times, management of risk is extremely important to keep the patient safe while enabling them to remain as independent as possible. Crisis teams operate in many areas of the UK, are available 24 hours a day and can see patients on a daily basis if necessary.

Prolonged admission is rarely helpful for people with a personality disorder as they lose their ability to function independently. It is, however, useful in the short term (often only a few days) to manage an acute increase in risk.

Prognosis

As personality disorders reduce in severity over time, approximately 50% of patients no longer meet the criteria for a personality disorder 10 years after diagnosis. The exception is patients with antisocial personality disorder, who do not experience remission but largely stop engaging in criminal behaviours by 50 years of age.

The treatment of co-morbid mental illnesses (see **Table 7.3**) is complicated by the symptoms of the personality disorder. This means that these conditions are often longer in duration and/or more severe. Schizotypal disorder evolves into schizophrenia for 50% of affected patients.

Patients with antisocial personality disorder often end up in prison or a specialist forensic unit. In borderline personality disorder, 3–10% of patients die by suicide.

Answers to starter questions

1. Narcissistic, histrionic and obsessive compulsive disorders are all over-represented in high-earning executives. People with a narcissistic personality disorder are egotistical, which motivates them to achieve. They also exploit others to achieve their own goals. People with histrionic personality disorder are adept at manipulating people, while those with obsessive compulsive personality disorder have a significant degree of perfectionism and attention to detail.

2. People with personality disorders are sometimes seen as choosing to behave antisocially. It remains a controversial diagnosis with some psychiatrists believing that it is not a mental illness. Personality disorders are chronic in duration and often resistant to treatments, which leads people to feel they are incurable.

3. Therapies that attempt to teach empathic skills to those with antisocial personality disorder are largely ineffective. Instead therapists focus on the consequences to the patient themselves to help reduce their antisocial behaviour.

Chapter 8
Substance misuse and addictions

Introduction. 185
Case 9 Excessive alcohol
      consumption. 186
Case 10 Heroin use. 189
Alcohol dependence 192

Drugs and psychoactive
    substances 197
Drug-induced psychiatric
    disorders. 201

Starter questions

Answers to the following questions are on page 202.

1. Why is it dangerous for people with alcohol dependence syndrome to suddenly stop drinking alcohol?
2. If a patient does not want to stop using alcohol or illicit drugs, can they be given any treatment?

Introduction

For centuries, people have used psychoactive substances, including alcohol and illicit drugs such as morphine. In some cultures, the use of such substances is currently considered acceptable. Psychoactive substances affect the central nervous system, producing changes in feelings, thoughts and behaviour. The resulting clinical features can be difficult to distinguish from psychiatric illnesses. In addition, patients with psychiatric illnesses such as depression, schizophrenia and anxiety sometimes use substances to help alleviate their symptoms.

It is difficult to detect illicit drug use or excess alcohol use because patients often deny or minimise their use of these substances. However, the type and severity of substance use must be determined to facilitate the provision of appropriate treatment. With support, people who are dependent on alcohol or illicit drugs can achieve abstinence, although this often takes several years during which there can be periods of relapse when the patient starts using the substance again.

Case 9   Excessive alcohol consumption

Presentation

Jeff Baines is a 40-year-old married man with no children, who visits his general practitioner, Dr Peterson, with concerns about feeling anxious, shaky, sweaty and nauseous each morning. Drinking cider relieves these symptoms. His wife, Tracey, who has accompanied him to the appointment, says they are having marital problems because Mr Baines drinks too much.

> **Express empathy and use a non-judgemental approach when speaking to patients about alcohol use.** This helps establish a rapport and to build a therapeutic relationship.

Initial interpretation

The initial history suggests that a further assessment of Jeff's alcohol intake is necessary to determine the severity of his alcohol use and any problems arising from his alcohol use.

History

Jeff started drinking at the age of 16 to fit in with his friends. He says his friends encouraged him to drink and that he felt more confident around them after consuming alcohol. At first, this was only on social occasions, but over the years his alcohol intake has steadily increased. In the last year, he has been drinking only cider and has been drinking increasing

Alcohol dependence: taking a history

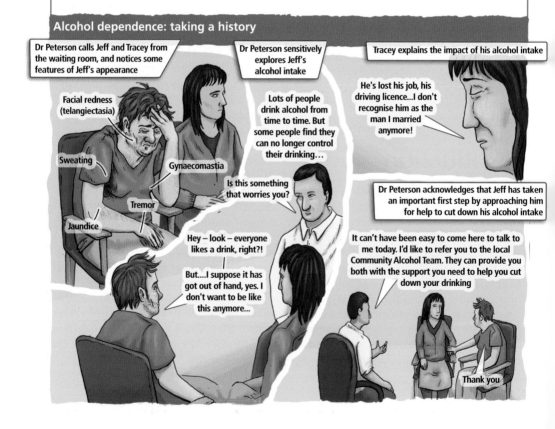

Case 9 *continued*

amounts to achieve the same effect. To avoid feeling shaky, sweaty, nauseous and anxious, he now has to drink a pint of cider before breakfast. His priority each day is to buy more cider.

He worries that his sweaty, shaky, nauseous, anxious spells are the result of his alcohol intake but feels unable to stop.

Interpretation of history

Jeff's symptoms are suggestive of alcohol dependence. A further history is necessary to assess the impact of these difficulties on his physical, mental and social well-being. This should also focus on the possibility of a primary psychiatric disorder that he is self-medicating with alcohol, e.g. depression or anxiety.

The initial history ascertained that Tracey is concerned about his alcohol intake. Obtaining a collateral history from her is vital because Jeff might minimise his alcohol use or deny adverse consequences.

> The adverse consequences of excess alcohol intake are best remembered by the '4 Ls': Liver, Livelihood (occupation), Love (relationships) and (getting into trouble with the) Law.

Further history

Jeff has not noticed any yellow discoloration of his skin or eyes (jaundice would indicate liver dysfunction). He has no abdominal pain and no episodes of vomiting blood or passing blood in his stools. He is embarrassed to admit that he has difficulties sustaining an erection, which has caused difficulties in his marriage.

On one occasion when he had been drinking more heavily than usual, he thought he could hear the voice of his deceased maternal grandfather, who died of chronic liver disease caused by excess alcohol intake. He has never had any other similar experiences and denies any symptoms suggestive of depression, anxiety or psychosis prior to the onset of his problem drinking. Apart from feeling anxious each morning before drinking, he has no other symptoms suggestive of an anxiety disorder, and no symptoms suggestive of a current mood disorder. He denies ever thinking of harming himself and denies suicidal ideation.

> The risk of suicide in people with excess alcohol consumption is 60–100 times greater than in the general population. Always ask about thoughts of self-harm or suicide.

Tracey tells Dr Peterson she is fed up with her husband's drinking and plans to divorce him if he cannot change. She reports that he was recently sacked from his job as a doorman at a local pub due to his alcohol problems, and has lost most of his friends because he has been rude towards them when drunk. He has lost previous jobs for the same reason. She says he was arrested for driving under the influence of alcohol 6 months ago.

> Excess alcohol consumption is a risk factor for domestic violence. Be alert for indicators of this and ask about it in a sensitive way.

Examination

A mental state examination is undertaken (**Table 8.1**). Of note, Jeff smells of alcohol and is unkempt. He does not appear depressed and does not appear to be responding to unseen external stimuli. He has some insight into his current difficulties.

Case 9 *continued*

Jeff's mental state examination

Category	Description
Appearance and behaviour	Unshaven, stained clothes, smells of alcohol Appears anxious Irritable when asked about alcohol, but no hostility or aggression
Speech	Slightly slurred
Mood	Appears euthymic Reactive affect
Perceptions	Not actively responding to unseen external stimuli
Thoughts	No formal thought disorder or delusions
Cognitions	No memory impairment
Insight	Feels he is no longer able to control his level of drinking, feels he might need help
Suicidal ideation	No suicidal ideas or thoughts of harming himself or others

Table 8.1 Jeff's mental state examination

> **Excess alcohol intake can result in fleeting hallucinations that resolve with abstinence from alcohol.** Delusions can also occur. In Othello syndrome, for example, patients have morbid jealousy, with delusions about their partner's infidelity.

CAGE screening questionnaire

1. Have you ever felt you should **Cut** down on your drinking?
2. Have you felt **Annoyed** when people criticise your drinking?
3. Have you ever felt **Guilty** about your drinking?
4. Have you ever had a drink first thing in the morning (an **Eye-opener**) to steady your nerves or get rid of a hang-over?

Table 8.2 CAGE screening questionnaire for alcohol misuse. Two or more positive replies identify those likely to be consuming excessive amounts of alcohol

A physical examination looks for for signs suggesting chronic liver disease resulting from chronic excess alcohol intake, e.g. jaundice, ascites or peripheral oedema. Jeff's physical examination shows the presence of gynaecomastia, suggestive of chronic liver disease.

Interpretation of findings

Jeff does not appear to have a co-morbid psychiatric disorder. His physical examination suggests chronic liver disease resulting from chronic excess alcohol consumption.

Investigations

Jeff scores 3 on the CAGE questionnaire (**Table 8.2**). A score of 2 or more indicates excessive use of alcohol.

Blood tests are requested, including a full blood count (which may reveal thrombocytopaenia in chronic liver disease), liver function tests, clotting screen (prothrombin time is an indicator of liver function) and γ-glutamyl transferase (GGT). A high GGT level is found, suggestive of alcohol use, but the liver function tests are otherwise normal.

Diagnosis

Jeff is shocked when Dr Peterson tells him he has the symptoms and signs of alcohol dependence (**Figure 8.1**). His wife is relieved when Mr Baines agrees to be referred to the local specialist alcohol service for further biopsychosocial support.

Case 9 *continued*

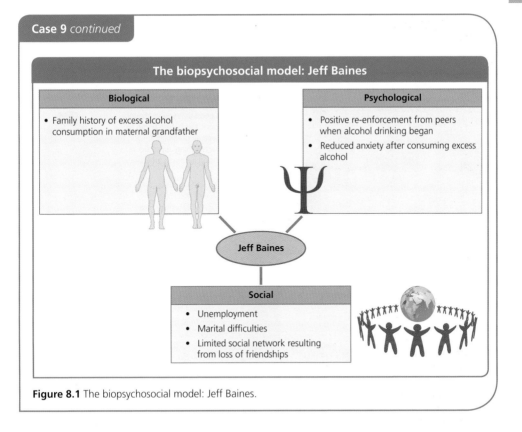

Figure 8.1 The biopsychosocial model: Jeff Baines.

Case 10 Heroin use

Presentation

Suzy Campbell is a 24-year-old unemployed, childless woman who lives alone. She is in a new relationship. She attends her GP surgery to ask for help to stop using heroin.

Initial interpretation

It is important to find out more about the heroin use, including how much she consumes (in terms of either a weight or how much she spends on heroin per day). As heroin is often used intravenously, she must be asked whether she takes any precautions such as abstaining from sharing needles with others. A full drug history should explore whether she uses any other substances, including alcohol.

An assessment must be made of how Suzy's drug use has affected her physical health, mental health and psychosocial well-being. A previous history of mental illness must be included. Current psychosocial circumstances, insight and motivation to change should be evaluated to help plan her management.

> **Always consider whether female heroin users are, or plan to become, pregnant.** Heroin use in early pregnancy reduces fetal growth. In later pregnancy, the fetus can become dependent on heroin. The baby then has serious withdrawal symptoms a few days after birth, including restlessness, irritability, tremor and a high-pitched cry.

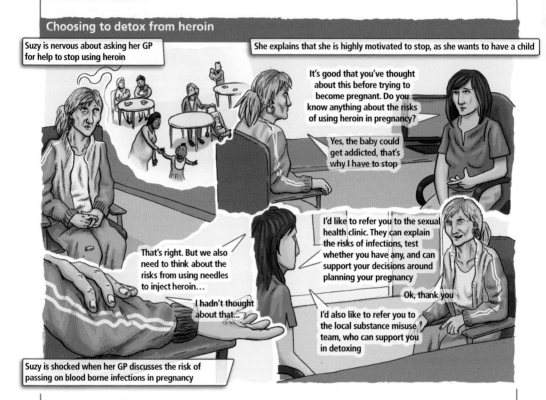

Case 10 *continued*

Choosing to detox from heroin

Suzy is nervous about asking her GP for help to stop using heroin

She explains that she is highly motivated to stop, as she wants to have a child

It's good that you've thought about this before trying to become pregnant. Do you know anything about the risks of using heroin in pregnancy?

Yes, the baby could get addicted, that's why I have to stop

That's right. But we also need to think about the risks from using needles to inject heroin…

I hadn't thought about that…

I'd like to refer you to the sexual health clinic. They can explain the risks of infections, test whether you have any, and can support your decisions around planning your pregnancy

Ok, thank you

I'd also like to refer you to the local substance misuse team, who can support you in detoxing

Suzy is shocked when her GP discusses the risk of passing on blood borne infections in pregnancy

Further history

Suzy says she has been using heroin for 2 years, and currently uses £20-worth per day. She injects into her arms and groin, and although she previously shared needles, she currently uses a needle exchange scheme. She initially used heroin at weekends with her friends. She now feels it has taken over her life as it is the first thing she thinks about each day. She feels restless and sweaty and has abdominal cramps and diarrhoea when she has not had heroin for some time.

Suzy admits to having previously used cannabis and amphetamines but she has not done so in the last 3 years. She drinks two glasses of wine per week.

Suzy says she was arrested last year for shoplifting to fund her heroin use. She now wishes to withdraw from heroin completely. She has tried to do this by herself but found it difficult as the peers she lived with in the hostel for homeless people pressurised her to start using it again. She now lives alone in a council flat with a steady partner who has never used heroin and will support her in trying to withdraw. She and her partner want to have a baby, and she knows heroin could harm her unborn child.

She has not experienced any symptoms suggestive of mental illness, although she feels low in mood between doses of heroin. She has no previous history of mental illness.

Examination

Table 8.3 shows the findings from Suzy mental state examination. Of note, she is unkempt with poor dentition, suggesting that she is neglecting her personal hygiene and dental health. She has no features suggestive of a pervasive low mood or psychosis, and has good insight into her current difficulties.

On physical examination, she is not keen to remove her cardigan to enable her blood pressure to be checked. When she eventually agrees, needle track marks are observed in her left antecubital fossa and wrist. There are no signs of surrounding infection.

Interpretation of findings

Suzy's history indicates heroin dependence. Her previous history of sharing needles puts her at risk of diseases such as HIV and hepatitis B and C. Her psychosocial circumstances have changed, and it seems that her attempt to withdraw from heroin will now be supported. She is planning to become pregnant and is motivated to stop using heroin before trying to conceive.

Suzy's mental state examination findings suggest an absence of co-morbid mental illness and a good insight into her heroin use. Her physical examination shows signs of intravenous drug use, consistent with her history.

Investigations

Suzy agrees to have a urine and blood drug screen, which confirms the presence of opiates.

Diagnosis

Suzy's GP informs her that although she is dependent on heroin, fortunately

Suzy Campbell's MSE	
Category	**Description**
Appearance and behaviour	Unkempt
	Poor dentition
	Needle track marks on left arm
	Calm
Speech	Normal rate, rhythm, tone, volume
Mood	Appears euthymic
	Reactive
Perceptions	Not actively responding to unseen external stimuli
Thoughts	No formal thought disorder or delusions
Cognitions	No memory impairment
Insight	Motivated to withdraw from heroin use with support
Suicidal ideation	No suicidal ideas or thoughts of harming himself or others

Table 8.3 Suzy Campbell's mental state examination (MSE)

she has not experienced any serious physical or mental health complications. Suzy accepts a referral to the local community drug team for support with detoxification from heroin.

She is shocked that there is a risk of passing on blood-borne infections during pregnancy and agrees to a referral to the local sexual health clinic for counselling and further tests. This will include blood tests for HIV and hepatitis B and C.

Alcohol dependence

Alcohol use is common, with many people drinking amounts that do not exceed safe daily limits (**Figure 8.2**). However, when substances such as alcohol are ingested in excessive amounts, there are a number of consequences (**Table 8.4**).

Alcohol dependence can develop after a significant period of hazardous or harmful drinking, with physical and psychological addiction. Alcohol dependence is associated with comorbid mental and physical illnesses that can lead to early death. Early detection is therefore important to facilitate the provision of effective interventions that can reduce, and ultimately stop, the excess alcohol intake.

Epidemiology

Excess alcohol consumption is the most common type of psychoactive substance misuse. Alcohol dependence affects 6% of men and 2% of women aged 16–65 years in the UK. The incidence of excess alcohol use is increasing among children and young people (**Figure 8.3**). Rates of alcohol dependence are higher in men, and lower in those aged over 45 years.

> **Doctors are at increased risk of excess alcohol use.** Other occupational groups with a higher risk include brewery workers, people who work in pubs, chefs, journalists and actors.

Aetiology

A number of biopsychosocial aetiological factors contribute to alcohol dependence. The risk of alcohol dependence is increased

Consequences of excessive psychoactive substance use	
Consequence	Description
Hazardous use	Pattern or quantity of use that puts user at risk of adverse consequences
Harmful use	Pattern or quantity of use that causes adverse consequences, including physical and mental health problems, without dependence
Dependence	Syndrome with physiological, psychological and behavioural symptoms resulting from continued excessive use
Intoxication	Acute, transient behavioural, psychological and neurological symptoms following intake
Withdrawal	Symptoms caused by reducing, or stopping intake, after a period of heavy use

Table 8.4 Consequences of excessive psychoactive substance use, e.g. alcohol or illicit drugs

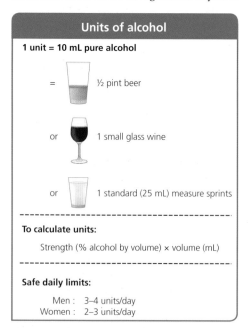

Figure 8.2 Units of alcohol.

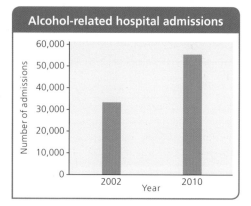

Figure 8.3 The number of alcohol-related hospital admissions in 15–24-year-old in the UK.

in those with alcohol-dependent relatives, reflecting both genetic risk factors and environmental factors including learned behaviours. Other risk factors for alcohol dependence include:

- Co-morbid psychiatric disorders such as depression, bipolar affective disorder, social phobia, panic disorder and schizophrenia because patients often use alcohol to cope with the symptoms of their psychiatric disorders
- Co-morbid antisocial or borderline personality disorder, associated with strong personality traits of impulsivity and risk taking
- Co-morbid physical illness

> **In the Japanese population an allele for faulty aldehyde dehydrogenase is common.** The result is accumulation of acetylaldehyde on drinking alcohol (see **Figure 8.7**). This leads to distressing flushing, nausea and tachycardia. Consequently, people from these groups are less likely to drink alcohol to excess.

Prevention

Public health strategies aimed at preventing alcohol dependence include health education on alcohol use and controls on the sale, advertising and pricing of alcohol to limit consumption.

Pathogenesis

The pathogenesis of alcohol dependence syndrome is incompletely understood. Multiple genetic and environmental factors, which are not clearly defined, increase vulnerability to alcohol misuse. Over time, people with these risk factors may struggle to manage their alcohol intake, leading to a gradual increase in the amount consumed. This eventually leads to problems in areas such as relationships and work. Alcohol may then be used to cope with these, leading to a vicious cycle that results in an inability to control alcohol intake and the emergence of alcohol dependence.

Clinical features

Alcohol dependence is diagnosed when three or more of the following ICD-10 criteria are present at some point during the previous year:

- A subjective awareness of a compulsion or strong desire to drink alcohol
- Difficulties controlling the onset, termination and levels of alcohol consumed
- Tolerance: increasing quantities of alcohol are required to produce the same effect
- Withdrawal symptoms such as tremors, nausea, sweating, anxiety, agitation and low mood when the alcohol intake is reduced or stopped, or continued use of alcohol to relieve or prevent withdrawal symptoms
- Persistent excess alcohol use despite clear evidence of harmful consequences, for example to physical health
- An increased salience of drinking: a neglect of other interests and activities as alcohol is given priority

A narrowing of repertoire, characterised by a tendency to drink the same type of alcoholic drink in a stereotypical pattern regardless of the social situation, is also characteristic of alcohol dependency.

> **Patients with chronic excess alcohol consumption often become deficient in thiamine (vitamin B1).** This is because of poor dietary thiamine intake and poor absorption of thiamine due to co-morbid gastritis.
>
> Thiamine helps maintain the normal structure of blood vessels. A deficiency can result in bleeding into the brain, causing damage to the thalamus and hypothalamus. This results in Wernicke–Korsakoff's syndrome (Wernicke's encephalopathy and Korsakoff's syndrome), a spectrum of alcohol-related brain damage. Wernicke's encephalopathy is characterised by a triad of confusion, ataxia and ophthalmoplegia (weakness of extraocular muscles controlling eye movement).
>
> Left untreated, Wernicke's encephalopathy progresses to Korsakoff's syndrome, with memory loss and confabulation – a falsification of memory with a clear consciousness, which leads the patient to give inaccurate and bizarre answers to questions they are asked.

Diagnostic approach

Doctors working in all specialities should routinely enquire about alcohol use. History-taking should include the type of alcohol used and pattern of use. It should also record other features of alcohol dependence and the consequences in terms of the 4 Ls (see page 187). Other substance misuse should be identified.

Previous or current co-morbid psychiatric disorders and other risk factors, including family history, should be evaluated. An exploration of the patient's current social circumstances will inform treatment decisions, for example whether detoxification in the community is suitable.

Screening questionnaires are used to identify those at risk of alcohol misuse. In addition to the CAGE questionnaire (see **Table 8.2**), the 10-item Alcohol Use Disorders Identification Test questionnaire is used to screen for hazardous drinking, harmful drinking and dependence (**Table 8.4**). Individuals scoring 20 or more out of 40 (equivalent to drinking over 15 units of alcohol per day) are offered detoxification.

The mental state examination aims to establish current symptoms of psychiatric illness and excess alcohol intake. Risk, in terms of thoughts of self-harm, harm to others and suicide, must be assessed. Risks to children and other dependents should also be considered. A sensitive enquiry should establish the patient's insight into their difficulties and whether they are ready to receive help for their alcohol intake.

> **As part of the risk assessment, remember to ask the patient whether they are a driver,** as alcohol use impairs driving skills and there are strict legal alcohol intake limits for UK drivers.

The physical examination should focus on detecting signs of complications of chronic liver disease such as jaundice, gynaecomastia and telangiectasiae. Signs of acute alcohol intake include slurred speech and ataxia. Signs of acute alcohol withdrawal include tremor, sweating and tachycardia.

Investigations

Although there is no single diagnostic test for alcohol dependence, abnormal results from a number of blood tests suggest the likelihood of alcohol misuse:

- GGT – levels of this liver enzyme are above the normal range in approximately 70% of patients who misuse alcohol
- Mean corpuscular volume – the mean volume of red blood cells is above the normal range in around 70% of those who misuse alcohol

Other investigations include:

- Breath alcohol level – this is often measured as a proxy for blood alcohol concentration, although high levels do not discriminate between acute and chronic alcohol use
- In those with a history of falls, CT scans of the head to assess the presence of a chronic subdural haematoma (**Figure 8.4**)

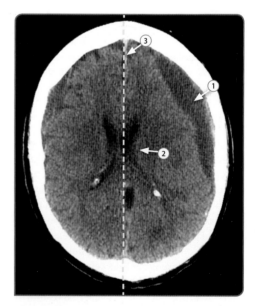

Figure 8.4 Axial CT scan showing a left-sided chronic subdural haematoma ① with crescent-shaped hypo-dense appearance. There is evidence of effacement of the left lateral ventricle ② and midline shift from left to right ③ indicative of raised intracranial pressure and mass effect.

Management

Patients who make excessive use of, or who are dependent on, alcohol must be advised not to suddenly stop drinking alcohol due to the risk of developing acute alcohol withdrawal (delirium tremens) which is life threatening (20% of cases die) and requires urgent medical treatment. Those who consume excess alcohol should be referred to specialist alcohol teams. Management strategies aim to help patients carefully detoxify from alcohol, manage associated withdrawal symptoms and then maintain abstinence from alcohol. The strategies are informed by Prochaska and DiClemente's stages of change model (**Figure 8.5**).

> Some patients with alcohol dependence are unwilling to aim for abstinence. In these patients, treatment aims to reduce levels of alcohol intake. It also explores patients' wishes around abstinence in more detail so that they may eventually be ready to aim for this.

Planned alcohol detoxification is ideally undertaken in the community, allowing the psychosocial factors perpetuating the patient's excess alcohol intake to be addressed. Inpatient detoxification is offered to patients who could not safely undergo a detox in the community (see Chapter 16). Once withdrawal from alcohol has been achieved, medications and psychosocial interventions are used to maintain abstinence.

Medication

In alcohol detoxification, medication is used to relieve withdrawal symptoms and reduce the risk of delirium tremens (acute alcohol withdrawal; see page 292). In acute alcohol withdrawal, benzodiazepines (e.g. chlordiazepoxide) are prescribed to treat withdrawal symptoms. The dose required is usually high initially and reduced as symptoms resolve over the following weeks.

Thiamine deficiency and low magnesium levels are common in people with alcohol dependence. These are corrected by prescribing

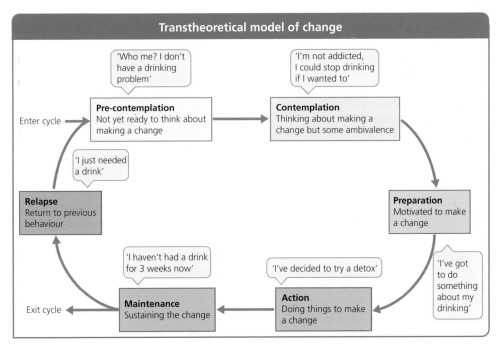

Figure 8.5 Prochaska and DiClemente's transtheoretical model of behavioural change. This model describes the stages of changing a health-related behaviour, such as drinking excess alcohol. Each stage is characterised by the types of thoughts the person has about changing their health-related behaviour.

magnesium and thiamine supplements, which are given orally or intravenously as Pabrinex.

Medications used to maintain abstinence from alcohol include:

- Acamprosate. This reduces the urge to drink alcohol by stimulating inhibitory neurotransmission involving γ-aminobutyric acid (GABA) resulting in reduced feelings of anxiety and reduced cravings for alcohol
- Disulfiram (Antabuse). This deters alcohol use by blocking aldehyde dehydrogenase, resulting in an accumulation of acetaldehyde (**Figure 8.6**). This causes unpleasant effects including facial flushing, nausea, vomiting, headache and palpitations when alcohol is ingested
- Naltrexone. This blocks opioid receptors, resulting in reduced cravings and a reduction in the pleasant effects of ingesting alcohol

Patients with alcohol dependence who also have symptoms of depression or anxiety should first be given treatment for their alcohol dependence as this sometimes reduces the symptoms of depression or anxiety. Antidepressants or anxiolytics are used to treat symptoms of depression or anxiety that persist after detoxification.

> Patients prescribed disulfiram must be warned that it also interacts with the alcohol in products such as perfume and aerosol sprays, which contain enough to cause its unpleasant effects.

Psychosocial interventions

Psychosocial interventions used to manage excess alcohol consumption and dependence include:

- **Motivational interviewing**, which is a style of patient-centred counselling informed

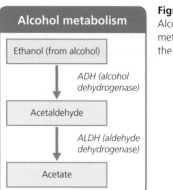

Figure 8.6 Alcohol metabolism by the liver.

by Prochaska and DiClemente's model of behavioural change (**Figure 8.6**). It helps patients to explore their ambivalence about changing their health-related behaviours
- **Cognitive behavioural therapy**, which focuses on behavioural responses to cues associated with alcohol ingestion, with the aim of preventing a relapse
- **Couples therapy**, which focuses on the impact of alcohol on relationships
- **Family therapy**, which may be offered to children or young people with alcohol dependence
- **Alcoholics Anonymous** which is a group-based, 12-step programme of spiritual and emotional support aimed at encouraging and maintaining abstinence from alcohol
- **Social support**, which helps with problems such as housing and manage debt, often required for patients with alcohol dependence

Prognosis

Patients often experience a number of relapses before achieving a sustained period of abstinence. Those with stable housing, relationships and employment, and patients who are motivated to change, have a better prognosis.

Drugs and psychoactive substances

In the UK, the Misuse of Drugs Act 1971 classifies which psychoactive substances are illegal – these are also known as illicit drugs. Penalties for possessing or dealing such substances include fines and imprisonment. As with alcohol misuse, the frequent use of illicit drugs can lead to dependence (**Figure 8.7**) and adverse consequences for patients and their family or carers.

Types of drug

The most commonly consumed illicit drug in England and Wales is cannabis. The most commonly encountered illicit drug in drug dependence is heroin.

Illicit drugs are available in different forms, including:

- Oral drugs such as 3,4-methylenedioxy-methamphetamine (MDMA) tablets
- Inhaled drugs such as cannabis or 'free-base' crack cocaine
- 'Sniffed' drugs such as glue and powdered forms of cocaine
- Liquids that are swallowed or mixed into drinks, such as liquid forms of amphetamine
- Intravenous drugs such as heroin

Epidemiology

Over a third of the adults in England and Wales have used illicit drugs at least once in their life. The highest prevalence rates of illicit drug dependence occur in those aged 16–24 years. Rates of illicit drug use and dependence are highest in the poorer areas of large cities, in men and among prisoners.

Aetiology

Multiple biopsychosocial factors contribute to illicit drug use. Certain personality traits, including impulsivity and sensation seeking are thought to be associated with an increased risk of illicit drug use. These may be evident from a personal history of a childhood conduct disorder. A history of mental illness or personality disorder in the patient or their family also increases

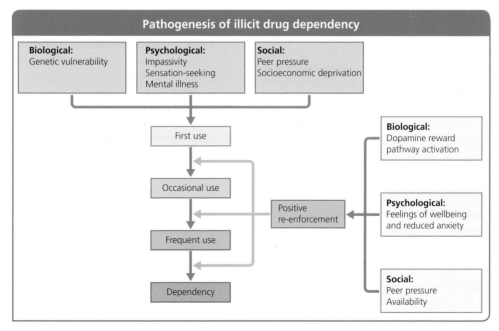

Figure 8.7 Pathogenesis of illicit drug dependency.

the risk. Predisposing social factors include social deprivation.

Prevention

Strategies to prevent illicit drug use include the provision of school-based education on the effects of drugs and legislation to discourage the supply and use of illicit drugs. Education on the risks of needle sharing and the provision of needle exchange programmes aim to reduce the physical health complications among intravenous users.

> Any patient can become dependent on medications prescribed by doctors, including opioids and benzodiazepines. These must be prescribed with caution.

Pathogenesis

The pleasant effects of illicit drugs, including reduced levels of anxiety and increased feelings of well-being, increase the frequency of their use – an example of positive reinforcement.

Illicit drug use activates mesolimbic dopamine pathways that connect the ventral tegmental area to the nucleus accumbens and pre-frontal cortex. This is known as the 'reward pathway' and results in pleasurable feelings when illicit drugs are used. With repeated use, the affected person is only able to feel pleasure from use of the illicit drug, and experiences withdrawal symptoms when the drug is no longer present in their body.

Over time, increasing amounts of the illicit drug are required to produce the original effect; this is known as tolerance and is a key feature of dependency.

Clinical features

The clinical features of different illicit drugs vary (**Table 8.5**).

Diagnostic approach

Illicit drug use is underdetected. Patients give misleading answers: some report using less than they actually do, while others overstate the amount used so that they can obtain extra supplies of prescribed medications such as methadone. They sometimes then sell these on. A collateral history from someone who knows the patient well is vital.

In the history, always ask about:

- Other substance misuse, e.g. excess alcohol consumption
- Whether the patient has ever injected substances. Also ask about the associated risk factors, e.g. needle sharing, which increases the risk of blood-borne diseases such as HIV and hepatitis B and C
- Psychosocial circumstances that help to inform treatment choices, e.g. whether or not community-based treatment would be appropriate
- Previous periods of abstinence and factors leading to previous relapse(s)
- Thoughts of suicide, harm to themselves or others, and whether any children or dependents are at risk

> As with excess alcohol use, ask whether the patient is a driver: illicit drugs impair driving abilities. In some countries, including England and Wales, driving under the influence of illicit drugs is illegal.

In the mental state examination, explore the patient's insight into their difficulties and feelings related to trying to achieve abstinence.

On physical examination, needle marks may be observed on the upper limbs, neck, groins or lower limbs of patients who use drugs intravenously. Look for signs related to the physical complications of injecting, including hot reddened areas of skin around injection sites, suggesting infection, or pitting oedema suggestive of venous thrombosis.

Investigations

Urine drug tests use immunoassays to detect the presence of illicit drugs or their metabolites in the patient's urine (**Figure 8.8**). Further investigations include testing for HIV and hepatitis B and C in patients who use intravenous drugs.

Clinical features of common illicit drugs			
Drug group	Examples (street name)	Psychiatric effects	Physical effects
Opiates	Codeine Dihydrocodeine Buphrenorphine (subutex) Morphine Diamorphine (heroin, smack, gear, brown) Methadone	Analgesia Euphoria Apathy Drowsiness Personality change	Miosis Conjunctival injection Pruritus Constipation Nausea and vomiting Bradycardia Respiratory depression Coma
Anxiolytics	Temazepam (downers, eggs) Diazepam (valium, vallies) Flunitrazepam (rohypnol, roofies) Gamma-hydroxybutyrate (GHB, geebs)	Reduced anxiety Euphoria Poor concentration Slowness of thoughts Confusion Drowsiness	Miosis Hypotension Respiratory depression
Anaesthetics	Ketamine (special K, vitamin K) Phencyclidine (PCP, angel dust)	Analgesia Feeling of detachment Hallucinations Paranoid ideas Confusion Aggression	Bladder dysfunction Abdominal pain Respiratory depression
Stimulants	Amphetamine (speed, whizz) Methamphetamine (crystal meth) Cocaine (coke, charlie, white) Crack cocaine, rock-like form of cocaine MDMA (ecstasy, e) Mephedrone (M-CAT, meow meow)	Euphoria Alertness Increased energy levels Hyperactivity Irritability Aggression Paranoid ideas Hallucinations Low mood	Sweating Tremor Mydriasis Hypertension Tachycardia Seizures Perforated nasal septum
Cannabinoids (from the cannabis plant)	Hash oil (hash) Cannabis (marijuana, pot, hash, weed, grass, skunk, dope)	Euphoria Altered time perception Paranoid ideas Hallucinations	Conjunctival injection Nystagmus Dry mouth
Hallucinogens	Lysergic acid diethylamine (LSD, acid, tabs, microdots, blotters) Psilocybe semilanceata/Liberty cap mushrooms (magic mushrooms, shrooms) Dimethyltryptamine (DMT, ayahuasca)	Hallucinations Flashbacks Paranoid ideas	Conjunctival injection Mydriasis Tachycardia Hypertension Fever Tremors
Inhalants	Glues (glue sniffing) Lighter fluids Petrol Aerosols Nitrous oxide (laughing gas)	Euphoria Disinhibition Hallucinations Delusions	Headache Slurred speech Muscle weakness Sudden death
Anabolic steroids	Anabolic steroids (roids)	Irritability Aggression Paranoid ideas Mood swings	Increased muscle mass Improved physical endurance Improved sports performance Hypertension Insomnia Acne Hair loss In men: gynaecomastia, erectile dysfunction In women: excess facial hair, menstrual abnormalities

Table 8.5 Clinical features of use of common illicit drugs

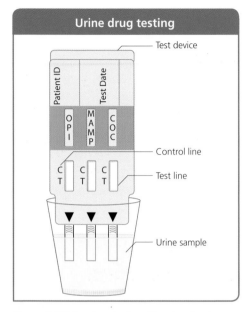

Figure 8.8 Urine drug testing. The absorbent strips of the urine drug test card are dipped into the urine sample for 10–15 seconds. The test is an immunoassay that uses antibodies against common illicit drugs or their metabolites including opiates (OPI), methamphetamine (MAMP) and cocaine (COC) to detect their presence. Within 5 minutes, test results are displayed as lines in the C (control) and T (test) results windows of the test card.

Management

Specialist community drug teams provide support to patients who use illicit drugs (see page 299). Prochaska and DiClemente's stages of change model (**Figure 8.5**) is used to inform the management of those using illicit drugs. Patients are offered treatment to encourage them to withdraw safely from the drug and maintain their abstinence.

Treatment may be offered in the community or in inpatient settings including general psychiatric hospitals or specialist 'detox' units. Patients treated in an outpatient setting should receive close supervision as there is a risk of depression and self-harm during withdrawal.

Intravenous illicit drug users are provided with education on minimising harm, including using clean injecting equipment, and on using condoms to reduce the transmission of infections such as HIV and hepatitis C.

Intravenous illicit drug users are at increased risk of hepatitis B, and should be offered hepatitis B vaccination.

Multidisciplinary management also addresses biopsychosocial factors perpetuating the patient's illicit drug use.

Medication

Some patients are not ready to stop using opioids such as heroin. Substitution therapy involves the prescription of methadone (a synthetic opioid receptor agonist) or buprenorphine (both a partial opioid agonist and an opioid antagonist) as an alternative to illicit heroin. Doses are tapered over time to gradually reduce illicit drug consumption.

This approach also aims to reduce the complications of heroin use and provide stability to the patient's life. However, some patients sell these medications to raise money for other illicit drugs, and others convert them into injectable forms. To reduce these risks, medications such as methadone are given under close supervision.

In those who are ready to withdraw from opioids, lofexidine (an α-adrenoreceptor agonist) is used to reduce the unpleasant effects of withdrawing from opioids, including sweating, chills and runny nose. Antiemetics, simple analgesia and antidiarrhoea medications are also given to treat withdrawal symptoms of nausea, vomiting, muscular and bone pain, and diarrhoea. In those with a higher use of heroin, methadone or buprenorphine is prescribed to reduce withdrawal symptoms of restlessness and poor sleep, and to help reduce cravings for heroin. Patients usually continue treatment with methadone or buprenorphine for several months and often years to help maintain their abstinence from heroin. Eventually, some patients are able to gradually reduce and discontinue methadone or buprenorphine, although many continue these medications to prevent a relapse of their heroin use.

In those withdrawing from anxiolytics such as benzodiazepines, gradual supported withdrawal is offered. Typically, doses are reduced over a period of 8 weeks to minimise the unpleasant effects of withdrawal, such as increased anxiety, low mood, poor sleep, headache, tremor and nausea.

Psychosocial interventions

Psychosocial interventions include group psychotherapy, which helps patients to gain insight into the effects of drug taking on their relationships. As with alcohol dependence, cognitive behavioural therapy is offered. This aims to alter the patient's response to triggers that would normally lead them to use illicit drugs.

Social care support is particularly important for helping those recovering from drug dependency to reintegrate into society away from their drug-taking social network.

Prognosis

Overall, between a quarter and a third of those who receive medication for illicit drug use or dependency achieve long-term abstinence. However, many patients relapse over time and some die from unintentional overdoses of illicit drugs. Others die from complications of drug misuse, including HIV and hepatitis B or C infection.

Drug-induced psychiatric disorders

Some people with pre-existing psychiatric disorders, such as depression, anxiety or schizophrenia, use illicit drugs to alleviate their symptoms. However, there are people with no pre-existing psychiatric diagnosis in whom psychiatric symptoms first occur after certain illicit drugs have been consumed. Culprits include amphetamines, cannabis, cocaine, ketamine, LSD, MDMA and mephedrone. These drug-induced psychiatric disorders have characteristic key features:

■ A temporal relationship in which illicit drug use precedes the onset of the psychiatric illness
■ Symptoms consistent with the type of illicit drug used
■ A remittance of symptoms after use of the illicit drug has ended

> **Symptoms of psychosis, including hallucinations and delusions, are a side effect of some prescribed medications.** These include levodopa, which is used in older adults to treat Parkinson's disease.

Clinical effects

Intoxication with alcohol or illicit drugs frequently results in psychiatric symptoms, such as hallucinations, delusions and mood changes (**Table 8.5**). Symptoms of psychosis, anxiety or mood disorder can occur during illicit drug or alcohol withdrawal.

Alcohol-related psychiatric disorders

Alcohol-related psychiatric disorders include alcohol-related psychotic disorder, alcohol-related mood disorder, and alcohol-related anxiety disorder. Excess alcohol use sometimes produces symptoms of psychosis, commonly:

■ Delusions – grandiose, persecutory or pathological jealousy (see Table 2.10)
■ Hallucinations – fleeting auditory or visual hallucinations during which insight is retained

These symptoms resolve with abstinence from alcohol. However, similar symptoms of psychosis can be seen as part of delirium tremens, where they are associated with cognitive impairment.

People using excess alcohol often experience low mood, which can be difficult to differentiate from depression.

Some people with pre-existing anxiety disorders drink alcohol to cope with their symptoms and to feel less anxious. However, withdrawal from alcohol can also produce symptoms of anxiety; a period of abstinence followed by reassessment of anxiety symptoms helps to assess whether an anxiety disorder is present.

Amphetamine-related psychiatric disorders

Amphetamine intoxication results in hyperactivity, characterised by repetitive behaviours such as cleaning or tidying. Amphetamine use, particularly when prolonged, sometimes results in symptoms of psychosis, including:

- Delusions – often persecutory, which can result in patients becoming hostile or aggressive towards those they believe are persecuting them
- Hallucinations – usually auditory or visual

These symptoms usually resolve upon abstinence. In some cases, however, they persist. It is not clear whether persistent symptoms of psychosis are drug-induced or whether amphetamine use has precipitated the onset of schizophrenia in these patients.

Individuals withdrawing from amphetamines often experience low mood, fatigue, anxiety and suicidal ideation. Again, it is difficult to distinguish a true depressive or anxiety disorder, and a re-evaluation should be undertaken once the patient is abstinent.

Cannabis-related psychiatric disorders

Cannabis intoxication results in short-term symptoms similar to those of psychosis, including hallucinations and delusions. These usually resolve upon abstinence. However, there is ongoing debate over whether such symptoms are the initial signs of schizophrenia in some people.

Cannabis use in adolescence leads to a twofold increase in the risk of developing schizophrenia. The risk is highest in those who used cannabis when they were younger than 15 years. In those who already have an established diagnosis of schizophrenia, cannabis use increases the risk of relapse.

Long-term cannabis use also results in symptoms of low mood, fatigue, decreased motivation and anhedonia. Differentiating these symptoms from depressive disorder requires assessment during abstinence.

Finally, there is evidence that cannabis can affect both short-term and long-term memory, although this is the subject of ongoing debate.

Answers to starter questions

1. People with alcohol dependence syndrome should not suddenly stop drinking alcohol without support due to the risk of acute alcohol withdrawal (delirium tremens) 24–72 hours after stopping use. This is a medical emergency with a high risk of mortality (20% of cases).

2. Management of patients who do not want to stop drinking alcohol focuses on minimising harm and on motivating the patient to consider addressing their excess alcohol intake. Those who do not want to stop using illicit drugs are offered substitution therapy, with medications being prescribed as an alternative to the use of illicit drugs to encourage gradual reduction and long-term abstinence once they are ready to change.

Chapter 9
Eating disorders

Introduction 203
Case 11 Rapid weight loss 204
Anorexia nervosa. 206
Bulimia nervosa 210

Starter questions

Answers to the following questions are on page 212.

1. Why are many patients with anorexia nervosa particularly difficult to treat?
2. Why should severely underweight patients only increase their weight very slowly?
3. Why are many patients with bulimia nervosa not diagnosed?
4. When is bulimia nervosa acutely dangerous?

Introduction

Eating disorders have become increasingly common in societies where food is readily available. They are not the same as ordinary concerns about weight and size. Anorexia nervosa and bulimia nervosa are psychiatric disorders characterised by deliberate, conscious and excessive efforts to reduce body weight. Patients go to extreme lengths to control their weight, including:

■ Severe food intake restriction

■ Extreme exercising
■ Abuse of purgatives
■ Self-induced vomiting

These behaviours are driven by overvalued ideas based on an excessive fear of fatness and an imposition of unfeasibly low target weights. There is also a disturbed body image in which patients continue to believe they are obese despite their very low body mass index (BMI).

Case 11 Rapid weight loss

Presentation

Kate Parker is a 15-year-old girl who reluctantly attends with her mother to see her general practitioner, Dr Brown. Kate insists that she is perfectly well but her mother is concerned that she has lost 12 kg, dropping from 54 to 42 kg in 4 months. Kate avoids eating with the family in the evening, saying that she has already eaten. Kate's best friend has said that Kate has been skipping meals at school. Despite the baggy clothes Kate is wearing, Dr Brown can see that Kate is indeed very thin.

Initial interpretation

Rapid weight loss as a consequence of a reduction in food intake in an adolescent suggests the possibility of an eating disorder. Physical disorders causing anorexia and/or loss of weight, including thyroid disturbances, inflammatory bowel disease, coeliac disease and diabetes mellitus, must also be considered. Other psychiatric disorders causing loss of appetite such as depression are also possible. However, the association of weight loss with a deliberate avoidance of meals in an otherwise healthy girl places eating disorders at the top of the differential diagnosis.

> Direct questions about weight and eating behaviours must be asked without alienating the patient, who may be quite resistant to treatment. Although the patient should be aware of the dangers of extreme weight loss, the initial assessment is not the place for lengthy lectures on these risks.

Rapid weight loss: taking a history

Dr Brown meets with Kate to discuss her recent weight loss

I'm only here because my mum wanted to me to come. She said I was losing too much weight

Have you been trying to lose weight?

Yeah, since the end of last term

Would you tell me a bit about it?

Some of the boys at school were laughing at the way I looked...

...and so I decided to do something about it...

...I started being healthy...

...you know, looking after myself

Look – I'm fine. I don't throw up or anything. I'm not ill

Apart from exercise, have you done anything else to lose weight?

Okay, but I understand mum's quite worried about you. Would it be okay for her to join us?

I suppose so...

In order to ascertain more information, Dr Brown decides to speak with Kate's mother

History

Dr Brown asks to speak to Kate on her own first. Kate reluctantly admits she has deliberately lost weight in the last 4 months after being teased by some of the boys at school during games lessons. She says she needed to lose weight as she was self-conscious about her thighs. She feels she would still like to lose another 5 kg.

Kate says she feels perfectly well. She admits that she has missed meals at school but denies feeling hungry, saying she is focusing on eating a healthy diet. She denies bingeing, making herself sick or using laxatives but admits to spending 40 minutes every night doing exercises before bed. She has joined a number of sports activities at school to get fit and now goes on a 3-mile run every evening when she gets in from school.

Kate denies having any other problems. In particular, she says she has no nausea or vomiting, and no excessive thirst or tiredness, making gastrointestinal disorders or diabetes unlikely. She says she is sleeping well, keeping up with her school work and enjoying life. She has not noticed any change in bowel habits. Her last period was 6 weeks ago, but her periods have always been erratic since her menarche aged 12 years. She denies any change in mood, although admits she can be 'moody', especially with her mother, who is always trying to persuade her to eat more. Kate is angry that her mother has made her come to the doctors and does not believe there should be any concern as she needed to lose weight.

Interpretation of history

Kate has no symptoms suggestive of any physical disorder to explain her significant weight loss. Her deliberate reduction in food intake in conjunction with a marked increase in her exercise level and her desire to lose more weight make anorexia nervosa the most likely diagnosis.

Examination

Kate is 160 cm tall and weighs 42 kg. Her ideal weight range is 51–64 kg. Her BMI is 16.4 kg/m^2.

Apart from the fact that Kate looks underweight, there are no abnormal physical findings. There are no abnormal findings on the mental state examination other than Kate's insistence that she is still overweight. She is resistant to any suggestion that she should eat more.

> **Body image may be extremely distorted in patients with anorexia nervosa.** A patient with an extremely low BMI may still indicate a specific part of their body that they consider to be disgustingly fat despite their extreme thinness.

Investigations

Dr Brown orders blood tests to exclude physical disorders and to assess Kate's current physical health. These include an erythrocyte sedimentation rate, a full blood count, urea and electrolytes, thyroid function tests and a pregnancy test (as Kate's period is overdue). The blood results are all normal and the pregnancy test is negative.

Interpretation of findings

Kate's test results make an underlying physical disorder unlikely. The fact that she still feels she has weight to lose despite her low BMI also makes a physical cause for her weight loss highly unlikely.

Kate fulfils the following criteria for an eating disorder:

- Her BMI is less than 17.5 kg/m^2

Case 11 *continued*

- Her weight loss is deliberate
- She expresses a desire to continue to lose weight and still feels fat
- She may be amenorrhoeic; her last menstrual period was 6 weeks ago

Diagnosis

On the basis of Kate's presentation with no physical signs or symptoms and a normal blood screen, Dr Brown diagnoses anorexia nervosa. Although it is of very recent onset, Kate has established a significant weight loss in a relatively short time through food restriction and excessive exercising. Kate started dieting because she felt fat, but her weight was still within the healthy range at that point.

Although Kate is otherwise functioning well, she remains convinced that she needs to lose more weight. As Dr Brown knows that the prognosis for patients with anorexia nervosa is better when they are treated early in the course of the disorder, she recommends a referral to the eating disorder service at the local hospital. Kate is distraught and resistant to the suggestion, saying she is perfectly healthy. Dr Brown spends considerable time persuading Kate, who eventually agrees to the referral.

Anorexia nervosa

Anorexia nervosa is an eating disorder characterised by abnormally low body weight associated with an intense fear of gaining weight and a distorted perception of body image. People with anorexia nervosa go to extreme lengths to control their weight.

Anorexia nervosa is often referred to as a culture-bound syndrome because it is much more common in developed societies, with a prevalence rate of around 1%. It is predominantly a disorder of young women, although the prevalence in young men appears to be rising and may account for up to 10% of cases (**Table 9.1**).

Aetiology

This is commonly attributed to the obsession with thinness that is particularly seen in developed countries, although other factors are also involved (**Table 9.2**). Although this is supported by the higher incidence of the disorder in individuals for whom appearance is a particular focus (e.g. models and dancers), many young women diet and control their weight without developing eating disorders.

Aetiological factors are very difficult to identify in any one patient. Anorexia nervosa has a powerful effect on the family and disrupts relationships to the extent that it is often impossible to assess how the family functioned before the disorder arose.

Clinical features

All four of the following clinical features must be present to establish a diagnosis of anorexia nervosa:

- Body weight maintained at least 15% below expected, or <BMI 17.5 kg/m^2
- Weight loss self-induced by food restriction and avoidance of fattening food. This may be augmented by self-induced purging or vomiting, excessive exercise and use of appetite suppressants or diuretics
- Distorted body image with an intense fear of fatness
- Endocrine disturbance with amenorrhoea or delayed puberty in premenstrual girls

In many patients, the most striking feature is excessive concern with body weight and

Epidemiology of anorexia nervosa and bulimia nervosa				
Condition	Gender	Age of onset	Groups affected	Prevalence
Anorexia nervosa	Women:Men >10:1	Peak age 15–16 years, uncommon after 30 years of age	Lower in Afro-Caribbean and other ethnic minority groups More common in dancers/models etc.	1% of school age/ young women
Bulimia nervosa	Women:Men 10:1	Teenage/early twenties	More common in models, ballet dancers, gymnasts, performers	3% in young women

Table 9.1 Epidemiology of anorexia nervosa and bulimia nervosa

Anorexia nervosa (AN): aetiological factors	
Factors	Effect
Genetic	Higher concordance for monozygotic twins, 60% than dizygotic twins, 25% Higher incidence of eating disorders in first degree relatives, 5% more than the general population
Biological	Raised comorbidity with depression and abnormalities of serotonin metabolites have implicated serotonin metabolism
Personality/psychological	Higher rates of AN in women with 'perfectionistic' traits and low self-esteem Raised prevalence in high-achieving girls More common in cluster C personality disorder
Sociocultural	Raised prevalence in western societies which promote thinness as desirable
Family	Theories have suggested AN arises more often in families where over-protection, over-involvement, rigidity and conflict avoidance are evident
Stressful life events	AN triggered by an acute event such as family separation, exam failure or a loss

Table 9.2 Anorexia nervosa (AN): aetiological factors

shape. This leads to an overwhelming fixation on all aspects of diet, activity and behaviour. Patients go to extreme lengths to lose weight, including avoiding all social activity at which food is consumed, and specifically avoiding high-calorie foods. They may hide food, lie about having eaten and refuse to eat with family members.

> **Constant hunger makes patients with anorexia nervosa entirely preoccupied with food.** They may spend many hours preparing food for others while avoiding eating themselves.

Establishing a good picture of the eating disorder is often difficult because patients avoid revealing the full extent of their behaviours. For example, for many patients, food restriction is inadequate to achieve their weight loss

goals so they exercise excessively, exhibiting distress if they are prevented from doing so.

Anorexia nervosa commonly co-occurs with other psychiatric conditions, particularly depression. In addition, a range of physical symptoms may develop in established anorexia nervosa (**Table 9.3** and **Figure 9.1**).

Diagnostic approach

All four key features must be present to make a diagnosis of anorexia nervosa. A thorough assessment of any patient with a suspected eating disorder must include:

- Exclusion of an underlying, causative physical disorder. This involves a full medical history (including the use of drugs, alcohol and medication), a physical examination and the investigations listed in **Table 9.4**. Any abnormal results must be investigated further

Physical symptoms and signs of anorexia nervosa

System	Symptom/sign
Skin	Dry skin
	Lanugo hair (fine, downy hair particularly on the face and upper body)
Musculoskeletal	Osteoporosis, muscle wasting, proximal myopathy
Cardiovascular	Bradycardia, hypotension and arrhythmias
	Peripheral oedema, congestive cardiac failure
	Mitral valve prolapse/dysfunction
Gastrointestinal	Constipation, abdominal pain and bloating from delayed gastric emptying
	Peptic ulceration
Endocrine	Amenorrhoea in women, and infertility due to ovarian atrophy, decreased libido and impotence in males and testicular atrophy
	Decreased free T3
Neurological	Seizures, peripheral neuropathies, autonomic dysfunction
Haematological	Iron deficiency anaemia, leucopaenia, thrombocytopaenia
Metabolic	Dehydration
	Hypoglycaemia/impaired glucose tolerance
	Hypokalaemia/hyponatraemia
	Hypercholesterolaemia
General	Intolerance to cold, lethargy

Table 9.3 Physical symptoms and signs of anorexia nervosa

Physical features and complications of anorexia nervosa

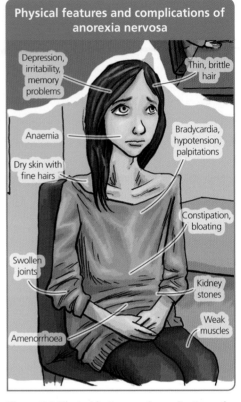

Figure 9.1 Physical features and complications of anorexia nervosa.

- A full psychiatric history, including a social and personal history and childhood development, to identify predisposing, precipitating and perpetuating factors

Assessment must include questions about:

- Strategies taken by the patient to lose weight, including food restriction, purging and vomiting, and excessive exercising
- Whether the patient ever loses control of the dieting with resultant binges and/or vomiting
- The patient's current body image
- Whether the patient wants to lose more weight and/or has a specific lower weight they are aiming for
- How the patient has changed their eating behaviour, such as avoiding eating socially or with the family
- Whether the changes in eating have caused any problems with family or partners
- Whether the patient has noticed any physical changes while losing weight

During your psychiatric assessment, consider other psychiatric disorders that are sometimes co-morbid with an eating disorder, including personality disorders, depressive disorders and substance misuse (including appetite suppressants).

Information from a close relative is valuable in clarifying the extent of abnormal eating

Investigations for eating disorder symptoms	
Investigation	Looking for
Full blood count	Anaemia in protracted starvation, leucopaenia and thrombocytopaenia
ESR	Screening test to exclude organic causes of weight loss. Should be low/normal in anorexia nervosa
Urea and electrolytes	Raised urea in patients with dehydration
	Potassium depletion occurs as a consequence of repeated vomiting or laxative abuse
	Hyponatraemia may also occur
Liver function tests	Hypoproteinaemia in protracted starvation
Thyroid function tests	Hypo or hyperthyroidism can cause significant weight changes
	Low T3 in established anorexia nervosa
Calcium and phosphate profile	Hypocalcaemia and hypophosphataemia in established AN/BN
Cholesterol levels	Hypercholesterolaemia in established AN/BN
DEXA bone density scan	Only indicated in patients with >2 years history of anorexia
ECG	Bradycardia may be present in protracted starvation plus arrhythmias as a consequence of electrolyte imbalances

Table 9.4 Investigations for patients presenting with symptoms of an eating disorder. AN, anorexia nervosa; BN, bulimia nervosa; ESR, erythrocyte sedimentation rate

behaviours, especially if the patient is particularly reticent or evasive.

> **Always start your assessment with the patient.** Many patients are resistant to seeking medical help and parents or partners are naturally very concerned. Avoid being drawn into conversation about the patient with relatives until you have established a rapport with the patient.

Management

Treatment should adopt a biopsychosocial approach. However, for any patient presenting with extreme life-threatening weight loss, physical needs must be dealt with as a matter of urgency.

Indications for urgent medical treatment include:

- BMI less than 13 kg/m^2
- Very rapid weight loss
- Significant cardiovascular symptoms – severe bradycardia and/or arrhythmias, cardiac failure or hypotension with a blood pressure less than 80/50 mmHg
- Electrolyte imbalances – low K$^+$, N$^+$ and PO$_4^{3-}$

- Severe depressive symptoms that are presenting a risk of suicide

> **Rapid refeeding can increase the risk of serious electrolyte imbalances.** This is a recognised cause of sudden death so patients must be treated under close medical supervision to avoid further decreases in K$^+$, N$^+$ and PO$_4^{3-}$.

The first major challenge with patients who are not acutely medically compromised is establishing a good therapeutic relationship despite their reluctance to cooperate. Conveying the serious risks of continued starvation must be balanced against a non-critical, non-judgemental, empathic approach that allows patients to feel understood and accepted.

Most patients can be effectively supervised as outpatients. For those who fail to respond to outpatient treatment or have severe, life-threatening weight loss or physical consequences of anorexia nervosa, treatment in a specialist inpatient unit is indicated. This often requires a protracted stay of several months before the patient is able to maintain a stable weight. Early relapses are common (**Table 9.5**).

Management for anorexia nervosa

Type	Management
Biological	Medication/treatment for any comorbid psychiatric disorders
	No psychotropic medication indicated for AN
	Gradual weight restoration of around 0.5–1.0 kg per week to an acceptable target weight using dietary planning with input from dietician
Psychological	Psycho-education covers consequences and risks of eating disorder and need for nutritional correction
	Supportive counselling for patient and family
	Psychotherapeutic treatments, e.g. interpersonal therapy, family therapy, CBT, psychodynamic psychotherapy
Social	Addressing consequences of abnormal eating behaviours on school, personal and family life During inpatient treatment academic education must continue.
	Attention to occupational, social and financial aspects of chronic illness

Table 9.5 Management options for anorexia nervosa (AN). CBT, cognitive behavioural therapy

Compulsory treatment under mental health legislation may be indicated for patients who are unable or unwilling to consent to informal treatment.

Prognosis

The prognosis of anorexia nervosa is extremely variable. Patients with the following have poor prognosis:

- A very low weight at diagnosis
- Additional bulimic symptoms
- Co-morbid mental disorders, e.g. depression or a personality disorder
- Poor interpersonal or family relationships

In general, one-fifth of patients make a good recovery, especially if they have a short history of symptoms. One-fifth develop chronic, severe illness. The remainder regain a normal weight but continue to exhibit abnormal eating behaviours for much of their life. Of note is the high mortality rate of 10–15%. The majority of deaths result from starvation but one-third occur as a result of suicide.

Bulimia nervosa

Bulimia nervosa is an eating disorder characterised by episodes in which huge volumes of food are consumed rapidly (binges). This is usually followed by behaviours which compensate for this, such as self-induced vomiting or purging with laxatives. It is more common than anorexia nervosa (**Table 9.4**) and the marked rise in incidence in recent years probably reflects a true rise in incidence rather than simply being due to increased reporting.

Aetiology

The aetiology of bulimia nervosa is unclear, and unlike anorexia nervosa genetic factors do not appear to contribute. General risk factors for psychiatric disorder are, however, implicated in the aetiology. These include stressful life events, a family history of substance misuse and depression and a history of physical or sexual abuse as a child. Bulimia nervosa is often co-morbid with alcohol and substance misuse, personality disorder and depression.

Perfectionist personality traits and low self-esteem appear to contribute to bulimia nervosa. Most patients have a past history of unsuccessful dieting and/or obesity, and 50% have a history of anorexia nervosa.

Clinical features

The following features must all be present to establish a diagnosis of bulimia nervosa:

- A persistent preoccupation with eating and irresistible craving for food with periods of overeating (binges) during which excessive amounts of food are quickly consumed

- Attempts to counteract the effects of bingeing by one or more of the following: self-induced vomiting, purgative or laxative abuse, periods of starvation or the use of appetite suppressants, thyroxine (taken to increase metabolism) or diuretics
- A morbid fear of fatness and a set threshold for desired weight that is below a healthy weight for the patient

The symptoms of bulimia (bingeing with or without vomiting) also occur in anorexia nervosa. In bulimia nervosa, there may never have been a specific weight restriction and many patients are within the normal weight range or slightly overweight. Some patients demonstrate dramatic fluctuations in their body weight. They are not usually amenorrhoeic but patients share the anorexic patient's abnormal concern with weight and shape.

Many patients go undiagnosed as they carry out their binge-eating rituals and vomiting secretively.

> **Patients with bulimia nervosa are generally more willing to seek help than patients with anorexia.** However, they are often embarrassed, ashamed and secretive about their abnormal eating behaviours so a non-judgemental and empathic approach is very important.

Patients' binge eating behaviours vary from planned, ritualistic behaviours to episodes of loss of control over eating restrictions precipitated by stress or life events. Patients usually binge in secret, consuming huge volumes of high-calorie foods followed by self-induced vomiting to relieve the guilt and fear of fatness as the binge comes to an end. Some patients do this several times in a day.

As most patients with bulimia nervosa are of normal weight, the physical consequences are mainly a result of repeated vomiting. These include:

- Severe dental erosion and cavities
- Dehydration
- Enlargement of the parotid salivary glands
- Calluses on the back of the knuckles from repeated trauma while inducing vomiting (Russell's sign)
- Muscle weakness due to electrolyte imbalances
- Oesophageal tears, gastric rupture and stomach ulcers
- Bloating and abdominal pain
- Arrhythmias due to hypokalaemia

In extreme cases repeated, frequent vomiting causes acute dehydration, electrolyte disturbances and cardiac complications.

Diagnostic approach

All three key clinical features must be present for a diagnosis of bulimia nervosa. As with anorexia nervosa, physical disorders must be excluded before making the diagnosis. In particular, physical causes of vomiting such as upper gastrointestinal disorders, intestinal obstruction and pregnancy must be excluded.

Other psychiatric disorders must also be considered, including personality disorders and depressive disorders, as these may be contributing to the clinical picture. They are more common than in patients with anorexia nervosa.

As for patients with suspected anorexia nervosa, the assessment must include a full physical and psychiatric examination. This must include careful questioning regarding eating behaviours and habits and a careful examination for the specific physical consequences of repeated vomiting. Investigations are ordered in line with the clinical picture (**Table 9.4**). Abnormal results should be investigated further. A pregnancy test may be indicated depending upon the history.

> **Ask specific detailed questions about the patient's daily eating behaviours.** Identifying the triggers for binges is crucial in helping patients to begin to take control of their disordered eating behaviours.

Management

The majority of patients with bulimia nervosa are managed as outpatient in a primary care setting using a range of treatment approaches (**Table 9.6**). Hospital treatment is occasionally indicated for acute physiological disturbances as a consequence of extreme repeated vomiting and purging.

Prognosis

Bulimia nervosa has a better prognosis than anorexia nervosa. Around 70% of patients make a reasonable recovery and no longer binge or vomit by 5 years, although many retain some abnormal eating behaviours. The mortality rate is not significantly increased compared to the general population. Poor prognostic indicators include low body weight, extreme, severe and frequent bingeing and purging and co-morbid depressive disorder.

Management options for bulimia nervosa	
Type	Management
Biological	Fluoxetine is effective at higher doses (60 mg once daily)
	Assess physical condition and address medical complications
	Treatment for comorbid psychiatric disorders
	Inpatient hospital treatment if physical complications are life-threatening (e.g. cardiac/electrolyte abnormalities)
Psychological	Supportive counselling
	Cognitive behavioural therapy (CBT)
	Interpersonal therapy
	Family therapy
Social	Education, patient and family
	Attention to occupational, social and financial consequences of abnormal eating behaviours, e.g. social avoidance of eating, debt as a consequence of binge-eating behaviours

Table 9.6 Management options for bulimia nervosa

Answers to starter questions

1. Patients with anorexia nervosa are often difficult to treat because their body image is so distorted and, despite their obvious extreme thinness, they maintain that they need to lose more weight. This means that they often do not co-operate with diets and develop very secretive food-avoiding strategies such as extreme exercising, vomiting or purging.

2. Suddenly increasing food intake in patients with very low body weight causes severe electrolyte disturbances within the first few days of refeeding. This causes neurological, endocrine and cardiac complications, such as arrhythmias, which can be fatal if not recognised. Patients with anorexia should have their food intake increased gradually with regular biochemical monitoring.

3. Bulimia nervosa often goes undiagnosed because most patients are within the normal weight range and are secretive about their disordered eating. The diagnosis is sometimes missed within a more complex picture, with more evident symptoms such as addiction, personality disorder or depressive illness being present.

4. From a physiological perspective bulimia nervosa is acutely dangerous if the patient repeatedly and frequently binges and vomits. This creates electrolytic disturbances, such as severe alkalosis and fatigue that cause weakness, constipation and fatigue, and can result in arrhythmias and cardiac arrest.

Chapter 10
Perinatal psychiatry

Introduction 213
Case 12 Low mood 6 weeks
     after delivery 214
Postnatal blues. 217
Postnatal depression 218
Postnatal psychosis 220

Starter questions

Answers to the following questions are on page 221.

1. Are 'baby-blues' clinically significant?
2. Why is the diagnosis of postnatal depression often missed?
3. Why is screening for suicidal ideation particularly important in patients with a postnatal psychiatric illness?

Introduction

Most women are psychologically healthy during and after pregnancy, but the prevalence of mental health problems increases after childbirth. Three main conditions occur in the first 12 months: postnatal blues, postnatal depression and postnatal psychosis (**Table 10.1**) – and the likelihood of being referred to the psychiatric services is greatly increased. The majority of women who develop serious mental illness after childbirth have been well during pregnancy. However, women with long-standing or recurrent psychiatric conditions sometimes experience significant psychiatric symptoms during pregnancy.

Psychosis is an uncommon postnatal presentation but has a 35-fold increase in incidence in the first month after delivery, 14-fold in the first 12 months.

Postnatal psychiatric presentations			
Presentation	Point of presentation	Incidence	Treatment
Postnatal blues	Peak symptoms evident 3–4 days postnatal, rapidly resolving	50–65%	None
Postnatal depression	First 2 months postpartum	10–15%	Psychosocial support with/without medication
Postnatal psychosis	Sudden onset within first 2 weeks	0.2%	Hospitalisation, close supervision and medication

Table 10.1 Postnatal psychiatric presentations

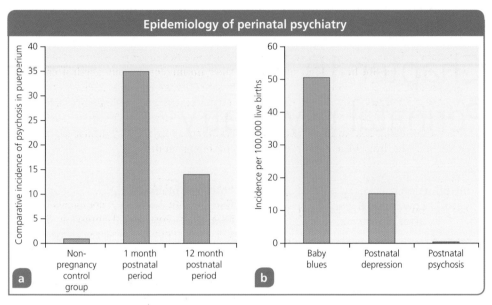

Figure 10.1 The epidemiology of perinatal psychiatry. (a) The likelihood of developing a psychotic illness during the postnatal period. (b) Comparative incidence of postnatal emotional changes.

Case 12 Low mood 6 weeks after delivery

Presentation

Natalie Billings brings Jason for his baby check with the health visitor. Natalie is 26 years old and delivered Jason 6 weeks ago after an uneventful, planned pregnancy. Natalie's labour was difficult. She was induced at 42 weeks, finally requiring an emergency caesarean section when fetal heart rate monitoring indicated that Jason was becoming distressed.

Natalie recovered well physically and she and Jason have no specific health problems. Jason is gaining weight appropriately, although Natalie says he seems unsettled and cries for hours, which she finds very distressing. She is certain something is wrong with him.

Initial interpretation

Although Natalie and Jason are both doing well physically, the difficult labour and Natalie's concerns about Jason's health should arouse concern about the possibility of postnatal depression.

History

The health visitor notices that Natalie and Jason are both well presented. However, Natalie seems flat, responding to questions with little enthusiasm. When the health visitor asks her how she is feeling, Natalie immediately bursts into tears. She feels she is a terrible mother and is finding everything a struggle. She feels tense, rarely enjoys anything and has been snappy with her husband.

Although Jason only wakes once in the night to feed, Natalie is unable to sleep, lying awake, feeling anxious and worrying about coping. She cannot relax when Jason is asleep, dreading the next time he will wake and need attention. She is finding it increasingly difficult to care for him.

Case 12 *continued*

Natalie's husband is supportive but works long hours. She has hidden her feelings from him as she knows he would be very disappointed as she had been so keen to start a family. Natalie has also found it difficult not being able to drive since the caesarean. She lives in a remote village with few facilities and is missing her work colleagues and friends.

Natalie feels at the end of her tether but has no thoughts of harming herself or Jason. Her mother has had recurrent depressive episodes throughout her adult life and Natalie dreads being the same.

Interpretation of history

Natalie is showing many signs of postnatal depression. She had a difficult labour and has become socially isolated since Jason's birth. Both of these are risk factors for postnatal depression, as is a family history of depression.

Natalie has no physical symptoms and takes no medication but physical causes must be excluded as precipitants for her low mood. These include infection, anaemia and thyroid dysfunction (such as Hashimoto's thyroiditis), which are more common after delivery.

Examination

The health visitor completes an Edinburgh Postnatal Depression Scale form with Natalie, who scores 18 out of 30. Scores above 13 may indicate depression so Natalie is referred to Dr Davies, the general practitioner, who carries out a mental state examination (**Table 10.2**).

Physical examination

A full physical examination shows that Natalie's caesarean section wound has healed well. She has no signs of infection, anaemia or thyroid dysfunction.

Postnatal depression: taking a history

Natalie meets with Dr Davies to discuss her concerns about her son, Jason

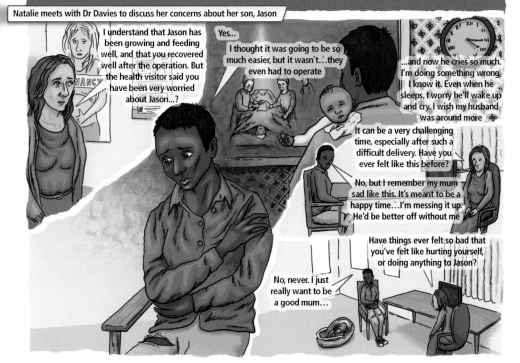

Case 12 *continued*

Natalie's mental state examination	
Category	Description
Appearance and behaviour	Well-dressed and presented, but appears rather flat in mood and becomes weepy when asked directly
Speech	Speech monotonous and diminished in quantity, but able to answer questions appropriately
Mood	Natalie feels anxious, agitated and tense. She describes feeling very guilty about being such a terrible mother and overwhelmed by the needs of her baby
	She describes irritability, loss of interest in her usual activities and difficulty motivating herself to do the things she needs to do. Objectively she appears low in mood
Perceptions	Natalie is not experiencing any abnormal perceptions.
Thoughts	Natalie's thoughts are focused on her failings as a mother and hopelessness about the future, feeling she will fail her new son and is fearful that she will feel as she does for the rest of her life
	She is also very concerned that there is something very wrong with Jason and is difficult to reassure
Cognitions	Natalie is not demonstrating any cognitive abnormalities
Insight	Premorbidly Natalie describes herself as a positive person who enjoyed her work and social life with friends and colleagues
	She cannot understand why she is feeling as she does and thinks it is just because she is no good as a mother. She feels she bonded well with Jason at first but is now struggling as she feels his demands upon her are unreasonable
Suicidal ideation	Although Natalie feels at times that her son would be better off without her, she strongly denies suicidal ideas or thoughts of harming herself or Jason

Table 10.2 Natalie's mental state examination

Investigations

Blood tests including a full blood count and thyroid function tests are all normal.

Diagnosis

Dr Davies diagnoses moderate postnatal depression (**Figure 10.2**). Natalie's symptoms have been increasing for 3 weeks and are interfering with her daily function, although she has been able to conceal this from others.

This is Natalie's first experience of mental health problems. Significant risk factors include the difficult delivery, her social isolation after the birth and her family history.

Natalie is relieved to be able to talk and to understand that this is a common,

treatable condition. She wants to avoid medication because she has been careful to avoid all drugs and alcohol while breastfeeding Jason.

Dr Davies agrees she will review Natalie in 2 weeks. During that time, Natalie and her husband will meet with the health visitor so Natalie can explain how she is feeling and begin to accept more help from her family. She can now drive again, so Dr Davies encourages her to have more contact with her friends.

As Natalie has no suicidal ideation, Dr Davies is happy to agree to conservative management. Natalie will have close contact with the health visitor and has agreed that she will contact her or the GP if things get worse.

Case 12 *continued*

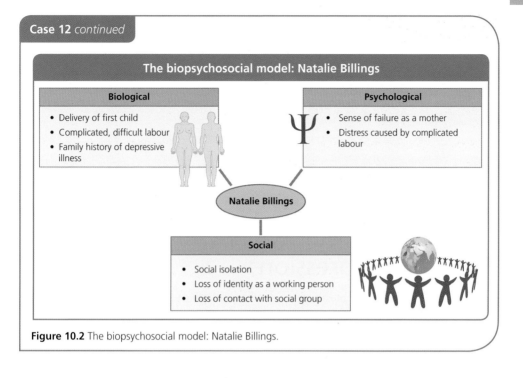

Figure 10.2 The biopsychosocial model: Natalie Billings.

Postnatal blues

Known as the 'baby blues', this is a normal experience. It occurs in at least 50% of new mothers, particularly after a first pregnancy.

The core characteristics of postpartum blues are:

- Irritability
- Tearfulness
- Lability of mood and affect
- A tendency to overreact

Management

Many women are surprised by this change in their emotional state as they are beginning to recover from the physical stresses of the delivery. Explanation, reassurance and plenty of emotional and practical support at home are usually all that is required. These mood changes usually settle spontaneously within 10 days postpartum.

There are a number of contributory factors (**Table 10.3**). There is no greater risk of developing postnatal blues if the woman has undergone adverse life events, has demographic variables that might put her at risk of developing postnatal depression (see below) or has a history of psychiatric illness.

> **Postnatal blues that do not rapidly resolve should be viewed with suspicion as this may indicate the development of a more serious postnatal depression.**

Factors contributing to postnatal blues	
Factor	Effect
Physical changes	Sex steroid levels plummet from elevated pregnancy levels following delivery
	Oxytocin levels rise to support breastfeeding
Psychological stresses of delivery	Particularly in first deliveries, many women feel stressed by the process, worrying about their own health and the health of their baby
Tiredness/exhaustion	Most deliveries result in sleep loss, followed by further disrupted sleep while looking after the baby
Anxiety/concern for the baby	Many new mothers are initially overwhelmed by the responsibility of caring for their new baby, but quickly adapt

Table 10.3 Factors contributing to postnatal blues

Postnatal depression

Postnatal depression is the most common postpartum psychiatric condition, occurring in 10–15% of new mothers (**Table 10.4**). It shares many symptoms with other types of depressive illness. Accordingly, the International Classification of Diseases 10th Revision (ICD-10) classifies it with other depressive disorders, stating symptoms must be present for 2 weeks to make a diagnosis.

Aetiology

Most of the psychosocial factors implicated in the aetiology of postnatal depression, also contribute to the development of other depressive illness:

- Recent stressful life events
- The lack of a close confiding relationship
- A poor marital relationship
- A young age during pregnancy

Risk of postnatal depression	
Patient group	Risk (%)
All pregnancies	10–15
Recurrence following a first episode of PND	33
Past history of bipolar disorder	50

Table 10.4 Risk of postnatal depression (PND) in specific patient groups

A past history of depressive illness, particularly previous postnatal depression increases the risk of postnatal depression. A family history of depressive illness and obstetric complications during the delivery are also risk factors.

Clinical features

The core clinical features of postnatal depression are the same as for other depressive disorders (see page 109). Other characteristic features are:

- Feelings of worthlessness, guilt and inadequacy
- Feeling ashamed about being unable to care for the child appropriately
- Overconcern about the baby's health despite the absence of any real health concerns
- A reduced ability to 'bond' with the child, saying that the child does not love them or they do not love the child
- Obsessional symptoms, including recurrent intrusive thoughts or images of harming the baby. These must be carefully assessed to differentiate them from suicidal thoughts
- Suicidal thoughts coupled with thoughts of harming the baby

Any expressions of suicidal ideation or urges must be taken seriously. Women who harm themselves during this period often choose a more violent method than is usual for women in general, and suicide is the leading cause of maternal death. Risk assessment is vital and must be revisited at every contact with the patient.

Diagnostic approach

This should follow the same approach as for other depressive illness (see Table 3.6). Some physical disorders, including infections after the birth, anaemia and thyroid disorders (e.g. Hashimoto's thyroiditis), are more commonly seen in this period and must be excluded.

Investigations

Depressive disorders must be considered by all those working with pregnant and post-natal women. Screening for depressive disorder is quick and easy with the widely used Edinburgh Postnatal Depression Scale (EPDS - see Case 12).

Many patients with postnatal depression conceal their true feelings as they are ashamed of how they feel when other mums appear to be coping so much better. Screening and a high level of suspicion are necessary to pick up this common condition.

Management

This should follow the approach taken for other depressive disorders, with additional specific considerations.

Family and friends should be involved to offer practical and emotional support by ensuring that the mother's sleep disturbance is minimised and that she has periods of respite from caring for the baby. Supportive community groups such as mother and baby activities provide social support, advice and structure and routine. Counselling can be offered, with partners attending to engage them in supporting their partner effectively.

Clear lines of access to support must be provided, such as providing a crisis number to call. Regular scheduled review appointments must be arranged by the medical team during the illness.

Postnatal depression is thought to result in delays in the infant's cognitive and emotional development. This may be because of difficulties in bonding in the early weeks. Screening, early recognition and effective treatment must be prioritised. Supportive family members should be closely involved to minimise the impact of the mother's illness on the child.

Moderate to severe depressive illness affects around one third of those with postnatal depression. Antidepressant medications are often necessary for this subgroup. Many of the medications are secreted into breast milk (**Table 10.5**). Therefore, although there is little evidence that they are harmful to the

Use of psychiatric medications postnatally	
Medication	Use
Lithium	Contraindicated: present in breast milk at 50% of maternal serum level and produces symptoms of toxicity in the baby
	If lithium vital, discontinue breastfeeding
Tricyclic antidepressants	Use with caution: secreted into breast milk in very small quantities, but little evidence of harm
Selective serotonin reuptake inhibitors (SSRIs)	No evidence of harm to baby
	Tricyclics preferable; longer track record, with little evidence of harm
Anxiolytics	Benzodiazepines cause neonatal sedation/lethargy (particularly long-acting compounds)
Antipsychotics	Excreted into breast milk in small quantities
	May be prescribed with caution, but avoid high doses
	Clozapine contraindicated

Table 10.5 Considerations in the use of psychiatric medications in the postnatal period

baby, they should always be prescribed with caution, seeking specialist psychiatric advice where necessary.

Hospitalisation is necessary for mothers with severe depression and evidence of suicidal or infanticidal thoughts or urges. This allows adequate supervision and care of the mother and baby. It also allows electroconvulsive therapy (ECT) to be given if required. ECT produces a much faster improvement than occurs with medication, minimising the negative impact on bonding and infant well-being.

Prognosis

Most patients recover completely, although there is an increased risk of recurrence in subsequent pregnancies.

Postnatal psychosis

Postnatal psychosis is the development of psychotic symptoms in the weeks after birth. It develops very quickly, nearly always within the first couple of weeks after delivery.

Postnatal psychosis is often viewed as a variant of bipolar affective disorder. In many patients, however, first-rank symptoms of schizophrenia predominate at presentation. The symptoms often revolve around delusions relating to the baby. Thoughts of self-harm or harming the baby appear against a background of insomnia and agitation, tearfulness and emotional lability.

Postnatal psychosis is rare (<0.2% of births) but the recurrence rate may be as high as 50% in subsequent pregnancies. A family or personal history of bipolar disorder also increases the risk of postnatal psychosis.

Nihilistic delusions often focus on the baby. The patient may believe the baby to be dead or deny the baby has been born, rejecting all contact with them. Hallucinations include instructions to self-harm or harm the baby. These must be taken extremely seriously as patients occasionally act on them with little warning.

Management

Postnatal psychosis is a psychiatric emergency requiring admission and close supervision in a mother and baby unit in a psychiatric hospital. Underlying physical disorders must be excluded. Antipsychotic, antidepressant and anxiolytic medications are then given as the circumstances indicate. This sometimes necessitates a discontinuation of breastfeeding. Electroconvulsive therapy should be considered early where life is at risk.

As the mother recovers, attention can be turned to addressing any contributory psychosocial issues. Counselling and support in the community can be established as indicated.

Most patients recover within 3 months but some develop subsequent episodes unrelated to pregnancy.

Answers to starter questions

1. 'Baby blues' (or postnatal blues) are common (50% of new mothers) that they are considered a normal psychological variant, which should settle spontaneously within a few days. If symptoms continue, the patient should be closely monitored as unresolved symptoms may indicate that a more significant postnatal depression is developing.

2. Postnatal depression is easily missed because many women find it very difficult to admit to how they are feeling. Some feel guilty about struggling with their new situation, have thoughts they are ashamed of or feel that everyone else expects them to be happy and positive. Active screening using the EPDS at the 6-week postnatal check up appointment allows women with postnatal depression to disclose their feelings and obtain appropriate professional help.

3. In addition to the usual risks associated with depressive illness, patients with postnatal psychiatric illness can find it particularly difficult to admit to suicidal ideas or ideas of harming their baby, of which they feel very ashamed. They are also more likely to choose a violent method of harming themselves which is more likely to be fatal.

Chapter 11
Physical and psychological co-morbidity

Introduction 223
Case 13 Chronic neck pain. 224
Somatisation and medically
unexplained symptoms 226
Conversion disorders. 228
Delirium 229
Psychiatric illness secondary to
physical illness 231
Organic personality change 233
Sleep disorders. 235
Psychosexual disorders 238

Starter questions

Answers to the following questions are on page 242.

1. Can emotional or psychological difficulties cause physical symptoms?
2. Is it possible to treat people who have physical symptoms but no underlying physical cause?
3. Is depression part of a normal response to a diagnosis of cancer?

Introduction

The relationship between the mind (psyche) and body (soma) is incompletely understood. Some physical illnesses, for example delirium, result in psychiatric symptoms such as hallucinations and confusion. Similarly, psychological difficulties sometimes present as physical symptoms – many of us have had a dry mouth or 'butterflies' in our stomach when feeling anxious. Many disorders, particularly sleep and sexual disorders, involve both physical and psychological factors.

In addition, patients with serious or chronic physical illness, such as cancer, can experience co-morbid psychiatric disorders, such as depression. These then negatively impact on the outcomes and prognosis of their physical illness. Understanding the complex interplay between bodily symptoms and a patient's state of mind is necessary so that inappropriate medical investigations are avoided and appropriate treatment is offered.

Case 13 Chronic neck pain

Presentation

Emma Robinson is a 31-year-old, divorced teacher who visits her general practitioner (GP). She tells him that her chronic neck pain has not improved despite physiotherapy and painkillers, and that she is still unable to work due to her pain. Physical examinations and investigations, including an X-ray and MRI scan of her cervical spine by specialists including neurologists and rheumatologists have revealed no abnormalities. Emma complains that no one is helping her and she wants to know which specialist will see her next.

Initial interpretation

It is important to assess whether there may be a physical cause for Emma's neck pain that has previously been missed. Further history taking should also examine the possibility that her symptoms may have a psychological basis.

History

Emma's neck pain started spontaneously 8 months ago. It worsens when she is teaching difficult classes and improves during school holidays. She has no other symptoms. She had similar neck pain 2 years ago. She felt that her GP did not help this as he offered her simple painkillers after nothing was seen on a radiograph.

Over the last 2 years, she has seen several GPs to discuss various problems, including shoulder pain, painful periods, abdominal bloating and leg pains. She has undergone numerous investigations and reviews by different specialists, but none

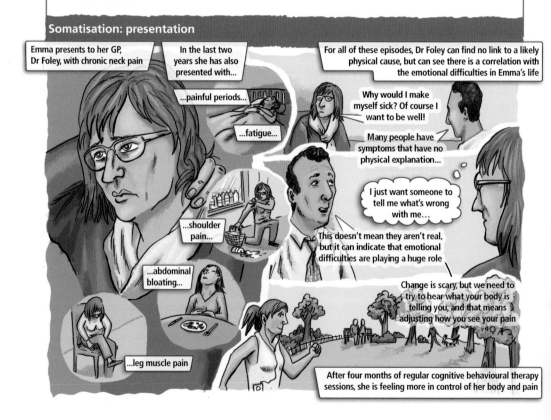

Somatisation: presentation

has shown a clear physical cause for her symptoms. She does not drink alcohol and denies ever using illicit drugs. She has no past psychiatric history and does not feel pervasively low in mood or anxious.

Interpretation of history

Emma has a long history of multiple, recurrent physical symptoms. No physical cause has been found for these or her current symptoms. Her beliefs about her symptoms must be explored, along with her current psychosocial circumstances to identify any potential stressors.

Further history

Emma explains that her neck pain started shortly after she received a warning at work due to her poor teaching performance. Around the same time, she discovered her husband wanted a divorce. He moved out of their home, leaving her to pay expensive household bills. She tells her GP she was 'carrying a huge weight' on her shoulders.

She is currently off work due to her neck pain. She has few friends and does not see her family as her mother was emotionally and physically abusive towards her during childhood. She regularly takes paracetamol and ibuprofen for her neck pain, with little effect. She feels her neck pain has a serious physical cause that has not yet been identified and from which she wants to recover. She asks her GP if there are any other scans she could have.

Examination

Emma's mental state examination does not suggest the presence of a mood disorder, psychosis or generalised anxiety disorder. However, it shows she is excessively worried about her neck pain (**Table 11.1**). A repeated physical examination of neck, including a musculoskeletal and

neurological examination, reveals no abnormalities.

Interpretation of findings

Emma has a history of multiple, recurrent physical symptoms that have caused her to worry and have affected her social functioning. Despite the previous extensive specialist investigations and reviews, there is no clear evidence of a physical cause. She is experiencing a number of significant psychosocial stressors and has a limited social network to help her cope. Her symptoms do not have an identifiable physical cause; instead, her psychological distress is being expressed as physical symptoms.

Emma's mental state examination	
Category	Description
Appearance and behaviour	Well-kempt, appropriately dressed, appears somewhat anxious, fidgeting with her hands at times
Speech	Normal in rate, rhythm, tone and volume
Mood	Subjectively 'ok', objectively euthymic with normal range of reactivity
Perceptions	No abnormal perceptions
Thoughts	Excessive anxiety regarding her neck pain, no delusions or formal thought disorder
Cognitions	Fully orientated to time, place and person
Insight	Feels there is an underlying physical cause for her chronic neck pain despite normal investigations and previous reassurance from specialists, and is requesting further investigations
Suicidal ideation	No suicidal ideas or thoughts of harming himself or others

Table 11.1 Emma's mental state examination

Case 13 *continued*

Investigations

None of Emma's previously investigations have shown any abnormalities. More recently, blood tests for inflammatory markers of rheumatological disorders, including full blood count, erythrocyte sedimentation rate, C-reactive protein and rheumatoid factor, have been normal. Her GP tactfully explains the aims and findings of these investigations and says no further investigations will be arranged at this time.

Diagnosis

Emma is initially annoyed that her GP is suggesting her symptoms might have a psychological rather than a physical cause. The GP sensitively explains how psychological and emotional factors, such as stress, can be expressed as physical symptoms. Emma eventually agrees to a referral to a psychiatry specialist to further explore the links between her physical symptoms and her emotional well-being.

Somatisation and medically unexplained symptoms

In somatoform disorders, patients experience physical symptoms that are inconsistent or cannot be explained by any detectable underlying physical pathology. Instead, it is thought that psychological or emotional distress is expressed as physical symptoms in a process known as somatisation. Somatoform disorders include somatisation disorder, persistent somatoform pain disorder and hypochondriacal disorder. They are difficult to diagnose; patients often undergo many investigations to rule out physical causes before eventually being diagnosed.

symptoms
■ Persistent refusal to accept reassurance from doctors that there is no physical cause of the symptoms

> **Patients with somatisation disorder disorder sometimes experience dismissive attitudes from health-care professionals.** A sensitive approach should be adopted, acknowledging that, although no physical cause has been found, the symptoms experienced by the patient are genuine and distressing for them.

Somatisation disorder

Somatisation disorder is a chronic condition lasting at least 2 years in which patients experience somatic symptoms which have no identifiable physical cause. It is characterised by:

■ Multiple, recurrent, frequently changing physical symptoms with no physical explanation
■ Functional impairment, e.g. affecting occupation or relationships, caused by the

Epidemiology

The prevalence of somatisation disorder is around 0.2%. The onset is usually before the age of 30 years. The prevalence is higher in women, those with a history of other psychiatric disorders, such as depression, and those with a personal history of sexual or physical abuse.

Aetiology

The cause of somatisation disorder is unclear. Patients misinterpret normal bodily sensations as indicative of disease. They focus on these sensations, leading to further anxiety and a need to seek symptom-relief advice and reassurance from health-care professionals (**Figure 11.1**). It is suggested that this is driven by underlying unconscious unmet needs for care, attention or closeness with others. Genes involved in neuroendocrine pathways within the hypothalamic–pituitary–adrenal axis have also been implicated in the aetiology of this disorder.

Clinical features

Patients with somatisation disorder report multiple and frequently changing physical symptoms (**Table 11.2**).

Diagnostic approach

Making a diagnosis of somatisation disorder is challenging. Physical causes for the patient's symptoms should be excluded before attributing them to a psychological cause. A thorough approach to diagnosis includes:

- History-taking to discover each symptom the patient has experienced over time, the investigations received and the patient's beliefs about their symptoms
- A physical examination to exclude physical causes

- Investigations to exclude physical causes according to the symptoms present
- A full psychiatric history to discover potential psychosocial stressors

Common symptoms of somatisation disorder	
System	Symptoms
Gastrointestinal	Nausea/vomiting
	Abdominal pain
	Bloating
	Difficulty swallowing
	Diarrhoea
Urogenital	Dysuria
	Dyspareunia
	Menstrual disorders:dysmenorrhoea, menorrhagia
	Erectile dysfunction
Musculoskeletal	Joint pain
	Back pain
Neurological	Headache
	Dizziness
	Double vision or blindness
	Muscle weakness or paralysis
	Amnesia

Table 11.2 Common symptoms of somatisation disorder

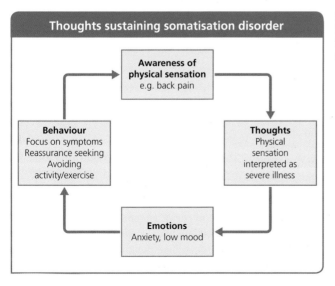

Figure 11.1 The relationship between physical sensations, thoughts, emotions and behaviour sustaining somatisation disorder.

- The investigation of features suggestive of underlying psychiatric conditions, e.g. depression or anxiety disorders, on mental state examination

Questions to explore potential psychosocial stressors contributing to the patient's difficulties include:

- 'Can you tell me some more about what is going on in your life at the moment?'
- 'How do you feel about it?'
- 'Have you noticed any links between what is going on in your life, how you feel and your symptoms?'

Management

Although there are no specific medications to treat somatisation disorder, medical treatment is offered for co-morbid psychiatric disorders. For example, antidepressants can be given for depressive disorder.

Psychological therapies, including cognitive behavioural therapy and mindfulness therapy, help patients explore and change their thoughts and behaviours around their interpretation of bodily sensations. Further psychological support related to stress management and problem solving improves functioning.

Prognosis

Outcomes are better for those with less complex symptoms of shorter duration. Those with multiple, recurrent symptoms of long duration often have a poorer prognosis and continue to experience fluctuating symptoms for many years.

Hypochondriacal disorder

In hypochondriacal disorder, patients misinterpret normal bodily sensations as being due to a serious physical disease and seek investigations to confirm an underlying disease. For example, they may suspect that a minor headache is caused by an underlying brain tumour. Despite repeated examination and investigations, they continue to fear that there is a serious underlying health problem. Patients will continue to seek investigations for what they believe to be the serious medical cause of their symptoms, unlike patients with somatisation disorder who seek relief from their symptoms.

Persistent somatoform pain disorder

This is a somatoform disorder in which the dominant symptom is severe, persistent pain with no identifiable physical cause. The pain is usually associated with psychosocial stressors.

Conversion disorders

In conversion disorders, patients experience symptoms which suggest disease of the brain or nerves, but which have no identifiable physical cause. Symptoms develop quickly in response to a stressful event or trauma. There are four types of conversion disorder (**Table 11.3**). The symptoms experienced by patients with conversion disorder are not under voluntary, conscious control, and are therefore not intentionally produced.

Conversion disorders should be detected so that appropriate interventions aimed at reducing symptoms can be provided and to ensure responses that perpetuate the patient's difficulties are avoided.

Aetiology

The aetiology of conversion disorder is incompletely understood. Current theoretical explanations hold that the brain reacts to the overwhelming anxiety caused by a traumatic event or potential threat by converting psychological distress into neurological symptoms. It is thought that this reduces the patient's levels of anxiety (primary gain). This

Types of conversion disorders

Type	Clinical features
With motor symptom or deficit	Impaired coordination
	Impaired balance
	Weakness or paralysis
	Difficulty swallowing
	Aphonia/loss of voice
With sensory symptom or deficit	Double vision
	Blindness
	Hearing loss
	Loss of touch sensation
	Loss of pain sensation
With seizures or convulsions	Seizures or convulsions
	With motor or sensory features under voluntary control
With mixed presentation	With symptoms from more than one of the above categories

Table 11.3 Types of conversion disorders and their clinical features

results in 'la belle indifference' – a state in which the patient is relatively unconcerned by their symptoms. The symptoms are reinforced by the benefits of being in the 'sick role', such as an avoidance of particular activities, such as going to work (secondary gain).

Diagnostic approach

The approach is similar to that of somatoform disorders; physical causes for the patient's symptoms must be excluded. History-taking should focus on temporal associations between stressful events and the onset of symptoms.

Conversion disorders can be comorbid with depressive or anxiety disorders, which must be excluded on a mental state examination. Investigations, e.g. brain CT scans, are arranged to exclude an identifiable physical cause of the patient's symptoms.

Management

Management aims to help patients understand the nature of their disorder and encourage a return to normal functioning, which may involve physiotherapy and occupational therapy. Patients are often offered psycho-analytic therapy to explore any painful or traumatic emotions or memories which are contributing to their conversion disorder. Medication is not used to treat conversion disorder, but appropriate drugs are prescribed to treat co-morbid depression or anxiety disorders.

Prognosis

In many patients, symptoms last no longer than 2 weeks. However, around 25% of patients experience a further episode of conversion disorder within one year. They have a poorer prognosis, continuing to have periods of conversion disorder for many years. Other indicators of a poor prognosis include a history of personality disorder.

Delirium

Delirium is a clinical syndrome characterised by the acute onset of fluctuating cognitive impairment in the presence of clouded consciousness. Patients with delirium experience mental symptoms, such as confusion and hallucinations, as a consequence of a range of physical problems, all of which affect brain functioning. Although it is common in patients admitted to general hospitals, delirium is often missed because the symptoms fluctuate. Additionally, in patients with dementia or an intellectual disability, symptoms of may be mistakenly attributed to their pre-existing dementia or intellectual disability. Prompt identification and treatment of delirium is important to reduce the complications, which include longer hospital stays, falls and death.

Delirium has many causes (**Table 11.4**).

Common causes of delirium	
Type	Examples
Acute infections	Urinary tract infection
	Pneumonia
	Meningitis
	Encephalitis
	Sepsis
Toxins	Alcohol: intoxication or withdrawal
	Illicit drugs: intoxication or withdrawal
	Prescribed medications: analgesia, anticholinergics, anticonvulsants, benzodiazepines, steroids
	Carbon monoxide poisoning
Metabolic disorders	Hypoxia
	Hypo/hyperglycaemia
	Hyponatraemia
	Hypercalcaemia
Vitamin deficiencies	Vitamin B_{12} deficiency
	Thiamine deficiency
Neoplasia	Primary brain cancers
	Metastatic brain cancer
	Paraneoplastic syndromes
Vascular disorders	Cerebrovascular disease
	Subdural haemorrhage
	Subarachnoid haemorrhage
	Vasculitis, e.g. systemic lupus erythematosus
Endocrine disorders	Hypo/hyperthyroidism
	Hypo/hyperparathyroidism
	Cushing's disease
	Porphyria
Trauma	Head injury
Others	Faecal impaction
	Urinary retention
	Postictally in those with epilepsy

Table 11.4 Common causes of delirium

Epidemiology

Around 10% of general hospital patients have a period of delirium, either developed during admission, or that they already had when they presented. The incidence increases with age and is higher in those with:

- Pre-existing dementia
- A head injury or stroke
- Terminal illness, e.g. terminal cancer
- Problems with vision or hearing
- Recent surgery, particularly emergency operations or hip fracture repairs
- Alcohol misuse
- Polypharmacy: being prescribed multiple medications, particularly opioid analgesics, benzodiazepines, antiparkinsonian medications and steroids
- A move to a new environment

Clinical features

Delirium is characterised by:

- An acute onset of confusion
- A fluctuating course
- Impaired, or clouded, consciousness
- Cognitive impairment, including impaired attention, concentration or short-term memory
- Abnormalities of the sleep–wake cycle
- Abnormalities of perception, which can include hallucinations
- Agitation
- Emotional lability

Diagnostic approach

A thorough history, mental state examination and mini mental state examination are vital to differentiate delirium from other conditions that present in similar ways. These include depression and, in older people, dementia (see Chapter 12).

A full physical examination should identify potential causes. These commonly include urine infection, chest infection, deydration and constipation.

Comprehensive investigations are required to exclude the many causes of delirium (**Table 11.4**):

- Urine dipstick and microscopy
- Bloods: full blood count, urea and electrolytes, calcium, magnesium, liver and thyroid function tests and blood glucose level
- Blood cultures and serology
- Pulse oximetry and arterial blood gases

- Radiographs of the chest and abdomen
- An ECG
- A CT scan of the brain

> **Patients with delirium** are acutely confused, making a collateral history from family, carers or staff who know the patient well, key to establishing the patient's pre-morbid level of functioning and their medical and psychiatric history.

Measures of cognitive functioning, such as the Abbreviated Mental Test Score, should be routinely completed for patients at risk of delirium. This allows for early detection and prompt remedial action.

Management

Management involves treating the underlying cause and environmental measures using physical, psychological and social strategies to reduce the patient's confusion and resulting anxiety. Environmental measures for patients with delirium include:

- Minimising noise
- Reassurance and reminders of what is happening and where they are
- Adequate nutrition
- Avoiding over- or understimulation
- Displaying a clock and calendar
- Ensuring accessibility to objects familiar to the patient
- The provision of normal aids, e.g. hearing aids
- Access to activities that help the patient to relax

Medication

The underlying cause of the delirium is treated with the appropriate medication.

Prognosis

Once identified and treated, symptoms of delirium can take weeks to resolve. In around one third of patients, symptoms of delirium persist for a period of months to around 1 year after the cause has been treated. As a result, some patients have to move into residential or nursing care.

Psychiatric illness secondary to physical illness

Up to one third of people with a chronic physical illness, such as cancer, cardiovascular disease, stroke, chronic obstructive pulmonary disease or multiple sclerosis, experience co-morbid psychiatric illness. This is usually a depressive disorder or anxiety disorder: both are more common in those with a physical illness than in the general population. Left untreated, co-morbid psychiatric illness results in poorer social functioning and a poorer quality of life. Furthermore, co-morbid psychiatric disorders interfere with a patient's ability to make decisions about treatment for their physical illness. They also increase the risk of non-concordance with treatment.

The clinical features of co-morbid psychiatric illness are broadly similar to those seen in patients with no concurrent physical illness. However, it is difficult to detect psychiatric disorders in people with chronic physical illness because its symptoms, such as fatigue and poor sleep, mimic those of the psychiatric disorder. Co-morbid psychiatric illnesses must be identified and managed to improve patients' abilities to cope with their illness and to improve the outcome of their physical disorder.

Aetiology

There are a number of ways in which psychiatric disorder arises secondary to physical illness (**Figure 11.2**):

- As a direct consequence of the effect of the physical illness, such as infection or malignancy, on the brain. It can also be a consequence of the psychological distress caused by the physical illness

- As a side effect of the treatment used for the physical illness. For example, beta-blockers prescribed to treat hypertension can produce depressive symptoms such as low mood and apathy. Psychologically distressing treatments such as radiotherapy are also associated with an increased risk of psychiatric disorder
- As a consequence of the psychosocial impact of the physical illness, for example, loss of social functioning and subsequent isolation

Psychiatric and physical disorders can also occur together by chance.

Diagnostic approach

The diagnostic approach to detecting psychiatric disorders in patients with chronic physical illness is similar to the approach in the general population: history-taking, physical examination, mental state examination and appropriate investigations are used to exclude differential diagnoses before a diagnosis of psychiatric disorder is made.

However, because somatic symptoms of psychiatric illnesses (e.g. insomnia, poor appetite, weight loss) can also present as a consequence of physical illness, psychological symptoms are more helpful for identifying psychiatric disorders in those with chronic physical health problems. For example, feelings of worthlessness or guilt, poor self-esteem, hopelessness, dysphoric mood, anhedonia and suicidal ideation in patients with cancer are suggestive of depression.

Questions you might ask to elicit features of depression in patients with cancer include:

- 'How have you been coping since you were given your diagnosis of cancer?'
- 'How has your mood been during your cancer treatment?' (mood)
- 'In spite of your cancer, are you still able to find pleasure in things in life?' (inability = anhedonia)
- 'Do you ever find yourself thinking that you brought your cancer on yourself?' (guilt)

Enquiring about thoughts of self-harm or suicide is vital. Suicide rates are higher in those with chronic or severe physical illness, such as cancer.

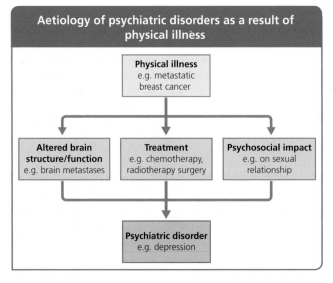

Figure 11.2 Aetiology of psychiatric disorders as a result of physical illness.

Investigations

Investigations are undertaken to detect physical abnormalities that may be contributing to the patient's mental state difficulties. For example, anaemia, hypercalcaemia, hypothyroidism, hyperthyroidism and vitamin B_{12} or folate deficiency all affect a patient's mental state. These should be corrected as far as possible before a diagnosis of a psychiatric disorder is made.

> **Always consider the patient's current physical health when prescribing.** For example, an impairment of kidney or liver function will impact on drug metabolism. To avoid drug interactions always check which other medications the patient is taking.

Management

The treatment is the same as that of patients without physical illness:

- Biological treatments include medications appropriate for the psychiatric disorder
- Psychological treatments include cognitive behavioural therapy
- Social interventions include referrals to appropriate support groups and to organisations that can help them obtain illness- or disability-related benefits. This ameliorates psychosocial stressors arising from a loss of income due to the disorder

Organic personality change

Organic personality change occurs when damage or disease of the brain causes a change in a patient's personality. It is especially seen with frontal lobe damage as this area controls many activities associated with personality, including motivation, making judgements about the consequences of current actions, making decisions about actions, learning rules and inhibiting socially unacceptable behaviour. The ensuing personality changes, including poor judgement and inappropriate sexual behaviour, leave patients at risk of exploitation or abuse. Identifying organic causes of personality change is necessary to institute appropriate treatment to ameliorate the effects of the underlying disease.

Aetiology

Damage or disease of the frontal lobe includes:

- Head injury
- Cerebrovascular disease
- Neoplasms
- Infections, e.g. resulting from abscesses
- Frontotemporal dementia (see Chapter 12)

Clinical features

Common clinical features in patients with frontal lobe disease or damage resulting in organic personality change include:

- Emotional instability
- Angry outbursts
- Inappropriate social behaviour
- Inappropriate sexual behaviour
- Apathy and loss of interest

Diagnostic approach

Symptoms and signs of personality change and frontal lobe dysfunction should be identified along with their causes, e.g. cerebrovascular disease or neoplasms.

Patients usually have poor insight into their personality changes; a collateral history from someone who knows the patient well is vital to complete psychiatric and medical history taking, and a thorough risk assessment.

History-taking should focus on obtaining a detailed account of personality changes, their onset and course, associated symptoms, risk factors for brain damage (e.g. a history of head trauma), and any temporal association with this and the onset of personality changes.

On physical examination, specific tests for frontal lobe function should be completed, as follows:

The go/no go test

Instruct the patient to hold up two fingers if you hold one and vice versa. A patient with frontal lobe impairment is unable to follow these instructions and holds up the same number of fingers as the examiner.

Letter fluency

Ask the patient to say as many words as they can think of beginning with 'F' in 1 minute. A patient with intact frontal lobes who completed secondary school education should be able to say at least eight words.

Motor test

Ask the patient to follow a series of three movements, such as making a fist, putting the palm of their hand on the table and then putting the side of their hand on the table. A patient with frontal lobe impairment is unable to follow these steps accurately and perseveres with only one or two of the movements.

Questions to ask during collateral history taking in suspected organic personality change

- 'Have you noticed any change in their manners?'

- 'Have you noticed whether they say things they would never have said before, for example "You look fat"?'

- 'Do they seem to be less interested than before in hobbies, friends or family?'

- 'Have you noticed any change in their temper?'

- 'Have you noticed any change in their interest in sex?'

Investigations

Investigations, including CT and MRI scans of the brain, are requested to detect possible causes of frontal lobe damage.

Management

Treatments are offered according to the underlying physical pathology, for example the surgical removal of a tumour, or the medical treatment of infections or dementia.

Psychosocial interventions, such as the provision of social care and support for carers, help to manage the risks to the patient and/or their carers that have arisen from the personality changes.

Prognosis

The prognosis depends on the underlying pathology, for example, patients who have had personality change due to dementia will show continued deterioration as the underlying dementia progresses.

Sleep disorders

Normal sleep is characterised by five distinct stages (**Table 11.5**). Sleep disorders can affect different stages of the sleep cycle and are characterised by abnormalities of the quantity and quality of sleep. Both physical and psychological factors contribute to sleep disorders.

Sleep disorders are categorised into primary and secondary:

- Secondary sleep disorders occur as a consequence of other physical health problems, mental health problems or substance use (**Table 11.6**)
- Primary sleep disorders: other sleep disorders, which do not arise as a consequence of these factors are divided into dyssomnias and parasomnias (**Table 11.7**). They are thought to be caused by dysfunction of the reticular activating system, the brain pathway responsible for regulating sleep and wakefulness

Sleep disorders are common, particularly primary insomnia which has a life-time prevalence of around 30% in primary care.

Detecting and treating sleep disorders is important because chronic poor sleep can have negative effects on mood, behaviour, social functioning and memory.

Diagnostic approach

Diagnostic assessment of sleep disorders involves history-taking, a mental state

Sleep cycle stages	
Stage	Features
Stage 1 (Non-REM)	Transition from wakefulness to sleep
	Eyes closed
	EEG shows theta waves: 4–7 Hz, low amplitude, spikes
Stage 2 (Non-REM)	Light sleep
	Muscle relaxation with spontaneous periods of increased tone
	Heart rate slows
	EEG shows sleep spindles (short 12–14 Hz clusters) and K^+ complexes (sharp negative wave followed by positive wave)
Stage 3 and 4 (Non-REM, slow wave sleep)	Deep sleep
	Abnormalities such as sleep terrors and sleepwalking
	EEG shows delta waves (high amplitude, <4 Hz waves), the intensity increases from stage 3 to stage 4
REM	Dreaming
	Occurs every 90 minutes during sleep
	Duration increases as length asleep increases
	Skeletal muscle paralysis and penile erection may occur
	EEG shows low-amplitude, high-frequency, saw-tooth pattern

Table 11.5 Stages of the sleep cycle. REM, rapid eye movement

Causes of secondary sleep disorders	
Type	Examples of causes
Caused by physical health conditions	Pain, e.g. gastro-oesophageal reflux disease, arthritis, cancer
	Nocturia, e.g. prostatism
	Orthopnoea (breathlessness on lying flat), e.g. pulmonary oedema caused by cardiac failure
Caused by mental health conditions	Anxiety
	Depression
	Mania
Caused by substance use	Alcohol
	Caffeine
	Illicit drugs, e.g. amphetamines
	Prescribed medications, e.g. some antipsychotics

Table 11.6 Causes of secondary sleep disorders

examination and physical examination to identify any underlying physical health, mental health or substance-related causes. A sleep history and a collateral history from the patient's sleeping partner can reveal further useful information. The Epworth Sleepiness Scale can also be used to measure the impact and severity of patients' sleeping difficulties.

Primary sleep disorders		
Type	Clinical features	Treatment
Dyssomnias		
Primary insomnia	Abnormalities in quantity, quality or timing of sleep	Sleep hygiene measures Limited use of sedative medications Cognitive behavioural therapy
Narcolepsy	Suddenly falling asleep at inappropriate times	Sleep hygiene measures Stimulant medications, e.g. modafinil
Breathing-related sleep disorders (e.g. obstructive sleep apnoea)	Repeated obstruction of the upper airway during sleep leading to repeated pauses in breathing and snoring	Advice on weight loss in obese patients Continuous positive airway pressure mask Tonsillectomy in those with enlarged tonsils
Circadian rhythm sleep disorders (e.g. jet-lag, shift work)	Disruption of circadian rhythm of sleep/wakefulness Difficulties falling asleep or waking up at the desired times Daytime sleepiness	Sleep hygiene measures Melatonin to regulate the brain's sleep/wake cycle
Parasomnias		
Nightmares	Intensely frightening dreams occurring during REM sleep; affected person is alert and orientated when they wake and can recall the details of the dream Can occur as a symptom of post-traumatic stress disorder	No specific treatment; most children grow out of them Those with nightmares as a symptom of PTSD are treated with appropriate medications and psychological therapies
Night terrors	Sudden waking from non-REM sleep in a state of panic, often with a loud scream, sweating, rapid breathing and disorientation Once fully awake, cannot recall episode	No specific treatment; children usually grow out of them
Sleepwalking	Complex motor behaviours, e.g. walking, looking in cupboards, eating, occur during non-REM sleep Affected person is difficult to waken and cannot recall the event	Safety measures, e.g. locking windows and using a stair gate, to reduce the risk of accidental injury whilst sleepwalking

Table 11.7 Primary sleep disorders. They are subdivided into dyssomnias (difficulties falling asleep, staying asleep, getting back to sleep or being unrefreshed by sleep) and parasomnias (abnormal episodes occurring during sleep). REM, rapid eye movement

Questions to ask when taking a sleep history are:

- 'What do you tend to do in the hour or two before you go to bed?'

- 'Do you go to bed at the same time each day?'

- 'Do you have a comfortable sleeping environment? For example, is your bed comfortable? Is the room quiet and a comfortable temperature?'

- 'Are you able to get to sleep straight away, or do you lie awake for some time before dropping off to sleep?'

- 'How long does it usually take you to fall asleep?'

- 'Do you wake up during the night?'

- 'Are you able to get back to sleep once you have woken up?'

- 'Do you wake too early in the morning and find you cannot get back to sleep?'

- 'Do you wake up at the same time each day?'

- 'Do you feel refreshed when you wake up?'

- 'Do you nap during the day?'

- 'Do other people ever mention that you snore?'

- 'Do other people ever mention any concerns about your breathing or other movements during sleep?'

Investigations

When the cause of a patient's sleep disorder is unclear, referral to a specialist sleep medicine clinic is arranged for further investigations. These include polysomnography – a process in which the patient spends a night in the sleep laboratory while various physical parameters are measured including:

- An electroencephalogram – to identify and measure the stages of the sleep cycle
- An ECG – to identify any abnormalities in cardiac rhythm
- An electromyogram – to identify any excessive muscular activity during sleep
- An electro-oculogram – to determine when REM sleep is occurring
- Pulse oximetry – to identify any abnormalities in blood oxygen saturation that may occur in obstructive sleep apnoea (a condition in which the muscles and soft tissues of the throat relax and collapse causing partial airway obstruction, resulting in episodes of apnoea during sleep)
- Mouth and nose air entry rates – to measures breathing rates and any respiratory interruptions
- Loudness of snoring – to help identify obstructive sleep apnoea

Management

Management options depend on the cause of the sleep disorder. Patients with primary insomnia should be offered sleep hygiene advice:

- Avoid daytime naps
- Avoid caffeine, alcohol and nicotine before bedtime
- Avoid stimulating activities before bedtime
- Develop a relaxing routine before bed, e.g. a warm bath or a milky drink
- Ensure the bedroom is quiet and comfortable
- Use the bed for sleeping and sex, and not for working, using a computer/smartphone or watching television
- Get up and do a relaxing activity if you have not fallen asleep within 15 minutes of being in bed
- Go to bed and get up at the same time each day

Medication

Sedative medications include benzodiazepines and 'Z' drugs such as zopiclone and zolpidem. These are useful for inducing sleep in those with primary insomnia but carry a risk of dependence. Their use should therefore be limited to a maximum of 2 weeks.

Psychological treatments

Cognitive behavioural therapy (CBT) is as effective as the short-term use of hypnotics in those with primary insomnia. During CBT, a formulation of the patient's thoughts, emotions, behaviour and physical reactions (**Figure 11.3**), and ways to make changes are explored.

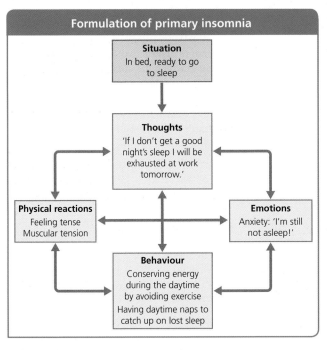

Figure 11.3 The relationships between thought, emotions, behaviours and physical reactions in a patient with primary insomnia.

Psychosexual disorders

Psychosexual disorders are sexual problems that have psychological rather than physical causes. These affect patients' self-esteem and relationships, but patients are often embarrassed about approaching professionals for support.

The three main groups of psychosexual disorders are:

- Sexual dysfunction
- Disorders of sexual preference (paraphilias)
- Gender identity disorders (gender dysphoria)

Patients are often very embarrassed about discussions relating to sex and relationships. Adopt an empathic approach. Appropriate terminology, such as penis, vagina and sexual intercourse should be used. Remember though that some patients, particularly those with intellectual disability, do not always understand these terms.

Sexual dysfunction

Both physiological and psychological responses to sexual stimulation are required for normal sexual functioning (**Figure 11.4** and **Table 11.8**). Difficulties at each stage of the sexual response cycle can result in sexual dysfunction, characterised by impaired sexual enjoyment or performance, and difficulties engaging in sexual activities, for example:

- A diminished desire to have sex or anxiety about having sex affects stage 1
- Impaired physical responses to sexual stimulation, including erectile dysfunction in men or vagismus in women, affects stage 2
- Disorders of stage 3 include premature ejaculation (ejaculation occurring before the man wants it to) and absent ejaculation (difficulty ejaculating despite sexual stimulation)

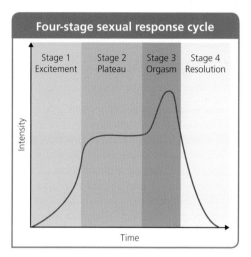

Figure 11.4 Masters and Johnson's four-stage sexual response cycle.

Sexual response cycle	
Stage	Features
1 Excitement	Desire to have sex
	Increased heart rate and breathing rate
	Increased blood flow to genitals
2 Plateau	Intensified sexual pleasure
	Erection in men
	Vaginal lubrication in women
3 Orgasm	Peak of sexual pleasure
	Release of sexual tension
	Ejaculation in men
	Contraction of outer third of vagina in women
4 Resolution	Muscular relaxation
	Sense of well-being
	Fatigue
	In men: refractory period during which further erection and orgasm cannot occur again
	In women: rapid return to orgasm phase with multiple orgasms possible

Table 11.8 Masters and Johnson four stage sexual response cycle

Epidemiology

Sexual dysfunction is relatively common, but prevalence rates vary between studies and depend on the nature of the problem. Erectile dysfuction is a particularly common type of sexual dysfunction; it is affects around half of men between the ages of 40 and 70 years.

Aetiology

Psychosocial causes of sexual dysfunction include:

- Anxiety. This may result from earlier traumatic experiences related to sex, such as sexual abuse or assault. Long-standing feelings of guilt or shame related to sexual intercourse and a fear of pregnancy or sexually transmitted diseases also lead to problems. Additional causes are concerns over sexual performance or attractiveness, and anxiety related to other psychosocial stressors, e.g. related to work or money
- Depression or fatigue
- Relationship difficulties such as underlying feelings of resentment or hostility, fear of rejection or lack of desire

Diagnostic approach

Sexual dysfunction disorders are diagnosed when the patient's problems are not solely due to physical causes and there is a clear psychological difficulty. Physical factors that are contributing to the patient's difficulties should be checked for and the patient's psychosexual history sensitively explored. Physical health conditions to rule out on history taking, physical examination and investigation include:

- Endometriosis and vaginismus (unconscious contraction of the vagina in response to touch), which can cause dyspareunia resulting in loss of sexual desire
- Diabetes, vascular disease and prostatectomy can all result in erectile dysfunction
- Low testosterone levels in men

Other causes that should be ruled out include:

- Prescribed medications, e.g. anticonvulsants, diuretics and antihypertensives, antidepressants, antipsychotics
- Alcohol and illicit drugs, e.g. cannabis, cocaine, opiates
- Mental disorders, e.g. alcohol dependence, depression and anxiety

Sexual history-taking should explore what the difficulties are, their onset, and changes over time, for example, whether similar difficulties have occurred with other partners. Asking about masturbation and morning erections is helpful in assessing whether the sexual response difficulties are pervasive or occur in the context of one particular relationship. It is also important to speak the patient and their sexual partner as individuals, and then as a couple to explore any relationship difficulties impacting on sexual functioning.

> **Psychological and physical co-morbidity may occur in patients with sexual dysfunction.** For example, erectile dysfunction can occur as a consequence of diabetes and lead to anxiety about sexual performance. This anxiety can in turn cause psychogenic erectile dysfunction.

Management

Psychological management options include:

- Reassurance and sex education
- Relationship counselling
- Sex therapy, in which the couple receive support to communicate openly about sex and receive education on the sexual response cycle. Guided behavioural tasks are introduced to gradually build pleasurable physical contact rather than focusing on achieving sexual arousal, intercourse or orgasm (**Figure 11.5**).

Medication

Oral sildenafil (Viagra) may be prescribed to counter erectile problems.

Surgery

Surgical options to correct erectile problems include intracavernosal injections and prosthetic implants.

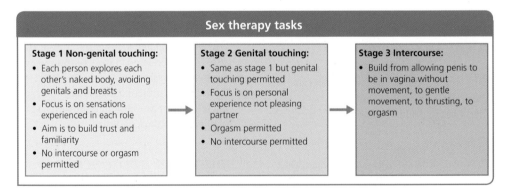

Sex therapy tasks

Stage 1 Non-genital touching:
- Each person explores each other's naked body, avoiding genitals and breasts
- Focus is on sensations experienced in each role
- Aim is to build trust and familiarity
- No intercourse or orgasm permitted

Stage 2 Genital touching:
- Same as stage 1 but genital touching permitted
- Focus is on personal experience not pleasing partner
- Orgasm permitted
- No intercourse permitted

Stage 3 Intercourse:
- Build from allowing penis to be in vagina without movement, to gentle movement, to thrusting, to orgasm

Figure 11.5 Guided behavioural tasks in sex therapy.

Prognosis

Difficulties such as premature ejaculation, psychogenic erectile dysfunction and vaginismus generally have a good prognosis. Loss of sexual desire is often difficult to treat and has a poorer prognosis.

Disorders of sexual preference

Disorders of sexual preference (paraphilias) are recurrent sexual fantasies, urges or behaviours that lie outside cultural norms and may result in suffering or harm to the person themselves or to others, such as children and other non-consenting individuals (**Table 11.9**).

Onset is usually around puberty and these disorders are often chronic, with periods of remission and relapse. It is not clear what causes the development of paraphilias. In some cases, patients have comorbid personality disorders and difficulties forming relationships with others.

Management

Paraphilias are difficult to treat. Management options include cognitive behavioural therapy, for example, to explore and challenge distorted beliefs around the object of sexual interest. Behaviour therapy is also used, in which the patient learns to associate paraphilic thoughts with an aversive stimulus, such as an unpleasant odour. Other psychosocial treatment options include interventions to promote victim empathy, and to address poor social and relationship skills. Male paedophiles and exhibitionists are often prescribed anti-androgens such as cyproterone acetate, which lower serum testosterone levels, resulting in reduced sexual urges and behaviours. Treatment in a forensic psychiatry setting is sometimes required to manage the risks of a sexual offence occuring.

Disorders of gender identity

Gender identity is the sense of being male or female, which usually matches the biological features associated with either gender, including genitalia, secondary sexual characteristics and sex chromosomes. However, patients with gender identity disorder have a strong conviction that they should be of the opposite gender to their chromosomes and biological features.

Types of paraphilias		
Type	Disorder	Features
Abnormalities of object of sexual interest	Paedophilia	Sexual interest in children
	Zoophilia (bestiality)	Sexual interest in animals
	Necrophilia	Sexual interest in corpses
	Fetishism	Sexual interest in parts of the body not usually thought to be erogenous, or inanimate objects
	Transvestic fetishism	Sexual interest in wearing clothing of the opposite sex
Abnormalities of act of sex	Exhibitionism	Exposing genitals to strangers
	Voyeurism	Observing unsuspecting people undressing or engaging in sexual activity
	Sadism	Inflicting pain, humiliation or suffering on others
	Masochism	Experiencing pain, humiliation or suffering oneself

Table 11.9 Types of paraphilias (disorders of sexual preference)

There is currently a debate over whether gender identity disorder is a mental disorder or not. 'Gender identity disorder' is a clinical term, but the term 'gender dysphoria' is less stigmatising and is usually preferred by patients.

Gender identity disorder usually starts before the onset of puberty. The individual often dresses as a members of the opposite gender as part of their desire to live as a member of this gender. In contrast, those with fetishistic transvestism dress as members of the opposite gender to produce sexual arousal.

The cause of gender identity disorder is unknown.

Always consider depression in those with gender identity disorder. Also remember that some patients have thoughts of wanting to alter their biological features themselves. They may also have suicidal ideation.

Management

People with this condition receive multidisciplinary treatment. The psychiatrist's role in this is to assess and treat any co-morbid psychiatric disorder that is a cause or a consequence of the gender identity disorder.

Further management includes real-life experience in which the person lives as fully as possible as a member of the opposite gender for at least 1 year. This is followed by hormone treatment to alter the person's biological features so they can live as a person of the opposite gender. Ultimately, surgical reassignment of gender may be carried out.

Answers to starter questions

1. The mechanism by which emotional or psychological difficulties cause physical symptoms is not fully understood. Most of us experience links between our thoughts and feelings and our bodily sensations, e.g. dry mouth or 'butterflies' in our stomach when we are anxious about something. In somatisation disorder it is thought that patients become excessively anxious about normal bodily sensations and seek excessive reassurance, advice and symptom relief from healthcare professionals, driven by unconscious unmet needs for care and attention. In conversion disorders, it is thought that the anxiety or distress caused by a traumatic event is 'converted' into physical symptoms to reduce levels of emotional distress.

2. It is possible to treat people with physical symptoms but no underlying physical cause when emotional or psychological factors are thought to be the cause. First, the patient's beliefs should be understood; then they should be sensitively introduced to the concept of the links between mind and body, and between emotional distress and physical symptoms. Cognitive behavioural therapy helps patients change their maladaptive patterns of response to normal bodily sensations.

3. When a patient is given a diagnosis of cancer a range of emotional responses occur, including anger and a period of sadness. However, these emotions are different to depression, which should not be considered normal for patients with cancer. Depression is not an inevitable consequence of cancer and can be effectively treated.

Chapter 12
Dementia and old-age psychiatry

Introduction 243
Case 14 Increasing forgetfulness . 244
Dementia 247
Alzheimer's disease 248

Vascular dementia 250
Other dementias 251
Mental illness in the elderly 255

Starter questions

Answers to the following questions are on page 257.

1. What is the difference between Alzheimer's disease and dementia?
2. Is dementia inherited?
3. Can dementia be cured?
4. Does depression present differently in the elderly?

Introduction

The global population is ageing, with the proportion over 60 years expected to double to 22% by 2050. Many people will enjoy the extra years brought to them by medical and social advances. However, the risk of dementia rises with age, so its prevalence is expected to continue increasing. Furthermore, some people experience psychiatric disorders such as depression and schizophrenia for the first time in old age.

Psychiatric disorders often present differently in older people, e.g. depression can present with memory loss. As forgetfulness is a common presenting complaint in older people, being able to differentiate between its causes is crucial to ensure appropriate treatment and care.

Treatment must also be adapted for the elderly population, e.g. lower doses of drugs must be used to accommodate age-associated changes in drug metabolism. Many older people are prescribed several medications for co-morbid physical health problems, and interactions with any psychiatric medications must be avoided.

In some countries, including the UK, specialist old age psychiatry teams provide mental health services to people aged 65 years and above. They work closely with other doctors, such as elderly medicine specialists.

Case 14 Increasing forgetfulness

Presentation

William Ainsley is a 71-year-old retired shopkeeper who has reluctantly come to see his general practitioner (GP). He is accompanied by his wife, who is concerned that he has become increasingly forgetful; for example, he recently forgot to pay the gas bill. Despite Mr Ainsley insisting he is well, he sometimes struggles to find the right word and forgets the GP's name during their conversation.

Initial interpretation

The many causes of forgetfulness in elderly people include normal age-associated memory changes, delirium, depression, potentially reversible physical causes (e.g. hypothyroidism, vitamin B_{12} deficiency anaemia) and dementia caused by primary neurodegenerative diseases.

Delirium is characterised by an acute onset of impaired cognition and has a fluctuating course and altered consciousness. It usually occurs with a new illness, such as a urinary tract infection. Dementia, on the other hand, has a gradual onset with progressive deterioration over months to years, usually without disruption of consciousness. More details of the onset, duration, progress over time and severity of the forgetfulness are needed.

History

Mr Ainsley says that he forgets the date but does not need to know it as he has retired. He is embarrassed to admit

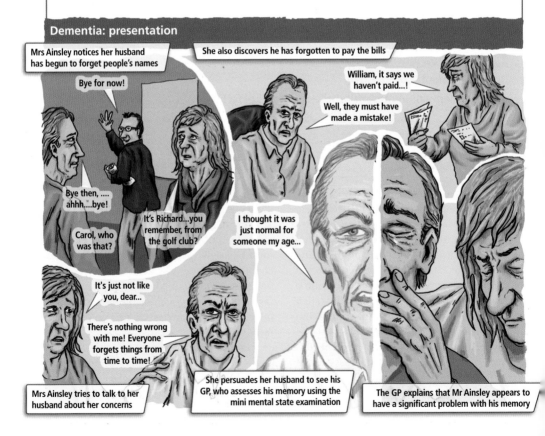

Dementia: presentation

Mrs Ainsley notices her husband has begun to forget people's names

Bye for now!

Bye then, ...ahhh....bye!

Carol, who was that?

It's Richard...you remember, from the golf club?

It's just not like you, dear...

There's nothing wrong with me! Everyone forgets things from time to time!

Mrs Ainsley tries to talk to her husband about her concerns

She also discovers he has forgotten to pay the bills

William, it says we haven't paid...!

Well, they must have made a mistake!

I thought it was just normal for someone my age...

She persuades her husband to see his GP, who assesses his memory using the mini mental state examination

The GP explains that Mr Ainsley appears to have a significant problem with his memory

Case 14 *continued*

that his wife often finds his keys in unusual places when he has misplaced them. He has to concentrate harder during conversations with his friends and has occasionally forgotten activities they have done together only the day before. He thinks these problems started gradually and have slowly worsened in the last few years.

Interpretation of history

Mr Ainsley's history of gradual-onset, progressive memory impairment with word-finding difficulties (dysphasia) is suggestive of a dementia. Other psychiatric and physical causes of memory impairment must be excluded to confirm the diagnosis. Further history taking may also identify other risk factors for dementia.

> **Patients with memory problems may not be aware of their difficulties or may try to cover them up.** A collateral history from someone who knows them is vital for making a diagnosis.

Further history

Mr Ainsley has not experienced any change in consciousness, hallucinations or mood changes. His wife confirms that he has shown no changes in personality. He has no family history of mental illness or memory problems. He is otherwise well, takes no medications, drinks one pint of beer per week and has never smoked.

> **Dementia may affect fitness to drive so always establish whether the patient is a driver.** Understandably, many patients will be reluctant to disclose their diagnosis to the relevant driving licensing authority, but they must be advised to do so.

Examination

A mental state examination (**Table 12.1**) and a mini mental state examination (**Table 12.2**) are carried out to assess Mr Ainsley's cognitive function. He loses a total of 8 marks on the MMSE, scoring 22/30. Scores of 24 or less are indicative of cognitive impairment (see page 66).

Mr Ainsley's mental state examination	
Category	Description
Appearance and behaviour	Well-kempt, but some of his shirt buttons are done up wrongly
	Mildly irritable when discussing his memory problems, otherwise calm and pleasant
Speech	Frequent pauses in speech
	Dysphasia (word-finding difficulties)
Mood	Appears euthymic
	Reactive affect
Perceptions	No abnormal perceptions
Thoughts	Takes more effort to think of how to put a sentence together
	No delusions
Cognitions	Experiencing memory problems
Insight	Thought that memory problems were part of normal ageing
Suicidal ideation	No suicidal ideas or thoughts of harming himself or others

Table 12.1 Mr Ainsley's mental state examination

Ainsley's mini mental state examination	
Category	Description
Orientation	Day, date and year incorrect (3 marks lost)
Recall	Recalls 1 of the 3 words he is asked to remember (2 marks lost)
Language	Unable to name 2 objects shown to him (2 marks lost)
Construction	Unable to accurately copy intersecting pentagons (1 mark lost)

Table 12.2 Mr Ainsley's mini mental state examination

Case 14 *continued*

A clock drawing test is carried out to identify more subtle cognitive impairments, including difficulties with executive function. Mr Ainsley makes mistakes when asked to draw the clock, add the numbers and set the hands to 10 past 11 (**Figure 12.1**).

Physical examination

The physical examination is normal apart from revealing mild word-finding difficulties. There are no signs of potentially reversible causes of memory impairment, such as anaemia or hypothyroidism, and no signs of risk factors for dementia, such as hypertension.

Interpretation of findings

Mr Ainsley has the following clinical features:

- A gradual onset of memory impairment
- Dysphasia
- Possible visuospatial difficulties (shown by the result of the clock-drawing test)
- No features suggestive of changes in mood or personality
- No features suggestive of perceptual abnormalities
- An otherwise normal physical examination

Together these features are suggestive of dementia.

Investigations

Blood tests are performed to rule out potentially reversible causes of memory impairment. The tests include urea and electrolytes, calcium, vitamin B_{12}, folate and thyroid function tests. All the results are normal (**Table 12.3**).

A CT scan of the brain is performed to look for potential causes of memory impairment, including cerebrovascular

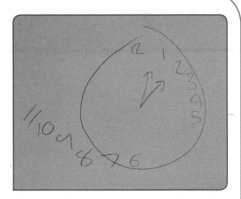

Figure 12.1 The result of Mr Ainsley's clock drawing test. The numbers are not in the correct place, nor are the hands set to the correct time. These abnormalities suggest a cognitive impairment.

Mr Ainsley's blood test results	
Test	Result (normal range)
Sodium	138 (135–145) mmol/L
Potassium	4.5 (3.5–5.3) mEq/L
Urea	6.2 (2.5–7.8) mmol/L
Calcium	2.28 (2.25–2.5) mmol/L
B12	411 (211–911) ng/L
Folate	14.9 (1.5–17.0) µg/L
Thyroid stimulating hormone	4.0 (0.4–4.5) mU/L

Table 12.3 Mr Ainsley's blood test results

disease, a chronic subdural haematoma, normal pressure hydrocephalus and neoplasms. The scan shows generalised cortical atrophy and ventricular enlargement, consistent with a diagnosis of dementia.

Diagnosis

Mr Ainsley is very upset to be told that he has signs of dementia as he thought his memory problems were part of normal ageing. The diagnosis and treatment options are explained to him, and he eventually agrees to be referred to the older people psychiatry service at the local hospital.

Dementia

Dementia is a neurodegenerative syndrome that generally affects adults >65 years old. It has a number of causes of varying prevalence (**Table 12.4**).

Clinical features

It is characterised by memory loss along with a deficit in one or more of:

- Language
- Judgement
- Planning
- Sequencing
- Abstract thinking
- Visuospatial skills personality

Patients experience a progressive deterioration in everyday skills such as washing, dressing or occupational tasks. Consciousness is not impaired (unlike in acute confusional state or delirium). Behavioural symptoms of dementia include:

- Aggression
- Wandering
- Inappropriate sexual behaviour
- Mood changes, e.g. irritability
- Symptoms of psychosis, e.g. hallucinations or persecutory delusions

Other conditions can also cause potentially treatable symptoms of memory impairment (**Table 12.5**). Some causes are potentially treatable, such as vitamin B12 deficiency with B12 supplements.

Causes of dementia	
Cause	Proportion of total dementia cases (%)
Alzheimer's disease	50–60
Vascular dementia	20–25
Mixed (Alzheimer's disease with vascular dementia)	10–20
Dementia with Lewy bodies	5
Other dementias, including frontotemporal dementia	2

Table 12.4 Prevalence of the different causes of dementia

Causes of memory impairment	
Cause	Examples
Primary neurodegenerative disorders	Alzheimer's disease
	Dementia with Lewy bodies
	Frontotemporal dementias, e.g. Pick's disease
	Parkinson's disease
	Huntington's disease
	Progressive supranuclear palsy
Vascular	Vascular dementia
	Multiple strokes
	Atrioventricular malformations
	Hyperviscosity syndromes
	Chronic subdural haematoma
Inflammatory	Systemic lupus erythematosus
	Neurosarcoidosis
	Multiple sclerosis
Infections	Variant CJD
	Neurosyphilis
	HIV
Neoplastic	Meningiomas
	Gliomas
	Lymphomas
	Metastatic disease
Trauma	Head injury, e.g. in boxers 'dementia pugilistica'
Metabolic/ Endocrine	Hypothyroidism
	Hypocalcaemia and hypercalcaemia
	Hypoglycaemia
	Uraemia
	Liver failure
	Hypopituitarism
	Cushing's syndrome
Nutritional deficiency	Vitamin B_{12} deficiency
	Folate deficiency
Toxic	Alcohol
	Heavy metals poisoning
	Carbon monoxide poisoning
	Organophosphates
Other	Normal pressure hydrocephalus
Mixed	Mixed pathologies also occur

Table 12.5 Causes of memory impairment. CJD, Creutzfeldt–Jakob disease; HIV, human immunodeficiency virus.

Diagnostic approach

Other causes of memory impairment should be rules out before a diagnosis is made; a collateral history, mental state examination, mini mental state examination, physical examination and any appropriate investigations should all be performed. If not other cause is identified, dementia is the most likely diagnosis. The type and severity are defined to ensure the correct treatment is given (outlined below).

Alzheimer's disease

Alzheimer's disease is the most common type of dementia, affecting around 15 million people across the world. Its prevalence is rising along with the expansion of the elderly population.

Alzheimer's disease usually affects people over the age of 65 years. The age-specific prevalence rates double every 5 years from 1% at the age of 65 years to around 40% at 90. It is rare in people under the age of 65 years.

Pathogenesis

Alzheimer's disease is characterised by the presence of widespread neurofibrillary tangles composed of abnormal tau proteins inside neurones and β-amyloid plaques between neurones (**Figure 12.2**). These lead to inflammation and widespread cortical atrophy with loss of cholinergic neurones. It is not known whether these changes are a cause or consequence of neuronal damage and generalised cortical atrophy, but it is thought that the degeneration of cholinergic neurones, resulting in a deficit of acetylcholine, leads to the development of cognitive impairment.

The main risk factor for Alzheimer's disease is age. Other risk factors include:

- A family history of Alzheimer's disease (Familial Alzheimer's disease is a rare inherited form, with onset of symptoms before the age of 65 years)
- A past psychiatric history of severe depression
- A past medical history of vascular risk factors, including smoking and diabetes, hypercholesterolaemia, coronary heart disease and cerebrovascular disease
- A previous head injury
- Down's syndrome

> Alzheimer's disease should be considered at a younger age in people with Down's syndrome as it presents earlier in these individuals.

Identified genetic risk factors include:

- The APOE ε4 allele at the apolipoprotein E gene locus on chromosome 19. Apolipoprotein E plays a role in the repair of nerve sheaths
- Familial Alzheimer's disease results from mutations in one or more of three genes:
  - Amyloid precursor protein (APP)

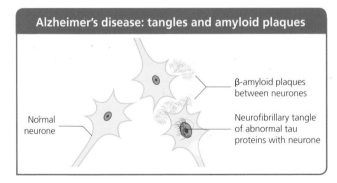

Alzheimer's disease: tangles and amyloid plaques

β-amyloid plaques between neurones

Normal neurone

Neurofibrillary tangle of abnormal tau proteins with neurone

Figure 12.2 Alzheimer's disease: aggregates of these abnormal proteins are found post-mortem within and between neurones in the brains of patients with Alzheimer's disease.

- Presenilin 1
- Presenilin 2

Clinical features

Alzheimer's disease is characterised by an insidious onset and progression of the clinical features of dementia (see page 247). There is a progressive impairment of the skills required for the activities of daily living.

Diagnostic approach

There is no single diagnostic test for Alzheimer's disease; a diagnosis is only definitively made by post-mortem examination of brain tissue, where the changes associated with Alzheimer's disease are seen (**Figure 12.2**).

The approach follows that of dementia in general (see page 247); in the UK these investigations are carried out by the patient's general practitioner. If Alzheimer's disease is suspected, the patient is then referred to a specialist old age psychiatrist for further evaluation, including CT or MRI imaging to investigate possible causes of memory impairment. Signs suggestive of Alzheimer's disease on brain imaging include widespread cortical atrophy, widened sulci and enlarged ventricles (**Figure 12.3**). If no other cause for the patient's memory impairment is found, they are diagnosed with 'probable Alzheimer's disease'.

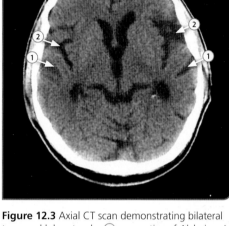

Figure 12.3 Axial CT scan demonstrating bilateral temporal lobe atrophy (1) suggestive of Alzheimer's disease. Note the prominence of Sylvian fissures (2) with increased sulcal spaces and cerebrospinal fluid spaces.

> In reminiscence therapy, patients recall and reflect on memories from their past using prompts such as photographs, music or objects. This helps provide a sense of continuity to their lives, and aims to optimise their cognitive function and quality of life.

Management

There is no cure for Alzheimer's disease. Psychological management is provided to slow the progression of the disease and to maximise the patient's quality of life. Multidisciplinary management includes:

- Psychological treatments
- Speech and language therapy
- Occupational therapy
- Physiotherapy
- Support from social services for patients and carers
- Other therapies used to reduce the patient's distress include reminiscence therapy, aromatherapy, animal-assisted therapy and music therapy.

Medication

Medication is cognition enhancing and aims to slow down the progression of symptoms. The acetylcholinesterase inhibitors donepezil, galantamine and rivastigmine are used in mild to moderate Alzheimer's disease (see Chapter 2). Memantine, an N-methyl-d-aspartate (NMDA)-receptor antagonist, blocks excess glutamate activity to reduce symptoms associated with Alzheimer's disease. It is used for patients with moderate disease who cannot tolerate acetylcholinesterase inhibitors and those with severe disease.

Other appropriate medications are used to target co-morbidities, including depression and anxiety.

Prognosis

Alzheimer's disease patients frequently move to permanent residential or nursing home care. The average survival from diagnosis is 5–10 years.

Vascular dementia

Vascular dementia is the second most common type of dementia. It is caused by various vascular diseases that result in areas of cerebral ischaemia or haemorrhage:

- Arteriosclerosis:
  - Large vessels
  - Small vessels
- Emboli
- Intracranial haemorrhage
- Amyloid angiopathies
- Genetic syndromes, e.g. cerebral autosomal dominant arteriopathy with subcortical infarcts and leukoencephalopathy (CADASIL)

The prevalence increases with age. It is also higher in men and in individuals of African-Caribbean and south Asian ethnicity. Other risk factors are:

- Smoking
- Diabetes
- Hypertension
- Hypercholesterolaemia
- A history of cardiovascular disease, cerebrovascular disease or coagulation disorders

> Distinguishing between vascular and Alzheimer's dementia is difficult. The Hachinski Ischaemic Score is a set of seven yes/no questions regarding clinical features that is used to identify whether there is a vascular component to the dementia. Approximately 50% of patients with Alzheimer's disease also have vascular dementia (mixed dementia).

Clinical features

Vascular dementia is characterised by an abrupt onset of dementia symptoms (which may occur after a stroke) with evidence of cerebrovascular disease on examination or brain imaging. There is stepwise progression, with distinct periods of worsening of symptoms that occur after further episodes of brain infarction.

The clinical features vary depending on which lobe of the brain has been affected. Unlike in Alzheimer's disease, mood and behaviour changes commonly occur early on.

On examination, there may be signs of cardiovascular risk factors, including hypertension. Focal neurological deficits may be noted on neurological examination.

Blood tests may reveal the presence of risk factors for vascular dementia, including a raised fasting glucose level (suggestive of diabetes) or hypercholesterolaemia.

Patients receive brain imaging with CT or MRI to exclude other intracranial causes of their symptoms, e.g. neoplasm. Vascular dementia is characterised by multiple infarcts on brain imaging (**Figure 12.4**).

Management

There is no cure for vascular dementia. Treatment focuses on the underlying vascular disease risk factors and on maximising the patient's quality of life.

Medication

Appropriate medication is prescribed to modify underlying vascular disease risk factors such as hypertension, diabetes, and hypercholesterolaemia. These reduce the risk of further episodes of brain infarction and slow the rate of progression of vascular dementia.

Other medications are used to treat co-morbid symptoms, including depression, anxiety and agitation.

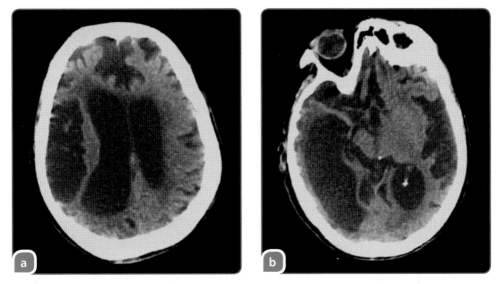

Figure 12.4 Axial CT scans at two levels demonstrating (a) bilateral infarcts (widespread low-density regions) and (b) cerebral atrophy consistent with vascular dementia.

Prognosis

The average survival from diagnosis is 4 years. One third of patients die from complications of vascular dementia, one third from cerebrovascular disease and one third from other causes, such as ischaemic heart disease or renal dysfunction.

Other dementias

Differentiating between Alzheimer's disease, vascular dementia and other types of dementia allows appropriate management to be instituted depending upon the underlying pathology.

Dementia with Lewy bodies

Dementia with Lewy bodies is the third most frequent cause of dementia. Its prevalence increases with age, although the cause of is unknown. There are no known modifiable genetic or environmental risk factors.

Pathogenesis

Lewy bodies, eosinophilic intracytoplasmic neuronal inclusion bodies that contain abnormal aggregations of α-synuclein, are found in the cerebral cortex and substantia nigra (**Figure 12.5**). This leads to a loss of cholinergic neurones (similar to Alzheimer's disease) and dopaminergic neurones (similar to

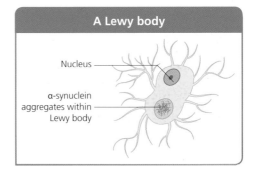

Figure 12.5 Lewy bodies are seen within neuronal cell bodies in both Parkinson's disease and dementia with Lewy bodies. They are composed of the protein α-synuclein.

Parkinson's disease). This results in reduced neurotransmission and areas of cerebral atrophy, which in turn cause cognitive decline.

Clinical features

The disease is progressive, with a gradual worsening of the key clinical features over a period of several years:

- Fluctuating levels of alertness
- Visual hallucinations that are usually recurrent, well formed and detailed
- Parkinsonism, including rigidity, bradykinesia, tremor, abnormal gait and balance difficulties
- Falls
- Sleep problems
- Mood changes including depression and apathy.

Diagnostic approach

The diagnostic approach is the same as for other causes of dementia. Early onset of of visual hallucinations and sleep problems, and signs of parkinsonism are suggestive of dementia with Lewy bodies.

Investigations

Specialised investigations are used to differentiate dementia with Lewy bodies from Alzheimer's disease and vascular dementia. Dementia with Lewy bodies is confirmed when a reduction in dopaminergic neurones is revealed by specialised brain scans, including:

- Dopaminergic iodine-123 radiolabelled 2β-carbomethoxy-3β-(4-iodophenyl)-N-(3-fluoropropyl) nortropane (FP-CIT) SPECT scans
- Meta-iodobenzylguanidine (MIBG) scintigraphy

Management

There is no cure. However, medication, social support, occupational therapy and physiotherapy are used to maximise the person's skills, functioning and quality of life.

Medication

Cholinesterase inhibitors such as rivastigmine help the cognitive decline and hallucinations. Antipsychotic medications should not be used to treat hallucinations because these can produce severe sensitivity reactions, including irreversible Parkinsonism, impaired consciousness and an increased risk of death.

Dopaminergic drugs, such as levodopa, are used to treat movement problems. Getting the right balance of drug treatments is difficult: medications given to improve cognitive abilities or hallucinations can worsen movement problems, and vice versa.

The average survival from diagnosis is around 8 years.

Frontotemporal dementias

Frontotemporal dementias are less common than the above-mentioned forms of dementia. They are characterised by atrophy and dysfunction of the frontal and temporal lobes. Pick's disease was previously used to describe all types of frontotemporal dementias, but it is now clear that this is one form of frontotemporal dementia.

Unlike other forms of dementia, frontotemporal dementias usually affect a younger age group, typically presenting between the ages

Clinical features of frontotemporal dementia	
Type	Features
Behavioural changes	Early disinhibition and loss of insight
	Impulsivity
	Hyperorality (e.g. craving sweet or fatty foods)
Mood changes	Emotional blunting
	Apathy
	Depression
Language abnormalities	Echolalia
	Perseveration
	Telegraphic speech
	Dysphasia

Table 12.6 Clinical features of frontotemporal dementia

of 45 and 60 years. The prominent clinical features (**Table 12.6**) develop gradually over several months.

Pathogenesis

The cause of most frontotemporal dementias is not known. However, a specific pathology is seen in Pick's disease, which is characterised by the presence of Pick bodies (abnormal aggregates of tau, ubiquitin and other proteins) within ballooned neurones (Pick cells) in the frontal and temporal lobes. This results in inflammation and atrophy of neurones in the temporal and frontal lobes.

Diagnostic approach

Pick's disease can only be definitively identified on autopsy, when Pick bodies are found in brain tissue. Therefore, in clinical practice patients with Pick's disease or other forms of frontotemporal dementia are given a general diagnosis of frontotemporal dementia. The diagnostic approach follows that of dementia in general (see page 247). Frontotemporal dementias are suggested by echolalia and perseveration on mental state examination.

A neurological examination may reveal rigidity and bradykinesia. Primitive reflexes are normally present only in infancy, and are an abnormal sign in adulthood. They include:

- **The palmomental reflex**, in which there is contraction of the ipsilateral chin muscle in response to stroking the patient's palm from the proximal to the distal thenar eminence
- **The palmar grasp reflex**, in which the patient's fingers flex in response to stroking the palm of their hand.
- **The snout reflex**, in which gentle pressure applied to the philtrum results in an upward movement of the chin and lips into a pouting position.

Investigations

Asymmetrical atrophy of the temporal and frontal lobes on CT or MRI scanning is suggestive of frontotemporal dementia.

Management

There is no cure, but a multidisciplinary approach is taken to optimise patients' quality of life. Speech and language therapy is particularly important to manage communication difficulties, which can frustrate and agitate the patient when their attempts to communicate with their carers or others are not understood.

Medication

No medications are yet available to slow the progression of frontotemporal dementia.

Prognosis

The average survival from diagnosis is around 8–10 years, although there is much variation.

Prion diseases

Prion diseases are a rare group of diseases in which abnormal prion proteins aggregate in the brain causing neuronal cell death. This results in small vacuoles in the brain that have a characteristic spongiform appearance on histology. Normal prion proteins help to protect neurones from injury; abnormal prion proteins are the result of a mutation to the prion protein gene on chromosome 20.

Creutzfeld–Jakob disease (CJD)

This is the main human prion disease. It is characterised by dementia which progresses rapidly over 6–8 months, with ataxia and myoclonic jerks. Around 85% of cases of CJD are sporadic. In these cases, it is thought that a normal prion protein spontaneously changes into an abnormal form, or that there is a spontaneous mutation of the prion gene leading to the production of abnormal prions proteins. Sporadic CJD usually affects adults in their 50s. There is no cure, and the average survival time from the onset of symptoms is around 6 months. In less than 5% of cases, CJD is inherited as an autosomal dominant disorder.

Iatrogenic CJD

This is very rare. Most cases are transmitted via contaminated tissue grafts, neurosurgery instruments or pituitary-derived growth hormone.

New-variant CJD

This is another rare form of CJD, thought to be transmitted via infected meat products. It tends to affect young adults, who present with mild depression or anxiety before developing dementia and ataxia. As with other forms of CJD, there is no cure. Survival is around 1–2 years from the onset of symptoms.

Huntington's disease

Huntington's disease, also called Huntington's chorea, is an inherited neurodegenerative disease and a rare cause of dementia, with a prevalence of between four and seven per 100,000. It has a mean age of onset of 30–50 years.

Aetiology

Huntington's disease is an autosomal dominant disorder caused by a trinucleotide repeat of the CAG codon within the huntingtin gene on chromosome 4 that leads to the production of abnormal huntingtin protein. It is unclear how this causes damage to brain cells, but its presence is associated with cell death, particularly in the basal ganglia, causing the characteristic motor symptoms. Non-affected individuals have fewer than 30 CAG repeats whereas those with Huntington's disease have 36 or more copies.

Clinical features

Huntington's disease shows almost complete penetrance, i.e. the disease develops in all carriers of the mutation. It also shows anticipation, which is an earlier age of onset in successive generations as the expansion length increases with each generation.

It is characterised by cognitive deterioration and choreiform movements. These may be subtle at first, presenting as fidgeting or fleeting facial grimaces, but progressively worsen over several years. Common behavioural features include:

- Apathy
- Low mood
- Irritability
- Poor self-care
- Social withdrawal
- Paranoia

Motor features include:
- Bradykinesia
- Spasticity
- Extensor plantar reflexes
- An inability to sustain tongue protrusion

Investigations

Genetic testing is used to confirm a diagnosis of Huntington's disease.

> **Genetic testing can be offered to affected families to predict Huntington's disease.** However, given the untreatable, progressive and familial nature of the disease, this requires extensive genetic counselling beforehand.

Management

There is no cure for Huntington's disease. It is hoped that treatments with neural and stem cell transplantation will eventually be developed.

Multidisciplinary management focuses on physical and emotional support for patients and carers. Symptomatic treatments include psychological treatments to address the often profound psychological symptoms. Speech and language therapy is used to improve communication. Physiotherapy and occupational therapy are used to improve movement and day-to-day living skills.

Prognosis

Prognosis varies, but average survival time is between 10–25 years from onset of symptoms.

Mental illness in the elderly

Common mental illnesses in older adults include depression, anxiety disorders and late-onset schizophrenia. For these disorders, there are often differences in presentation in older and younger age groups.

Furthermore, many elderly people take a combination of medications for co-morbid health problems, and these can also affect their mood and behaviour.

> **Always consider underlying mental illness in elderly patients presenting with somatic symptoms that cannot otherwise be explained.**

Clinical features of memory loss in depression and dementia	
Depression	Dementia
Acute onset	Insidious onset
Biological symptoms of depression	Short-term memory particularly poor
Family or personal history of depression	Flat/blunted effect on MSE
Patient's subjective reports of memory loss worse than objective measures	Patient minimises memory problems, carers more concerned than patient
'Don't know' answers on MMSE	Attempts to give answers on MMSE

Table 12.7 Clinical features of memory problems in depression (pseudodementia) and dementia

Depression

Rates of depression in older adults in the community are similar to those in younger people. However, they are higher in elderly people in hospital with physical health problems. Untreated depression in these patients can slow their recovery and rehabilitation.

Clinical features

Depression in older adults may present with the same features as in younger patients (see page 109). However, some elderly patients present atypically with more somatic symptoms, such as fatigue, insomnia, hypochondriasis and pseudodementia. In the latter, severely depressed patients report difficulties remembering and concentrating, but have no major objective memory impairment. Differentiating between depressive pseudodementia and dementia is difficult (**Table 12.7**).

> **Always ask about suicidal ideation in elderly people in whom the diagnosis of depression is a possibility,** as the risk of suicide is particularly high in this population.

Diagnostic approach

Physical disorders and dementia must be excluded. Mood changes can occur as a side effect of medications. An alcohol history is vital for detecting alcohol misuse.

> **Do not assume that older people are unlikely to drink alcohol.** Physical ill-health, bereavement, social isolation and boredom are common in elderly people who drink alcohol to cope with these difficulties.

The Geriatric Depression Scale can be used to screen for depression in older adults. It is a set of 30 yes/no questions, each scored as 0 or 1. Scores of 0–9 are normal; scores of 10 and above indicate depression.

Management

A biopsychosocial approach to management is vital. Antidepressants should be started at a low dose and increased slowly because age-related changes in glomerular filtration rate, plasma albumin levels and body fat composition affect drug metabolism, resulting in higher tissue concentrations in elderly patients.

Psychological interventions, such as cognitive behavioural therapy, may be offered. Electroconvulsive therapy is considered for those with life-threatening stupor or severe agitation. It is also used when drug treatment has been ineffective. Psychosocial factors perpetuating depression, such as isolation and a lack of support, must also be addressed.

Prognosis

Older adult patients take longer to respond to antidepressants, with improvements in symptoms usually taking up to 6–8 weeks to begin. Prognosis is better in those with an onset before the age of 70 years. Indicators of a poorer prognosis include poor concordance with antidepressant treatment and co-morbid physical illness. Older adults with depression also have a high risk of suicide.

Anxiety

Anxiety disorders can present for the first time after the age of 65 years. In this age group, features of anxiety disorders and depression may overlap. Medications, alcohol abuse and physical disorders may also mimic symptoms of anxiety. Differentiating these requires a thorough physical and psychological evaluation.

Elderly patients with anxiety disorders often present with hypochondriasis.

Diagnostic approach

The medical causes of symptoms of anxiety, for example thyroid disorder or arrhythmias, must be excluded (see page 153). Side effects of medication and an excessive use of alcohol must also be ruled out.

Depression is an important differential diagnosis as symptoms of anxiety can arise secondary to depression in elderly people.

Management

Psychological interventions such as cognitive behavioural therapy, and medications such as selective serotonin reuptake inhibitors, are used to manage the symptoms.

Late-onset schizophrenia

Late-onset schizophrenia is a rare condition in which symptoms of psychosis develop for the first time in people over the age of 60

years. It accounts for around 0.5% of all cases of schizophrenia.

Aetiology

The cause of late-onset schizophrenia is unclear. Personality traits, including a paranoid or schizoid personality disorder, and social isolation are more common in those who go on to develop late-onset schizophrenia. Sensory impairments, such as deafness or visual loss, are also more frequent.

> **Elderly patients with impaired eyesight may develop florid, well-formed visual hallucinations as a consequence of visual loss with no other symptoms of psychosis, delirium or dementia.** This is Charles Bonnet syndrome and must be distinguished from late-onset schizophrenia as it does not require treatment with antipsychotic medication, but responds to behavioural techniques, such as performing series of particular eye movements

Clinical features

Patients with late-onset schizophrenia have fewer negative symptoms than younger people with the disorder (see page 133). There is also less evidence of formal thought disorder. Features commonly seen in late-onset schizophrenia include:

- Delusions – typically persecutory or grandiose
- Partition delusions – a fixed false belief that objects, people or radiation can pass through things that would normally be a barrier to them, e.g. walls
- Auditory hallucinations (e.g. third person, derogatory, running commentary)
- Visual hallucinations
- Tactile hallucinations
- Olfactory hallucinations

Diagnostic approach

Dementia and disorders that cause symptoms mimicking first-episode schizophrenia in elderly people (e.g. delirium) must be excluded.

Brain imaging is used to exclude other intracranial pathology, such as space-occupying lesions. A careful mental state examination is needed to exclude other psychiatric diagnoses, for example mood disorders with psychotic features and delusional disorder.

Management

Patients with late-onset schizophrenia can be hard to engage. A key task of community psychiatric nurses working with the patient is therefore to develop a therapeutic rapport, with the aim of improving concordance with medications and psychosocial interventions.

As in younger adults with schizophrenia, antipsychotic medication is used (see page 85), taking into consideration the physiological changes affecting drug metabolism in elderly people.

Answers to starter questions

1. Dementia is an umbrella term used to describe a syndrome characterised by memory impairment with additional cognitive deficits, and it has many causes. Alzheimer's disease is the most common cause.

2. Genetic factors play a role in some forms of dementia. Inherited autosomal dominant mutations in one of three genes (APP, presenilin 1 and presenilin 2) can result in familial Alzheimer's disease, a rare form of Alzheimer's disease. Other genetic risk factors for Alzheimer's disease include the APOE ε4 allele and Down's syndrome (trisomy 21). Huntington's disease can also cause dementia and genetic testing is available for members of affected families.

3. There is no specific cure for dementia. However, medications are prescribed in addition to psychosocial interventions to slow the progression of some types of dementia, such as Alzheimer's disease, (e.g. acetylcholinesterase inhibitors) and, in some cases, to treat associated mood and behavioural symptoms (e.g. antipsychotics and antidepressants).

4. Although some of the features of depression that characterise it in younger people are seen in the elderly, presentation is often atypical in those over 65 years of age. In this age group, patients with depression present with more somatic symptoms, such as insomnia, fatigue, or with hypochondriasis or pseudodementia-subjective memory impairment not confirmed on examination and investigation.

Chapter 13
Child and adolescent psychiatry

Introduction 259
Case 15 Disruptive behaviour in a
      5-year-old 260
Developmental disorders 262
Behavioural disorders 265
Emotional disorders. 269

Starter questions

Answers to the following questions are on page 270.

1. Why is disruptive behaviour in a child suggestive of abuse?
2. Why is ADHD diagnosed more frequently in boys?
3. Why are autism spectrum disorder and ADHD difficult to tell apart?
4. What is the difference between a child behaving badly and conduct disorder?

Introduction

Many children experience behavioural or emotional problems that lead their parents to seek advice. In preschool age children (under 5 years), these concerns often revolve around tantrums, potty training and sleep. In older children, anxiety, problems with school, hyperactivity and conduct disorders become more prevalent. Teenagers experience similar problems to adults, but often with different presentations.

It should be remembered during the assessment that it is usually the parents or carers who seek help rather than the child. It may in fact be the parents who need support rather than the child. All children should also have a developmental assessment when considering what could be abnormal behaviour for their age.

The treatment of children is often different from that of adults. Fewer medications and more behavioural interventions and psychological therapies are used. Very few psychotropic medications are licensed for children; for many medications, such as most antidepressants, the risk of side effects outweighs the benefits.

> If a child's problems only manifest at home, it is likely to represent problems with parenting rather than a formal mental health condition in the child.

Case 15 Disruptive behaviour in a 5-year-old

Presentation

Jake Stevens is a 5-year-old boy who is brought to the general practitioner's surgery by his mother, Carol, who is concerned about his behaviour. Jake is in his first year at school and is frequently in trouble for being disruptive and ignoring instructions. At home, he is chaotic and difficult to manage. Carol has stopped taking him out to the shops because she is worried he will run off or damage something. While she is speaking, Jake is climbing on the furniture and exploring the room.

Initial interpretation

A history of disruptive behaviour, restlessness and poor attention starting in early childhood suggests that attention deficit hyperactivity disorder (ADHD) is the most likely diagnosis. There are, however, other possible causes that must be ruled out (**Table 13.1**).

> For a diagnosis of ADHD, the symptoms should be noticeable in more than one environment, for example both at home and at school.

History

Carol's pregnancy and Jake's birth were uncomplicated. Jake achieved his developmental milestones appropriately, and his eating, weight and sleep have all been good. As a toddler, Jake was friendly and

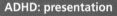

ADHD: presentation

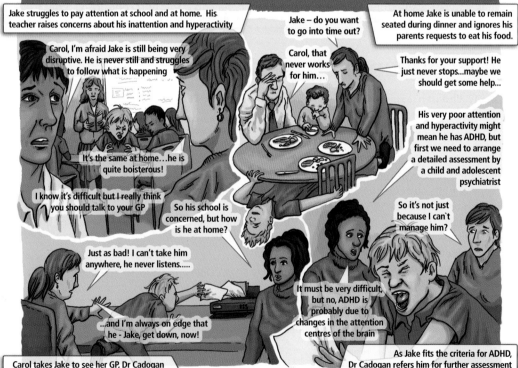

Case 15 *continued*

Differential diagnoses for ADHD	
Psychological	Physical
Anxiety	Hyperthyroidism
Abuse	Epilepsy
Sleep disturbance	Diabetes
Autism spectrum disorder	Neurological conditions, e.g. neurofibromatosis

Table 13.1 Differential diagnoses for attention deficit hyperactivity disorder (ADHD)

affectionate but 'boisterous'.

Carol first started to think Jake was different from other children when he was 3. There was no sudden change in his behaviour and no incidents that could have been considered stressful.

She noticed that Jake climbed and jumped around much more than other children, especially when they were eating or reading a story. Jake never sat down for more than a few minutes and would wriggle and tip over his seat when required to sit still. He is not aggressive and plays energetic games happily with other children. Carol feels he is quite bright for his age but will not focus, so she worries he might fall behind at school.

Jake lives with his mum, older sister and father. There is no history of mental illness or similar problems in the family. Jake has no medical problems and is not taking any medications.

Interpretation of history

Jake has no developmental delay, which could indicate autism spectrum disorder (ASD) or a neurological condition. He is not overly aggressive and has no symptoms of anxiety, making a conduct or emotional disorder unlikely. His restlessness and hyperactivity started at an early age without a particular trigger, such as an unstable family life, so ADHD remains the most likely diagnosis.

Many parents ask whether food allergies, additives and excess sugar cause ADHD. There is inadequate evidence to suggest that reducing the intake of sugar or additives will reduce symptoms of ADHD in a child who has no clear evidence of an allergy. However, a healthy diet should always be encouraged.

Examination

Jake is on the 50th centile for weight and height. On examination, there are no unusual bruises or marks suggestive of physical abuse. His cardiovascular, neurological and abdominal examinations are unremarkable. This reduces the possibility of his behaviour being due to a physical cause.

Diagnosis

On the basis of the history and physical examination, ADHD is the most likely diagnosis (**Figure 13.1**). The GP refers Jake to the child and adolescent mental health unit for further assessment. She requests a school report on Jake's behaviour because for a diagnosis to be made ADHD should be present in more than one setting. She also discusses with Carol behavioural strategies to help Jake, such as breaking tasks into smaller parts that do not require sustained attention.

Case 15 *continued*

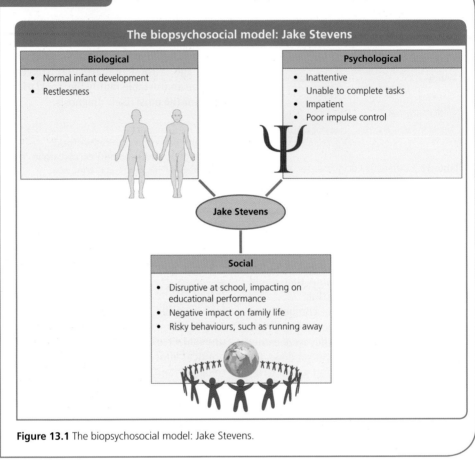

Figure 13.1 The biopsychosocial model: Jake Stevens.

Developmental disorders

Disorders of psychological development cover specific difficulties which only affect one area, for example with speech, movement, and scholastic skills such as reading, writing and maths (**Table 13.2**). Developmental disorders also include more pervasive conditions, the most common being autism spectrum disorder (ASD).

Autism spectrum disorder

ASD affects a range of areas including communication, intelligence and social abilities.

Epidemiology

ASD affects approximately 5–15 people per 1000, with men four times more likely to be diagnosed than women. The prevalence of ASD has been increasing significantly over the last 30 years – in 1990 only one person per 1000 was diagnosed.

The increase in ASD is probably due to improved public and clinical awareness. However, it has also been suggested that the increase is linked to environmental factors such as the increasing use of chemicals in farming.

Types of developmental disorders				
Condition	Prevalence (UK)	Aetiology	Signs and symptoms	Treatment
Dyslexia	10%	Genetic changes in the left hemisphere of the brain	Difficulty in reading, spelling and processing words	Educational support, reading from coloured paper
Dyscalculia	5%	Some genetic link. Environmental factors, e.g. alcohol consumption in pregnancy	Difficulty in conceptualising or manipulating numbers, poor spatial awareness	Educational support
Dyspraxia	4–6%	Abnormal motor neurone connections	Delayed motor milestones, poor co-ordination, slow and/or unsteady movements	Occupational and speech therapy

Table 13.2 Common types of specific developmental disorders

Aetiology

ASD has no single cause but is the result of a complex interaction between genes and the environment. Genetic factors place a large role: if one child in a family has ASD, the chance of a sibling having it is 20–40 times higher than average. ASD can also occur as a result of genetic syndromes such as Rett's, fragile X or Down's syndrome. Environmental factors include:

- Exposure to certain chemicals in utero, e.g. the anti-epilepsy medication sodium valproate or alcohol
- Premature birth (before 35 weeks)
- Hypoxia at birth

Patients with ASD have been found to have abnormally high numbers of connections between their cerebral cortex (which processes thoughts and consciousness) and their limbic system (which processes emotions). This could result in people with ASD having an extreme emotional response to minor changes in their thoughts.

> **Vaccination rates fell sharply when a media scare linked the mumps–measles–rubella (MMR) vaccine with development of ASD.** Massive epidemiological studies disproving any link were given little coverage by much of the media until the original study that had prompted the alarm was demonstrated to be flawed and unethical. The vaccine does not raise risk of ASD.

Clinical features

Mild ASD is known as Asperger's syndrome (**Figure 13.2**). Patients may have average or above average intelligence and have no

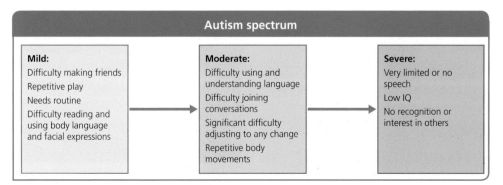

Figure 13.2 The spectrum of autism. Symptoms range from mild (Asperger's syndrome) to severe.

speech delay. They often have a good level of functioning. Children with more severe ASD have below average intelligence and have delayed or little speech, requiring a significant level of care.

Features of ASD should always be present from before the age of 3. To be diagnosed with Asperger's syndrome, there must be no cognitive or language delay. Otherwise the symptoms are the same as for ASD (**Table 13.3**). Only one of the core features has to be present for a diagnosis of ASD to be made, and there is no one symptom that is pathognomonic.

Diagnostic approach

There is no one test for ASD. The diagnosis should always be made by a specialist paediatrician or psychiatrist. An assessment is made of the child's interactions and play activities. **Figure 13.3** shows an abnormal way of playing with farm animals, lining them up along the edge of a play mat. This contrasts with **Figure 13.4**, where the play is more appropriate: the farm animals are being played with imaginatively using the play mat.

A detailed history should be taken from the parents. This should include the pregnancy, birth (looking for complications such as hypoxia at birth or postnatal depression in the mother), development and current symptoms. Consider the possibility of abuse or severe neglect as this can cause similar symptoms.

> **Severe neglect and/or abuse from a very early age can cause a child to have many of the symptoms of ASD.** Depending on the length of the neglect, these may be only partially reversible even with support and removal from the abusive situation.

Investigations

There is no specific investigation for ASD. Assessment employs the Autism Diagnostic Interview-Revised, Autism Diagnostic Observation Schedule and often an intelligence quotient test.

A full examination is conducted to look for dysmorphic features and disorders such as neurofibromatosis and tuberous sclerosis which can cause autism spectrum disorder. Any

Symptoms of autism spectrum disorder	
Core features	**Symptoms**
Abnormal social interaction	Poor eye contact or use of facial expressions
	Difficulty making or keeping friends
	Doesn't respond to emotions
Abnormal communication	Delayed or absent speech
	Difficulty holding a conversation
	Repetition of words/phrases
	Abnormal pitch or rhythm
Abnormal behaviour	Repetitive or intense interest in restricted patterns of 'play' or parts of a play object
	Compulsion to observe rituals or routines
	Repetitive movements
	Distress over small changes in environment

Table 13.3 Symptoms of autism spectrum disorder

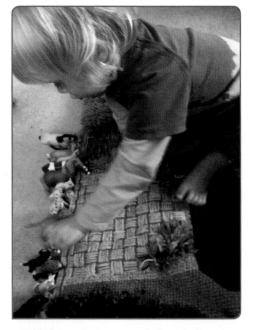

Figure 13.3 Play with farm animals that could indicate ASD. The child lines up the animals on the edge of the play mat and shows no imaginative play.

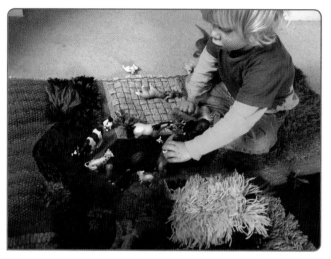

Figure 13.4 Appropriate play with farm animals. The child uses the animals to play imaginatively, assigning characteristics to the animals and making them interact.

evidence of abuse should be noted. Impaired hearing can cause speech delay so a hearing test and speech and language assessment are usually conducted. A diagnosis is made after excluding other conditions or disorders such as anxiety or attachment problems.

Management

There is no cure for ASD (including Asperger's syndrome), therefore, the aim of management is to improve the child's quality of life using interventions to target the biopsychosocial aspects of their condition.

Social interventions aim to improve social interactions, reduce stress on the family and reduce problem behaviours. They are tailored to the child's needs. For example, a child with Asperger's syndrome may be managed with extra support in school. Conversely, a child with severe ASD may require a residential placement with 24-hour care.

Psychological interventions include behavioural therapy and training in social skills. This can be at a basic level such as eating habits or at a more complex level such as peer relationships. Children with ASD often receive speech therapy to improve their communication skills.

Biological interventions include medications such as low-dose risperidone to help manage associated problematic behaviours, for example aggression or self-harm. However, they do not reduce the severity of the ASD.

Some ASD symptoms reduce in severity with targeted treatment or as the person adapts to their condition.

Behavioural disorders

Many parents have some difficulties with their child's behaviour. Behavioural disorders are, however, more pervasive and have a significant impact on the child's ability to function and their family's ability to cope.

The two most common disorders seen in children and adolescents are:

- Conduct disorder
- Attention deficit hyperactivity disorder (ADHD)

ADHD is now thought to be a developmental behavioural disorder reflecting a large underlying genetic component

Conduct disorder

Conduct disorder is characterised by a pervasive and repetitive disregard for social norms beyond what would be considered 'bad behaviour' compared with peers of the same age. Conduct disorder often develops into antisocial personality disorder in adulthood (see page 181). Oppositional defiant disorder is a milder version of conduct disorder that involves no criminality or cruelty to animals.

Epidemiology

Conduct disorder (including oppositional defiant disorder) occurs in 5% of children aged between 5 and 16 years. It is three times more common in boys than girls. Around 40% of these children have suffered abuse or significant disruption of their family life.

Aetiology

Conduct disorder shows evidence of a genetic link, with heritability around 40–50%. However, there is a stronger association with environmental factors, including:

- A reduction in time the parent is able to dedicate to the child
- Poor or unpredictable boundary setting
- Inadequate supervision of the child
- Experienced or witnessed abuse

> **Having a difficult temperament is linked to the development of conduct disorder.** However, it is difficult to demonstrate a cause and effect relationship as the child's temperament is, at least in part, dictated by the parenting style.

Clinical features

Conduct disorder can start in young children, usually with severe tantrums and a persistent challenging of boundaries (**Figure 13.5**). However, it usually does not manifest until late childhood or early adolescence. Behavioural features include:

- Being very argumentative or deliberately disobedient
- A short temper
- Appearing spiteful or vindictive in their actions
- Physical acts of cruelty to others or animals
- Stealing, damaging property and arson, which may result in juvenile detention

Diagnostic approach

A history from the child and their parent or carer should exclude other psychiatric conditions such as schizophrenia, bipolar disorder or ADHD. Drug and alcohol use must also be assessed, although misuse of substances does not necessarily rule out a diagnosis of conduct disorder as the two often occur together. Any signs of ongoing abuse must also be identified.

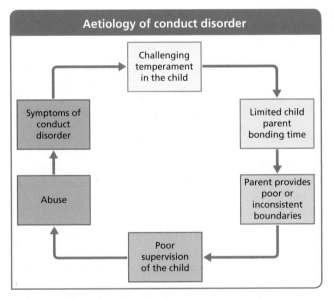

Figure 13.5 Aetiology of conduct disorder.

> **Conduct disordered behaviour will usually precede any drug or alcohol abuse.** If there were no signs before the drug or alcohol abuse, this may be causing the behavioural problems. Alternatively, the need to acquire drugs or alcohol may be leading the child to behave in this way.

Investigations

An examination should be conducted to identify any medical conditions that cause similar symptoms like disruptive or oppositional behaviour. These include hyperthyroidism, diabetes or neurological conditions such as epilepsy. A urinary drug screen can be useful if drug use is suspected.

Management

As conduct disorder does not have a significant biological basis, management focuses on psychological and social interventions. The two main focuses are:

- Parent training, which focuses on improving interactions and providing consistent boundaries
- Child-focused interventions, which use cognitive behavioural therapy to help the child improve their self-control and positive social skills

Attention deficit hyperactivity disorder

ADHD is characterised by pervasive inattention and hyperactivity. Symptoms present from 3–4 years old but are usually not detected until the child needs to show sustained attention, for example when they start school. The symptoms of ADHD usually reduce with age as children gain more control over their actions and thoughts. However, 25–33% of people with ADHD require treatment into adulthood.

Epidemiology

ADHD has a prevalence of around 3% in 5–15-year-olds in the UK. There is a 3:1 ratio of boys to girls. This could in part be attributed to cultural bias and also to how ADHD presents in girls. In many cultures, girls are encouraged from an early age to be less disruptive or active than boys. As they are encouraged to have interests that encompass nurturing and socialising, the symptoms of ADHD are more likely to go undiagnosed.

Aetiology

ADHD has a strong genetic component: the siblings of a child with ADHD are four to five times more likely than average to develop it themselves. Other risk factors include:

- Exposure to chemicals in utero, e.g. cigarette smoke and alcohol
- Premature birth
- Birth complications, e.g. hypoxia or a low birth weight

Clinical features

The three core features of ADHD are:

- Impulsivity
- Inattention
- Hyperactivity

The signs of these are shown in **Table 13.4**. In girls, the symptoms may be more subtle, such as disorganisation or a propensity to daydream.

> **ADHD is more common in the USA.** This may be because the Diagnostic and Statistical Manual, used in the USA, requires only signs of inattention or of hyperactivity with impulsivity to make a diagnosis. In contrast, the International Classification of Diseases, used in Europe, requires all three criteria to be present.

Diagnostic approach

The mainstay of diagnosis is a detailed developmental history and assessment of current symptoms. The symptoms must be present in more than one setting, so the child's behaviour in school is usually also observed.

Symptoms and signs of ADHD	
Symptoms	Signs
Inattention	Easily distracted
	Changes play frequently
	Tasks unfinished
Hyperactivity	Excess running/climbing
	Fidgeting
	Leaves seat often
Increased impulsivity	Can't wait in turn
	Interrupts

Table 13.4 Signs and symptoms of ADHD

Investigations

A full physical examination must rule out other possible medical causes, including problems with hearing (which could explain inattention). There is no specific test for ADHD, although a questionnaire (the Connors questionnaire) is often used to aid diagnosis. Using this, teachers and parents rate the child's behaviour on a series of scales that are then scored. The score indicates how likely it is the child has ADHD.

A school assessment will show the child's behaviour in a different setting. It can also help to know which behaviours are a particular problem at school when considering treatment.

> Using stimulant medication in an overactive child seems counter-intuitive. However, it works by stimulating the child's attention centres, therefore increasing their ability to focus.

Management

Initially, psychosocial interventions are used, including support for the parent and school to minimise the impact on the child's functioning. This can involve teaching techniques such as:

- Giving the child frequent breaks from tasks to exercise
- Breaking large tasks into smaller chunks (**Figure 13.6**)
- Managing behavioural problems, e.g. aggression or impulsivity

Older children may also receive some skills training to help them control some of their symptoms and improve their understanding of ADHD.

Medication

Methylphenidate (Ritalin) is used for symptom control when the interventions above have not prevented significant disruption. It increases dopamine in the brain thus strengthening the signals of neurones involved with attention. Methylphenidate is a derivative of amphetamine, which means it may be abused or sold on the black market. An alternative is atomoxetine, which is not an amphetamine derivative, and therefore has less potential to be abused or resold.

The side effects of medication include poor appetite, growth retardation and changes in heart rate or blood pressure. Before starting medication, the child's height, weight, pulse and blood pressure should be measured. These should be monitored regularly while the child remains on the medication to ensure any side effects are identified before they cause harm.

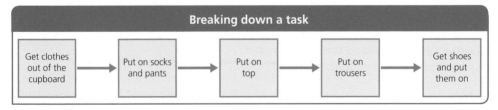

Breaking down a task

| Get clothes out of the cupboard | → | Put on socks and pants | → | Put on top | → | Put on trousers | → | Get shoes and put them on |

Figure 13.6 Breaking down the task 'get dressed' to help a child with ADHD.

Emotional disorders

Emotional disorders encompass all anxiety and mood disorders (such as depression). Between 5% and 15% of children develop an anxiety disorder before the age of 18 years. Some emotional disorders are specific to childhood (**Table 13.5**).

The type of attachment a child forms with their parent or carer can increase their risk of developing an emotional disorder (**Table 13.6**). Ambivalent (and to some extent avoidant) attachment is associated with the development of anxiety disorders.

Clinical features

Many of the symptoms that adults experience in emotional disorders are also seen in children and especially adolescents (see Chapters 3 and 4). However, they can present in other ways such as mutism in certain settings or as tantrums in a young child. Older children can become withdrawn or self-harm. Children of all ages can be disinhibited or aggressive when emotionally disturbed.

The child's stage of development is important when considering what is abnormal behaviour.

Types of emotional disorders specific to childhood				
Condition	Prevalence (%)	Aetiology	Signs/symptoms	Treatment
Separation anxiety	4	Insecure attachment, cold or over anxious parenting style	Extreme worry about harm coming to the parental figure Refusal to allow separation	Behavioural therapy, in older children CBT
Sibling rivalry disorder	2	Being first born and a different gender to the new sibling. Parents not preparing the child for a new sibling	Extreme, abnormal negativity towards a new younger sibling Oppositional behaviour or tantrums	Parenting interventions
Elective mutism	1	Social anxiety	Normal speech and language but mute in certain social situations	Behavioural therapy and educational support
Reactive attachment disorder	0.5	Early neglect, abuse or separation from the care giver	Apparent lack of emotions Aggression in response to distress. Onset before 5 years of age	Parenting interventions
Enuresis	15	Anxiety, abuse, post infection, developmental delay, genetics	Involuntary urinating 1–2 times a month after 5 years old with no organic cause	Alarms and bladder training Desmopressin
Encopresis	1–4	Diet, post constipation, anxiety, developmental delay, abuse or neglect	Involuntary passing faeces in inappropriate places after 4 years old with no organic cause	Toileting routine, improved diet, parenting interventions
Pica	5–20	Developmental delay, brain injury, anxiety, mineral deficiencies, e.g. anaemia	Frequent ingestion of inedible substances, e.g. hair after 2 years old	Behavioural therapy, CBT
Tic disorders	3	Genetic predisposition, anxiety, developmental delay	Muscle contractions that are partially involuntary, e.g. blinking	Exposure response prevention (form of CBT)

Table 13.5 Types of emotional disorders specific to childhood. CBT, cognitive behavioural therapy

Types of attachment		
Attachment	Child's behaviour	Parents' behaviour
Secure	Distressed when parent leaves, but easily comforted. Happy to be reunited with parent	Consistently provides for the child's needs
Ambivalent	Extreme distress when parent leaves, but refuses affection when reunited	Does not consistently meet the child's needs.
Avoidant	Little or no distress when parent leaves and little interest when they return.	Child may not get a response when emotionally distressed
Disordered	A mix of the above. Child seems scared of the parent or can 'freeze'	Child does not have its needs met and receives conflicting information on how to react. Often associated with abuse

Table 13.6 Types of attachment

For example, clinging to a parent and refusing to speak is normal behaviour in a 2-year-old but demonstrates anxiety in a 10-year-old.

Management

In younger children, play therapy, behavioural therapy and improving parenting skills are the mainstay of treatment. In older children, cognitive behavioural therapy has the strongest evidence base for treating emotional disorders. Other therapies, such as interpersonal therapy or cognitive analytical therapy, are also used depending on the child's needs and preferences. Family therapy is of benefit as the parent can have a significant impact on the course, duration and severity of emotional disorders (e.g. if the patient refuses to engage with the therapy or is unable due to an intellectual disability).

Medication, usually an antidepressant, is considered only if talking therapies do not work or the child or family are unable to work with them. The only antidepressant licensed for use in under-18s in the UK is fluoxetine.

Answers to starter questions

1. Disruptive behaviour is often a sign of insecurity and distress intolerance in a child. A child that was settled suddenly becoming disruptive is a possible sign of abuse, which should be considered in all children presenting with possible mental illness.

2. Attention deficit hyperactivity disorder (ADHD) has a genetic component that appears more prevalent in boys. It is also argued that, in Western cultures, boys are encouraged to be more active and less attentive, therefore making any symptoms of ADHD easier to detect.

3. Both autism spectrum disorder and ADHD present with behavioural problems and difficulty concentrating. Both sets of patients can have difficulty making friends and managing classroom activities. In ADHD, look for restlessness and an increased need to be active, which is different from the repetitive movements autistic children exhibit. Children with ADHD can empathise and play with peers appropriately, albeit in short bursts; those who have autism spectrum disorder often show little interest in playing with others and have difficulty empathising.

4. All children occasionally have difficulty with behavioural problems to some degree. Conduct disorder is more pervasive and involves more abnormal behaviours than is normal. A child may occasionally engage in some of the behaviours that appear conduct-disordered, but most of the time behave appropriately. Simple interventions given consistently will usually correct problem behaviours.

Chapter 14
Psychiatry of intellectual disability

Introduction 271
Case 16 Angry outbursts at work. . 272
Intellectual disability 275

Mental illness in the context of
intellectual disability 278

Starter question

The answer to the following question is on page 280.

1. Why is mental illness more common in people with an intellectual disability?

Introduction

People with an intellectual disability have a reduced ability to understand complex information, learn new skills and cope on their own. They often require considerable support and are vulnerable to exclusion and neglect.

A number of demeaning terms have been used to describe people with lower than average intelligence, such as 'mental subnormality', 'mental handicap', and 'mental retardation'. The latter is, however, used as a clinical term in the International Classification of Diseases 10th Revision , in the Diagnostic and Statistical Manual of Mental Disorders, 4th edition, and in clinical practice in several countries including the USA. As these terms have become associated with significant stigma, they have been replaced in the UK by 'learning disability'. This has more recently been superseded by the term 'intellectual disability'.

'Intellectual disability' and 'learning disability' are not the same as 'learning difficulty'. A person with a learning difficulty has problems with a specific aspect of learning. For example, someone with dyslexia may have difficulties with reading. Intellectual disability indicates a more global impairment of learning, understanding and doing new things.

People with an intellectual disability face significant social exclusion. In some countries, people with intellectual disability are still segregated from the general population, where they are at significant risk of neglect and abuse. In others, such as the UK, they are more integrated into society, living in group residential or nursing homes or independently with support from the social and health care services. Many live with their parents or family carers, who themselves require support to care for the person. This is particularly so at challenging times, such as periods of illness or bereavement in the family.

Case 16 Angry outbursts at work

Presentation

Martin Colman is a 44-year-old man with mild intellectual disability and Down's syndrome who lives at home with his mother, Jean. Jean takes him to see their general practitioner, Dr Fonseca, as she is worried his behaviour has changed.

Jean tells Dr Fonseca that he is usually sociable and content but has recently become increasingly irritable and withdrawn. He usually spends three mornings a week working in a supported employment placement at a local café. However, he has now been suspended for a week after shouting at one of his colleagues who asked him not to eat the crisps on sale at the café.

Initial interpretation

Martin's behaviour has changed and a number of different possibilities must be considered. His behavioural changes must be categorised further in terms of their onset, duration and progress over time, any associated symptoms and whether they change in different settings.

Aids to communication

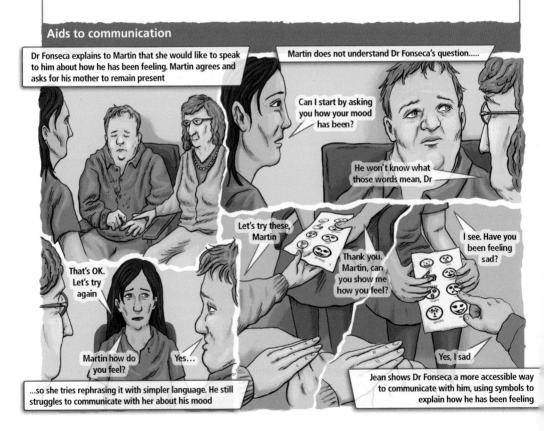

Dr Fonseca explains to Martin that she would like to speak to him about how he has been feeling. Martin agrees and asks for his mother to remain present

Can I start by asking you how your mood has been?

Martin does not understand Dr Fonseca's question.....

He won't know what those words mean, Dr

Let's try these, Martin

Thank you. Martin, can you show me how you feel?

I see. Have you been feeling sad?

That's OK. Let's try again

Martin how do you feel?

Yes...

Yes, I sad

...so she tries rephrasing it with simpler language. He still struggles to communicate with her about his mood

Jean shows Dr Fonseca a more accessible way to communicate with him, using symbols to explain how he has been feeling

Case 16 *continued*

Physical health causes must be considered. For example, hypothyroidism, which can result in mood changes, is more common in people with Down's syndrome. Changes in behaviour are also sometimes the only way a person with an intellectual disability can express physical pain. A thorough systems review is therefore required.

Mental health problems, such as depression, should be considered as differentials, especially as these can present differently in people with an intellectual disability compared with the general population. In addition, people with Down's syndrome have an increased risk of Alzheimer's dementia, with a younger age of onset, so further history taking must include an assessment of Martin's memory.

History

Jean tells you his weight has steadily increased over the last few months as he has been eating chocolate and crisps between meals, which is unusual for him. He used to take pride in dressing smartly, but in the last 5–6 months has gradually become less interested in choosing his clothing. She has also had to persuade him to bathe regularly.

Martin used to ask to help with household chores and enjoyed watching television, but now spends his time at home in his bedroom doing nothing in particular. He no longer wants to go to the weekly evening club he used to attend with his friends. Jean has noticed him crying at times for no discernible reason. He now sleeps until mid-morning despite previously being an early riser.

Jean has not noticed any changes in his memory, and tells you Martin has not recently complained of any physical pain. There is no family history of mental illness and he does not take any other medications.

> Do not assume that a person with an intellectual disability is unable to participate in a consultation. Speak directly to the person themselves rather than only to their carer.

Interpretation of history

Martin's collateral history suggests depression. The relevant features are the gradual onset of increasingly irritable and withdrawn behaviour, loss of interest in previously enjoyed activities, episodes of tearfulness and changes in diet and sleep pattern. The possibility of depression should be explored in further history taking with Martin and in his mental state examination. Physical causes must also be excluded.

> People with an intellectual disability are vulnerable to neglect, exploitation (including financial exploitation), verbal abuse, physical abuse, sexual abuse and hate crime. All of these must be considered in patients with intellectual disabilities who present with a change in mood or behaviour.

Further history

Dr Fonseca explains to Martin that she would like to speak to him about how he has been feeling. He asks if his mother can stay in the room with him and Dr Fonseca reassures him that this is fine. Martin answers 'no' when asked if he drinks alcohol, smoke or uses any illicit drugs.

Dr Fonseca finds it difficult to word some of her questions so that Martin understands her. However, he is able to explain that he feels tired and hungry all the time. He uses symbols to indicate that he has been feeling sad. He is able to explain

Case 16 *continued*

that he has felt this way since his father's death 1 year ago. He has not told anyone about this before as he was worried his mother would cry.

Examination

Dr Fonseca completes a mental state examination (**Table 14.1**). She notes that Martin appears unkempt and withdrawn. He has a flattened affect and quiet, monotonous speech.

Physical examination

Martin is overweight, but his cardiovascular, abdominal and respiratory examinations are all normal. There are no signs of anaemia, thyroid dysfunction or infection.

Interpretation of findings

The clinical features of a gradual onset of Martin's behavioural changes in the context of the death of his father 1 year ago, alongside a normal physical examination, are suggestive of a depressive disorder.

Investigations

Although the physical examination appears normal, Dr Fonseca arranges blood tests to exclude other physical health problems which may not be apparent on examination, but which might be contributing to Martin's symptoms. These include a full blood count, urea and electrolytes, liver and thyroid function tests and calcium, vitamin B_{12} and folate levels. Martin says he does not like needles but, after reassurance from his mother, eventually agrees to the blood tests.

When the results return, they are all normal.

Diagnosis

Dr Fonseca explains to Martin and to his mother that his history, mental state examination, physical examination findings and blood test results are suggestive

Mr Colman's mental state examination	
Category	Description
Appearance and behaviour	Martin has with unwashed hair and stained clothing. He is withdrawn, with poor eye contact. He is tearful when discussing his father's death
Speech	Martin frequently pauses before answering questions, checking with his mother when he does not understand what has been asked. His speech is quiet and monotone
Mood	Martin describes his mood as 'sad'. Objectively, he appears low in mood with flattened affect
Perceptions	He does not describe experiencing any abnormal perceptions
Thoughts	Martin struggles to understand Dr McGinty's questions around his thoughts, but has no clear delusions or ruminations
Cognition	Martin is orientated in place and person, but not in time, which his mother states has always been normal for him
Insight	Martin demonstrates insight into his current difficulties with his mood
Suicidal ideation	Martin says he has never thought about harming himself or about ending his life

Table 14.1 Martin's mental state examination

Case 16 *continued*

of depression. This may have been precipitated by the loss of his father.

Dr Fonseca finds it difficult to explain
depression to Martin. However, when she
explains that she would like to refer him to
the local community team for people with
an intellectual disability for more in-depth
assessment and further support for him
and his mother, he is pleased and agrees
to this.

Intellectual disability

Intellectual disability is characterised by
three core features:

- A reduced ability to understand new or
  complex information or learn new skills
  (impaired intelligence)
- A reduced ability to cope independently
  (impaired social functioning)
- An onset before the age of 18 years

The severity of intellectual disability varies
from mild to profound (**Table 14.2**).

Epidemiology

The global prevalence of intellectual disability is around 2%, with around 1.5 million
affected people in the UK. The male-to-female
ratio is approximately 3:2. The majority of
cases are mild (**Table 14.2**).

Aetiology

There are many causes of intellectual disability, all of which result in varying degrees

Classification of intellectual disability			
Severity	IQ score	Functioning	Proportion of intellectually disabled population (%)
Mild	50–69	Independent self-care and social skills Good language abilities Usually able to work Many people with mild intellectual disability are not formally identified	85
Moderate	35–49	Require some support with self-care Often have better receptive than expressive language abilities May be able to work in supported employment Often live in residential settings	10
Severe	20–34	Limited self-care abilities Limited communication May be able to undertake simple tasks with close supervision Often live in residential settings	3–4
Profound	<20	Severely limited communication, mobility, communication and self-care skills Often have comorbid visual and/or hearing impairment Require constant support, usually living in residential or nursing settings	1–2

Table 14.2 Classification of intellectual disability

of impaired intellectual, social and adaptive functioning. In around one third of people with an intellectual disability, no clear cause can be established. This may change in the future if there is an increase in the availability of genetic tests for less common genetic syndromes that result in intellectual disability. Current identifiable causes of intellectual disability can be broadly grouped into genetic, prenatal, perinatal and postnatal causes (**Table 14.3**).

Causes of intellectual disability	
Type	Examples
Genetic	Aneuploidy, e.g. Down's syndrome (trisomy 21)
	Deletions, e.g. cri du chat syndrome
	Sex chromosome anomalies, e.g. fragile X syndrome, Klinefelter's syndrome, Turner's syndrome
	Other: associated tuberous sclerosis, neurofibromatosis, phenylketonuria, Tay–Sachs disease, other enzyme-deficiency diseases
Prenatal	Congenital infections, e.g. TORCH (toxoplasmosis, rubella, cytomegalovirus, herpes simplex and zoster), AIDS, syphilis
	Toxins, e.g. prescribed drugs with teratogenic effects (such as phenytoin), alcohol (leading to fetal alcohol spectrum disorder)
Perinatal	Maternal pre-eclampsia, antepartum haemorrhage
	Prematurity, with associated intraventricular haemorrhage, hyperbilirubinaemia
	Prolonged labour, with associated birth trauma, asphyxia, intracranial haemorrhage
Postnatal	Endocrine, e.g. hypothyroidism
	Infections, e.g. meningitis, encephalitis
	Injury or accident , e.g. accidental/non accidental head injury, near drowning, asphyxia
	Metabolic, e.g. iodine deficiency, hypoglycaemia, severe jaundice
	Toxins, e.g. carbon monoxide, lead
	Other: status epilepticus, severe neglect

Table 14.3 Causes of intellectual disability

Clinical features

People with an intellectual disability often present with delayed development. For example, they may be slow to learn to sit, stand, walk or talk in childhood, leading their parents to consult a doctor.

Although each person with intellectual disability is unique, specific syndromes, such as Down's syndrome and fragile X syndrome (two of the most common genetic causes of intellectual disability) are characterised by particular clinical features (**Table 14.4**).

Diagnostic approach

The detection of intellectual disability starts prenatally, for example testing for Down's syndrome in pregnancy (**Figure 14.1**). In the UK and other developed countries, routine screening of newborn babies for phenylketonuria using a heel prick blood test forms part of primary prevention by allowing the early detection and management of the associated metabolic abnormality that results in intellectual disability.

In some cases, intellectual disability is not suspected until later in childhood, at which time referrals are made to the local child and adolescent mental health specialist team for further psychological testing. This includes an assessment of intelligence quotient (IQ) using standardised intelligence tests such as the Weschler Intelligence Scale for Children, which does not rely on ability to read or write. Individuals with an intellectual disability have an IQ score of under 70 – which is 2 standard deviations below the population mean of 100 (**Figure 14.2**).

Babies or children with suspected intellectual disability may also be referred to paediatricians, to arrange further diagnostic tests including brain imaging with CT or MRI scans. Changes suggestive of particular causes of intellectual disability include areas of intraventricular haemorrhage or structural abnormalities such as cortical tubers in tuberous sclerosis. Genetic counselling and genetic testing can be completed when a genetic cause is suspected.

Management

Intellectual disability cannot be cured. In more developed countries, such as the UK,

Clinical features of genetic syndromes associated with intellectual disability

Syndrome	Genetic abnormality	Facial features	Other features
Down's	Trisomy 21 (extra copy of all or part of chromosome 21)	Low set ears Eyes that slant upwards and outwards Flat nasal bridge Protruding tongue Brushfield spots (white spots on iris)	Hypotonia Single transverse palmar creases Broad hands Short fingers Congenital heart defects, e.g. atrioventricular septal defect
Fragile X	Repeat expansion in fragile X mental retardation (FMR1) gene on X chromosome	Elongated face Broad forehead Large or protruding ears Strabismus	Hypotonia Hyperextensible finger joints Macro-orchidism (large testicles) in men Mitral valve prolapse

Table 14.4 Clinical features of common genetic syndromes associated with intellectual disability

Genetic testing for Down's syndrome

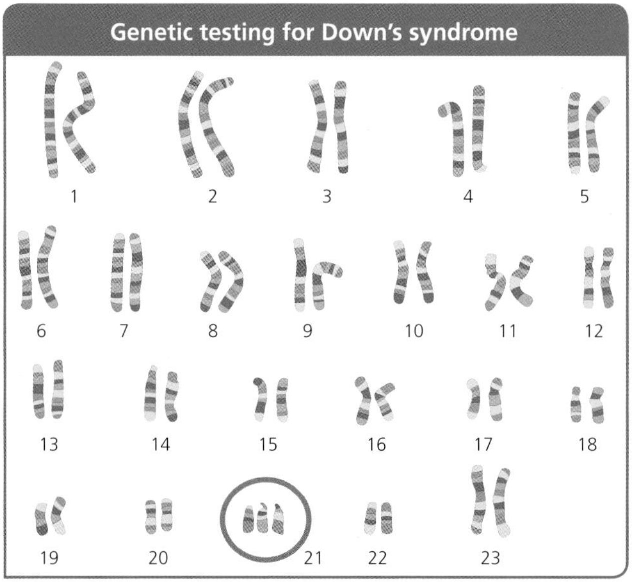

Figure 14.1 Genetic testing: karyotype showing three copies of chromosome 21 (trisomy 21) causing Down's syndrome.

multidisciplinary management involving health-care, social care and education services focuses on supporting the individual with an intellectual disability to maximise their skills, opportunities, health and quality of life. Young people may require an assessment of their special educational needs to get extra support in school or college. Some attend mainstream schools with additional support, while others attend schools or colleges exclusively for pupils with special educational needs. It is also vital to provide support for families and other carers.

> **Carers, particularly family carers, often experience stress as a consequence of their role.** It is important to enquire sensitively about whether carers feel able to manage. Also ensure they know about the sources of support available to them.

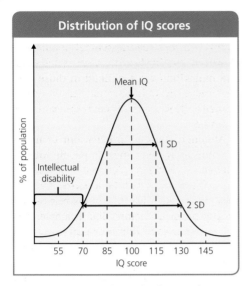

Distribution of IQ scores

Figure 14.2 The population distribution of intelligence quotient (IQ) scores. SD, standard deviation.

In some cases, a person with an intellectual disability does not have the mental capacity to make a decision about treatment proposed as part of their management (see page 29). In such cases, the team involved in supporting the person, along with their carers, may be involved in discussions to determine which course of action would be in the individual's best interests.

Prognosis

As they age, people with an intellectual disability may encounter problems specific to their situation. For example, if they live with elderly parents, they may experience significant distress when the parents die; they will have to cope with bereavement at the same time as adjusting to living somewhere new. Elderly parents who care for a person with an intellectual disability often themselves find it increasingly difficult to cope with the demands of caring as they age, and they worry who will look after their child when they die.

Although life expectancy has improved in the last few decades, people with an intellectual disability continue to die at a younger age than people in the general population, often 15–20 years earlier in the UK. The reasons for this are complex, and include discrimination by health-care professionals and delays in access to diagnosis, investigations and treatment.

Mental illness in the context of intellectual disability

People with an intellectual disability experience the same range of mental illnesses as the general population, but detecting it is challenging. Clinicians experience significant difficulties communicating with individuals with limited language skills. Furthermore, people with an intellectual disability can find it difficult to understand words spoken to them or to describe the symptoms they are experiencing. In addition, mental illness is difficult to recognise because it can present atypically in people with an intellectual disability, for example, with changes in behaviour that may be attributed to other factors.

Epidemiology

Mental illness is more common in people with an intellectual disability. Up to one third of people with an intellectual disability have a co-morbid mental illness such as depressive disorder. The most common mental illness in people with an intellectual disability is schizophrenia, with a higher prevalence (3%) than in the general population (1%). Similarly, Alzheimer's disease and autism spectrum disorder occur more often in those with intellectual disability.

Tips for communicating with people with an intellectual disability:

- Allow extra time
- First talk to the person to assess their ability to engage in the consultation
- Use short, simple sentences
- Avoid jargon and abstract language
- Do not make assumptions – people with an intellectual disability can smoke, drink alcohol, use recreational drugs and have sexual relationships
- Obtain a collateral history from a carer who knows the person well but do not talk only to the carer – include the person with the intellectual disability as far as possible
- Be aware of the risks of abuse and neglect; make it clear that the patient can ask the person accompanying them to leave at any time
- Provide information in simple, easy-to-read English and consider using pictures or symbols
- Check the person's understanding of what has been discussed

Aetiology

The aetiology of mental illnesses in people with an intellectual disability is unclear. In some people the underlying brain damage leading to intellectual disability may also be associated with the development of a mental illness. In addition, people with an intellectual disability are likely to have one or more of the risk factors associated with mental illness, such as poverty and social exclusion.

Clinical features

Mental illness should be considered in the differential diagnosis in those people with an intellectual disability who present with changes in mood, or changes in behaviour, including:

- Worsening social functioning
- The onset of any new unusual behaviour

In those with a mild intellectual disability, mental illness presents with similar clinical features to those in the general population. However, eliciting features such as delusions and hallucinations is difficult in those who have more severe intellectual disability and limited ability to verbally communicate their symptoms.

Although changes in behaviour or mood can indicate mental illness in people with an intellectual disability, it is vital to remember that such changes may be a person's way of communicating frustration or distress caused by psychosocial factors. For example, angry outbursts can occur when others cannot understand their attempts to communicate or when the environment is too noisy or too boring. They can also result from significant changes in the person's life or routine, such as the loss of a carer.

Diagnostic approach

When considering a differential diagnosis of a change in mood or behaviour, remember that, as a population, people with an intellectual disability have an increased prevalence of:

- Mental health problems, such as schizophrenia
- Physical health problems, such as constipation, gastro-oesophageal reflux disease, dental caries, epilepsy, mobility difficulties and incontinence
- Sensory impairments, such as visual or hearing impairment
- Autism spectrum disorder

In a person with an intellectual disability a change in behaviour or mood may be the only way of communicating pain and distress caused by an underlying physical health problem. Therefore, it is particularly important that physical causes of changed mood or behaviour are excluded.

The challenges of communicating with a person with an intellectual disability mean that diagnosis of suspected mental illness is usually carried out by a specialist community intellectual disability team. A multidisciplinary approach to assessment is used. In addition to psychiatric assessment, a speech and language therapist assesses how well the person is able to communicate with their carers, and an occupational therapist will assess whether the person's environment is suitable.

Management

A biopsychosocial approach is taken to managing mental illness in people with an intellectual disability. People with mild intellectual disability and co-morbid mental illness are often managed alongside individuals from the general population by mainstream mental health services. However, adjustments are required, for example, longer appointments so that people have enough time to understand what is being said to them and to express themselves, and providing information in an easy-to-read format. In the UK, people with more severe intellectual disability and mental illness or autism spectrum disorder with behaviours that challenge others or their environment are managed by specialist community intellectual disability teams. These comprise psychiatrists, nurses, speech and language therapists, occupational therapists and psychologists who work closely with social care services.

People with an intellectual disability may find it difficult to understand standard written health materials. Instead, clinicians should provide the same information in an easy-to-read format which:

■ uses short, clear sentences

■ avoids jargon

■ provides an explanation of difficult words

■ provides pictures and photographs

Medication

Medications used to treat mental illness in people with an intellectual disability are similar to those prescribed for patients in the general population. However, people with an intellectual disability are sometimes particularly sensitive to the effects of medication, and close monitoring for side effects is required.

Epilepsy is a common co-morbidity affecting up to 25% of people with intellectual disability. Antidepressants and antipsychotics can lower seizure threshold, increasing the risk of seizures. Medications should be started at low doses and increased slowly, with close monitoring of seizure frequency and severity.

Psychological therapies

Some people with an intellectual disability are able to engage with psychological therapies, such as cognitive behavioural therapy, if this is appropriately modified to meet their needs. Psychologists also work with carers to understand how to modify their responses to a patient's behaviour to bring about change. Family therapy and psychoeducation is offered to patients who live with their family.

Prognosis

The prognosis of mental illness in those with an intellectual disability has received little research attention. However, it is thought to be similar to that of the general population.

Answer to starter question

1. It is thought that the underlying brain damage that causes intellectual disability may be a common aetiological factor in the development of mental illness. Other shared risk factors include socioeconomic deprivation and social exclusion.

Chapter 15
Psychiatric emergencies

Introduction 281
Case 17 Refusal to be admitted
        to hospital 281
Case 18 Acute psychotic
        symptoms 284
Case 19 Acute confusion 286
Case 20 Suicidal behaviour 287

Case 21 Agitated and violent
        patient 289
Case 22 Acute alcohol
        withdrawal 290
Case 23 Fever, muscle stiffness
        and tremor 293

Introduction

Psychiatric emergencies often present in a non-psychiatric medical setting or in the community. Assessing patients who present this way is complex and requires assessment for underlying physical disorders and intoxication with drugs or alcohol as well as for psychiatric disorders. Patients may initially come to the attention of community services such as the police, presenting additional challenges in management of the acute situation. Patients may not be aware of their own illness and its effect upon their behaviour, and their lack of insight may mean they are unwilling or unable to co-operate with medical services. In these circumstances, legislation regarding mental capacity and mental health are used to ensure the patient receives the treatment they require, for example the Mental Capacity Act 2005 and the Mental Health Act 2007 in England and Wales.

Case 17 Refusal to be admitted to hospital

Presentation

Anna Miller, a 23-year-old woman, is reluctantly brought in to the emergency department by her husband who says she has taken a large overdose of paracetamol and ibuprofen. However, once in the hospital she asks to go home and refuses receive any treatment.

Initial interpretation

Anna needs a physical examination to assess for the effects of overdose and for any underlying medical conditions. She also needs blood tests to assess the effect of the overdose and indicate the need for treatment. However, Anna has the right to leave the hospital at any time

Case 17 *continued*

unless she is deemed to lack capacity or is detained under mental health legislation. She has taken a significant overdose, so it is in her best interest to receive treatment, but she can refuse if she has the capacity to make that decision, even if it results in her death. The only exception is if the overdose was directly caused by a significant mental illness, in which case Anna could be treated under mental health legislation.

Further history and examination

Anna admits planning to die by suicide and to that end bought a large amount of medication. She has taken approximately 60 paracetamol and 30 ibuprofen, with alcohol, approximately 8 hours ago. She has been feeling low for some time and was prescribed an SSRI 2 weeks ago after being diagnosed with depression. There are no significant findings on physical examination. She is quiet and occasionally tearful, frequently asking to be left alone to die. She does not engage with questions, instead talks about having no future and feeling there is no point in living.

Working diagnosis

Anna's depression has led to her attempting suicide. She does not want to receive treatment because she feels she has no future. Although she allowed an examination she refuses blood tests. An assessment of her capacity should be undertaken urgently.

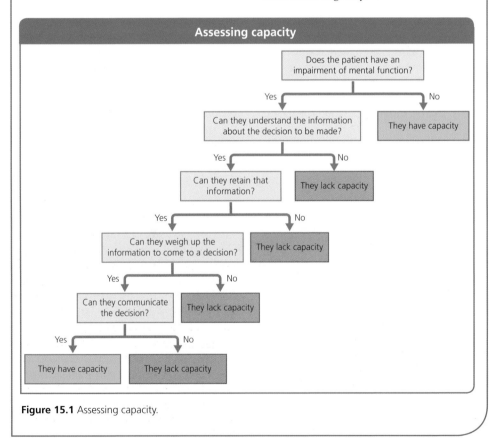

Figure 15.1 Assessing capacity.

Case 17 *continued*

Immediate intervention

Initially you try to establish a rapport with Anna and see if there is anything that could help her change her decision. As Anna is refusing assessment and treatment it is vital to ascertain whether she has capacity to make this decision (**Figure 15.1**). She is suffering from severe depression and therefore does have an impairment of mind; as a result of this she is also unable to understand and weigh up the information given to her. Taken together, these facts signify that she does not have capacity to make a decision about treatment and therefore can be treated in her best interests without her consent. The local mental health team are consulted about this decision and asked for their input during her treatment for the overdose.

Capacity assessment

Refusal to be admitted after overdose is relatively rare because many patients can be persuaded to stay by establishing a rapport and helping them to overcome any anxieties they may have about admission. However, when refusal does occur it is critical that a careful assessment is undertaken to ensure the patient has the capacity to make that decision.

> **Try to find out why the patient is refusing help** and what has led them to this point. Then consider the positives in their lives that could lead them to change their mind.

An assessment of capacity (**Figure 15.1**) requires there to be a mental impairment, otherwise the patient is assumed to be able to make a decision even if that decision is unwise. A mental impairment can be from physical, medical or mental illnesses (**Table 15.1**).

An assessment of capacity is decision specific; therefore it should be assessed for each decision the patient makes. For example a patient may not have capacity to refuse admission but may have capacity to make choices about treatment for a physical illness that is not the reason for their admission.

If the patient is deemed to have capacity but is thought to be suffering from a significant

Conditions that commonly affect capacity	
Type	Condition
Physical conditions	Stroke
	Tumour
	Brain injury
Medical conditions	Septicaemia
	Hypoglycaemia
	Thyrotoxicosis
	Epilepsy
Mental illnesses	Schizophrenia
	Severe depression
	Bipolar disorder
Ingesting substances	Alcohol
	Sedatives
	Amphetamines

Table 15.1 Conditions that commonly affect capacity

mental illness that has directly contributed to the need for admission, then an assessment from a psychiatrist is required because the patient may need to be detained for treatment under the appropriate mental health legislation (e.g. the Mental Health Act 2007 in England and Wales). Occasionally a patient may have an advance directive that states they do not wish to have treatment in certain situations, such as post overdose. Such a statement should be adhered to regardless of capacity, however it should be reviewed (often by a legal specialist acting for the hospital) to ensure it is legally binding.

Case 18 Acute psychotic symptoms

Presentation

22-year-old Nathan Dale is picked up by the police after throwing a brick through a local shop window. He did not resist arrest and asked the police to help him saying he had done it because he knew that the owner of the shop had put the dummies in the window to watch him and he was sick of them spreading rumours about him to all of the shoppers. Nathan cannot be reassured that the window dummies cannot speak. He is unable to understand the police who explain that the dummies are not speaking.

Initial interpretation

Nathan is clearly experiencing auditory hallucinations and is describing his delusions and hallucinations increasingly insistently. These features indicate an acute psychotic illness (**Table 15.2**).

History and examination

Nathan is agitated and cannot be reassured. He is adamant that the dummies are speaking and that he can see their lips moving. He says that he has heard them speak about him occasionally before but noticed this morning that they were laughing and pointing as well. Nathan is well dressed, clean and tidy but clearly anxious and over-aroused, insisting that others should believe him. He believes that the owner of the shop had decided to monitor his behaviour as they had heard that he was infected with a contagious disease and wanted to know where he was going. He does not believe that he is infected but feels that the rumour is being spread deliberately to prevent him from studying for his degree and graduating.

Differential diagnoses for acute psychotic episodes		
Disorder	Characteristics of psychotic symptoms	Associated features
Schizophrenia	Extensive psychotic symptoms with well-developed delusions constructed around hallucinations	Often seen without apparent precipitant, in young adults
	Characteristic auditory hallucinations may discuss the patient as if they aren't there	Psychotic symptoms are associated with changes in behaviour and social withdrawal
Affective disorders	Mood congruent delusions and hallucinations, e.g. in depressive psychoses patient may believe they have committed a terrible wrong in their past	Marked mood change: symptoms of either depression or hypomania
Substance misuse	Onset of symptoms is acute and florid, resolving quickly on discontinuing the relevant drug	Some characteristic psychotic symptoms, e.g. formication (sensation of insects crawling under skin) in cocaine abuse
		Psychotic symptoms present on withdrawal of substances, e.g. alcohol
Organic disorders	Florid psychotic symptoms, including visual hallucinations	Acute confusional states with signs and symptoms of acute physical illness
		Common in some dementias, Parkinson's disease and with some medications, e.g. steroids

Table 15.2 Differential diagnoses for acute psychotic episodes

Further history and examination

The police surgeon examines Nathan for any signs of infection, such as pneumonia, because this can cause hallucinations as part of a delirium. Cranial nerve and peripheral nerve examinations are conducted to look for signs of brain injury, epilepsy or tumor that could be the cause of his symptoms.

Immediate intervention

Nathan is taken to the police station as a place of safety as he is behaving irrationally, has already committed a criminal act and does not appear to be able to take responsibility for his own actions. The duty psychiatrist is called to the police station and interviews Nathan, during which Nathan gives a full account of his psychotic symptoms which have developed over the last 3 days. As he is unable to understand that he is unwell, and remains insistent that he must go back to the shop to get rid of the dummies, he is admitted to the local psychiatric hospital under Section 2 of the Mental Health Act 2007 for further assessment.

Acute psychosis

Acute psychosis is a common psychiatric emergency and can present to any health service. Many patients present late for psychiatric attention, when the episode is already severe, or come to the attention of psychiatric services via a route initiated by others such as the police or medical staff in general hospitals.

It commonly presents with co-morbidities, particularly in older patients, so assessing for physical and other mental disorders is essential.

> In acute psychosis, a single antipsychotic drug should be given at the lowest effective dose. For first episodes of psychosis, atypical antipsychotics are usually better tolerated. Benzodiazepines can be added in the acute phase for additional sedation.

A patient experiencing an acute psychotic episode should be seen and assessed by a specialist multidisciplinary psychiatric team which can deliver psychosocial interventions as essential adjuncts to drugs. Early assessment must include both a detailed mental state examination (MSE) and medical history, including details of any medication and alcohol and substance misuse.

Organic causes should be ruled out by relevant investigations, followed by appropriate treatment of any contributory medical conditions.

Over 70% of patients with a first episode of non-organic illness are admitted for treatment in a psychiatric hospital. When patients decline voluntary treatment, assessment under mental health legislation is considered if the patient appears to be at risk of self harm or harm to others.

Case 19 Acute confusion

Presentation

76-year-old Martha Winfield is brought to the emergency department by her neighbour as she was found wandering outside in her nightdress, disorientated and talking to herself.

Initial interpretation

Martha's confusion could be caused by medical, physical or mental causes (**Table 15.3**). These should be sought via a history, including a collateral history, a full examination, observations and blood tests. An ECG, chest X-ray and a head CT should also be considered. It is important that modifiable causes are sought first, before considering other possibilities such as dementia.

Further history and examination

Martha is unable to give a history and talks incoherently about a relative. Her neighbour, John, states that Martha has been living alone for a number of years and has recently had a diagnosis of vascular dementia. She has high blood pressure and used to smoke but otherwise is usually healthy and well. Her dementia was diagnosed after she was noticed often forgetting what to buy when shopping; however, it had not affected her ability to look after herself. John calls in on Martha regularly and noticed yesterday that she did not seem well. She had not done the washing up and had slept on the sofa. John thought she might have had a fever as she was complaining of feeling

Causes of acute confusion	
Cause	Examples
Infection in the body	Urinary infection, pneumonia
Infection in the brain	Meningitis, encephalitis
Physical abnormality in the brain or spinal cord	Hydrocephalus, stroke
Heart conditions	Atrial fibrillation, myocardial infarction
Respiratory conditions	COPD, effusions
Abdominal/pelvic conditions	Pancreatitis, constipation
Hormonal abnormalities	Diabetes, hyperthyroidism
Tumours	Bowel cancer, lung cancer
Toxic substances and drugs	Sedatives, carbon monoxide, alcohol (or alcohol withdrawal)
Trauma/surgery	Head injury, appendectomy
Other	Pain, epilepsy

Table 15.3 Causes of acute confusion. COPD, chronic obstructive pulmonary disease

Martha's investigation results		
Investigation	Result (normal)	Conclusion
Full blood count	WBC 17 x10^9/L (3.5–11.0)	Indicates infection
Urea and electrolytes	Urea 9 mmol/L (3–9) Creatinine 1.5 mg/dL (0.6–1.3)	Probably resulting from her dehydration
C-reactive protein	38 mg/L (<6)	Indicates infection
Liver function tests	ALT 12 U/L (5–21) AST 13 IU/L (6–40) ALP 58 U/L (42–128)	Normal
Thyroid	Free T3 4 pg/mL (3–7)	Normal
Glucose	6 mmol/L (4.4–7.8)	Normal
Urine dipstick	Positive for nitrates and leucocytes	Indicates urinary tract infection

Table 15.4 Martha's investigation results. ALP, alkaline phosphatase; ALT, alanine transaminase; AST, aspartate transaminase; WBC, white blood count

Case 19 *continued*

cold despite the house being very warm. Examination reveals some generalised abdominal tenderness and some evidence of dehydration as her mouth is dry.

Working diagnosis

Although Martha has had a diagnosis of dementia, which could be contributing to the current presentation, she is most likely to be suffering from delirium given the acute onset of her disorientation and confusion. This is not a diagnosis in itself and will need further investigation to assess for the underlying cause.

Immediate intervention

A full set of observations are taken, including a blood glucose, urine dip and culture. She also has blood tests to assess for signs of infection, kidney or liver conditions (**Table 15.4**). Blood cultures are requested if she develops a temperature again. A chest X-ray and ECG are also ordered to help rule out conditions such as myocardial infarction and pneumonia.

Martha is nursed in a side room with adequate lighting and minimal staff changes to help her remain orientated. As she does not have severe dehydration she is encouraged to drink frequently; if this fails she would be hydrated intravenously. If it was felt absolutely necessary to prescribe something reduce her agitation a low dose of an antipsychotic could be used.

Delirium

Delirium has multiple causes. A patient with delirium should always have a careful history taken from someone familiar with the patient because the patient may forget recent symptoms or changes in medications. Contacting the patient's GP can be helpful to obtain an up-to-date list of conditions and medications.

> **Sedating benzodiazepine medications are generally avoided in delirium** as they can increase the risk of falls and, paradoxically, often increase agitation.

Investigations should be tailored towards the condition that has caused the delirium, but screening all cases for signs of infection and heart conditions can be useful. All patients should be nursed appropriately to prevent falls and reduce disorientation. Fluid and dietary intake is monitored. Occasionally dementia or other mental illnesses, such as schizophrenia or mania, can present as acute confusion but this should only be suspected if the history is suggestive and other causes have been excluded.

Case 20 Suicidal behaviour

Presentation

The ambulance service is called to 32-year-old Helen Barclay. Her husband had returned early from a business trip to find Helen vomiting; finding empty paracetamol packets, he questioned her and she admitted taking 30 tablets with some vodka. When the ambulance arrives, Helen refuses to get in, saying that she has been sick and does not need further help.

Case 20 *continued*

Initial interpretation

An untreated overdose of paracetamol confers a high risk of liver damage, which may be fatal. Immediate treatment is essential and patients must be assessed in hospital because early symptoms may not reflect the severity of overdose or the risk of organ damage.

History and examination

Helen admits that she only took the overdose 30 minutes before her husband arrived. She now regrets overdosing saying she only did it because she was feeling sorry for herself having recently lost her job. Although she has had some vodka she is not overtly intoxicated and is conversing lucidly with ambulance staff. She has no symptoms other than nausea and is otherwise fit and well.

Immediate intervention

The history indicates that Helen has taken a potentially fatal overdose of paracetamol. Although she has been sick, further treatment is required. Plasma paracetamol concentration should be measured at 4 hours or later after ingestion (earlier concentration measurement is unreliable).

Ambulance staff call the local mental health team to assess Helen's competence to decline treatment. The impact of alcohol upon her ability to make competent decisions must also be considered. However, her husband persuades her to go to hospital voluntarily.

As the overdose was taken less than an hour ago, treatment with activated charcoal is given. Plasma paracetamol concentration is measured 4 hours after ingestion of the overdose (earlier concentration measurement is unreliable).

The plasma paracetamol level indicates that treatment with *N*-acetylcysteine is required and this is administered intravenously. This may be used up to 24 hours after ingestion of paracetamol, with maximum protective effect being obtained up to 8 hours post-ingestion, declining rapidly after this point.

Attempted suicide

The acute assessment of a patient who has harmed themselves or taken a deliberate overdose can be a complex and challenging process, especially in a community setting, where there may be no witnesses and no ascertainable history. The degree of suicidal intent associated with such acts is extremely variable and the possibility of the patient continuing to completed suicide must always be assessed. All patients who harm themselves deliberately should receive a full biopsychosocial assessment by an appropriately trained clinician because suicide is the third largest contributor to premature death in the UK. The rates of mental illness are much higher in patients who have attempted suicide.

Acute assessment of patients who have harmed themselves includes:

- Immediate assessment of the patient's physical condition, with appropriate physical treatments instituted as quickly as possible
- Psychosocial and mental state assessment, including consideration of alcohol and drug misuse
- Careful assessment of ongoing, immediate suicide risk
- Referral for psychiatric treatment where appropriate
- Consideration of medicolegal issues during emergency management including consent to treatment and assessment of capacity where indicated

Many patients refuse consent to treatment in the acute situation; this may be caused by intoxication with drugs or alcohol, acute emotional distress or genuine lack of insight into an underlying psychiatric illness or a conscious and considered disagreement with the doctor's point of view. Assessment of capacity to refuse treatment may be necessary during acute assessment (**Figure 15.1**).

Case 21 Agitated and violent patient

Presentation

Louise Salter is a 23-year-old who was recently admitted under mental health legislation to a psychiatric hospital with symptoms of mania. Initially she was settled, but following an argument about which television show to watch she has become very agitated and has hit another patient, fortunately not causing any significant injury.

Initial interpretation

The trigger for Louise's increased agitation is probably the argument she had, but there are many other causes of increased disturbance, including medication, psychosis and physical illnesses such as infections. The safety of patients and staff is paramount, therefore isolation and de-escalation is implemented as soon as it is possible to do so without causing injury. The patient assaulted by Louise also has an assessment for injuries that require treatment.

Further history and examination

Louise is brought to her bedroom and chaperoned while a history and examination are undertaken. She states that she hit the patient because she realised he was part of a conspiracy to send her messages through the television. She then talks rapidly and at length on various topics loosely connected with the television programme she was watching. While talking she is pacing in her bedroom, unable to sit down. She refuses to be examined and tries to hit the doctor when an examination is suggested.

Immediate intervention

Louise is restrained by nursing staff until it is felt that she is calm enough to be released without causing injury to herself or others. She is reassured by staff who explain what is happening and try to de-escalate the situation through talking to her. When it is evident that this will not work without pharmacological intervention lorazepam is offered orally to Louise. She refuses to take any medication and continues to try to harm the members of staff holding her, therefore the lorazepam is given as an intramuscular injection. After this Louise is monitored closely to ensure she is not over sedated. She is examined and her pulse, blood pressure and respiratory rate monitored regularly. She is not left alone during this time.

Agitation

Severe agitation or violent behaviour often occurs in the context of mental or physical illness. When possible it should be treated without the need for pharmacological intervention, through use of de-escalation techniques (**Figure 15.2**). These include:

- taking the person into a quiet room
- discussing the incident or distracting them as felt appropriate.

If restraint is required it should be done by trained professionals and the patient should be told what is happening and why. Restraint or tranquillisation without patient consent can only be done if the patient has been detained under mental health legislation, in an emergency situation or when the patient lacks capacity and it is in the patient's best interests.

> **Traditional physical restraints** such as tying patients to their bed and straitjackets are no longer used due to safety concerns and ethical considerations.

If rapid tranquillisation is needed it should be at the minimum dose necessary and only one drug should be used if possible. A short-acting benzodiazepine such as lorazepam or an antipsychotic such as olanzapine can be used. If possible the patient should take this orally, however, if they refuse it can be given intramuscularly. In the case of intramuscular administration, blood pressure, pulse and respiratory rate are closely monitored and resuscitation equipment must be readily available.

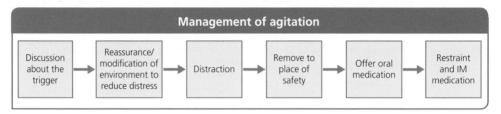

Management of agitation

Discussion about the trigger → Reassurance/modification of environment to reduce distress → Distraction → Remove to place of safety → Offer oral medication → Restraint and IM medication

Figure 15.2 Management of agitation. patient require close monitoring and continued discussion and reassurance.

Case 22 Acute alcohol withdrawal

Presentation

Harry Bucknall is a 57-year-old who had surgery on a broken foot 2 days ago. He is due to be discharged soon but is now acutely confused, is having visual hallucinations and is agitated. He admits to having drunk heavily for many years before coming into hospital but has not had any alcohol since admission.

Initial interpretation

Severe withdrawal from alcohol (delirium tremens) is the most likely cause of Harry's symptoms. However, there are many other causes that should be excluded through further investigations before this diagnosis is made. Alcohol withdrawal can be fatal due to autonomic instability and risk of seizures. Harry should be treated promptly and monitored closely while withdrawing.

Further history and examination

Harry is disorientated and keeps asking to see his deceased wife. He occasionally states he can see snakes slithering across the floor and up the curtains, which he finds very distressing. His son is contacted and acknowledges that his father does drink heavily, usually about a bottle of whiskey per day and has done for a number of years. On examination he has a tremor, is tachycardic and tachypneic. He does not have a fever or other symptoms of infection.

Working diagnosis

A tremor along with transient hallucinations, agitation and autonomic instability supports a diagnosis of delirium tremens. However, infection and other conditions

Case 22 *continued*

should be excluded through observations, blood tests and a urine dipstick test.

Immediate intervention

A member of staff sits with Harry to reassure him and reduce his level of agitation. Blood test results (**Table 15.5**) rule out infection or other causes. An ECG is completed to ensure the withdrawal is not causing arrhythmias. A Clinical Institute Withdrawal Assessment for Alcohol scale (CIWA-A) score is taken to measure the severity of the withdrawal (**Figure 15.3**). Harry scores 37, which indicates a need for benzodiazepine treatment.

Harry's investigation results		
Investigation	Result (normal)	Conclusion
Full blood count	Hb 118 g/L (120–175) Platelet 110 x10⁹/L (140–450) WBC 8 x10⁹/L (3.5–11.0)	Thrombocytopenia and anaemia can occur in alcoholism. Normal WBC indicates no infection
Urea and electrolytes	Urea 5 mmol/L (3–9) Creatinine 1 mg/dL (0.6–1.3)	Normal
C-reactive protein	2 mg/L (<6)	Indicates no infection
Magnesium	0.60 (0.60–0.95 mmol/L)	Can be low in alcoholism
Liver function tests	ALT 20 U/L (5–21) AST 49 IU/L (6–40) ALP 128 U/L (42–128) GGT 189 U/L (5–78)	Common in alcoholism
Thyroid function tests	Free T3 4.5 pg/mL (3–7)	Normal
Glucose	5.4 mmol/L (4.4–7.8)	Normal

Table 15.5 Harry's investigation results. ALP, alkaline phosphatase; ALT, alanine transaminase; AST aspartate transaminase; GGT, gamma-glutamyl transferase; Hb, haemoglobin; WBC, white blood cell

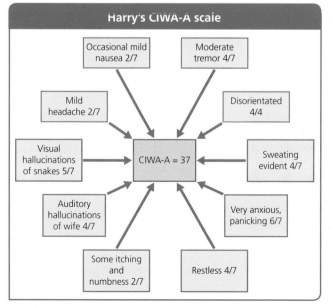

Figure 15.3 Harry's CIWA-A scale (see **Figure 15.4**). Harry scores 37, which indicates a need for treatment with benzodiazepines.

Withdrawal

Withdrawal from most substances is extremely unpleasant (**Table 15.6**) but with a few exceptions is not life threatening. Most withdrawal symptoms can be managed with symptomatic relief only, such as simple analgesia and antinauseants. Treatment with other addictive substances should be avoided where possible (with a few exceptions, for example the treatment of alcohol withdrawal using benzodiazepines).

Alcohol withdrawal

Delirium tremens, or alcohol withdrawal delirium, occurs 24–72 hours after cessation of alcohol in people with a long history of heavy drinking (**Figure 15.4**). It is characterised by severe agitation, altered consciousness, disorientation, hallucinations, insomnia, tremor and autonomic disturbance (resulting in sweating, tachycardia and hypertension), with dehydration and electrolyte imbalance. This is a medical emergency with a high risk of death (20% of cases) and urgent hospital treatment is needed. Alcohol-dependent patients should therefore be encouraged not to suddenly stop drinking without additional support. Complications of withdrawal include:

■ Seizures
■ Arrhythmias
■ Hallucinations
■ Wernicke–Korsakoff syndrome
■ Dehydration
■ Ketoacidosis
■ Pancreatitis

Magnesium and thiamine levels are often low in alcohol withdrawal and need supplementation. Correcting the magnesium level reduces the risk of seizures while thiamine correction reduces the risk of Wernicke–Korsakoff syndrome.

Benzodiazepines are the mainstay of treatment, the dose is dependent on the severity of the symptoms which can be quantified using the CIWA-A scoring system (**Figure 15.5**). A score of 20 or more indicates a need for benzodiazepines. The dose of benzodiazepine should be tailored to the response, usually starting high and then reducing as the symptoms (and CIWA-A score) reduce.

Symptoms of acute substance withdrawal	
Substance	Symptoms
Alcohol	Insomnia, agitation, nausea, hypertension, tachycardia/arrhythmias, tremor, delirium, seizures
Benzodiazepines	Insomnia, anxiety, nausea, tremor, headache, hallucinations, delirium, seizures
Heroin/opiates	Agitation, insomnia, pain, sweating, runny nose, diarrhea, dilated pupils, vomiting
Cocaine	Agitation, fatigue, nightmares/vivid dreams, increased appetite, low mood, suicidal thoughts
Ecstasy	Insomnia, anxiety, low mood, psychosis
Amphetamine	Hypersomnia, anxiety, mood swings, increased appetite, tachycardia/arrhythmias, tremor, seizures
Cannabis	Insomnia, nausea, low mood, anxiety, headaches
Tobacco	Insomnia, anxiety, sweating, abdominal cramps, headaches

Table 15.6 Symptoms of acute substance withdrawal

Symptoms of alcohol withdrawal	
Time since last alcoholic drink	
12 hours	Insomnia / Anxiety / Nausea / Headache
24 hours	Hallucinations / Authonomic instability / Tremor
48 hours	Delirium / Seizures

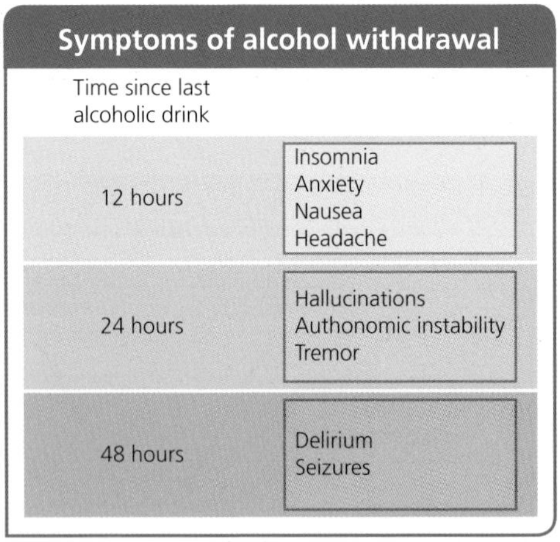

Figure 15.4 Symptoms of alcohol withdrawal.

Although many patients withdrawing from heroin request opiates such as methadone, it is important that this is only prescribed as part of a managed withdrawal programme and not given in the acute setting as a one-off.

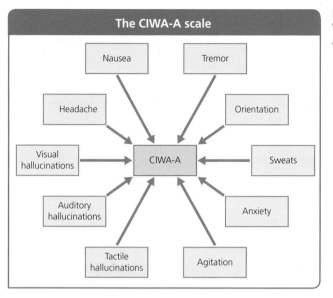

Figure 15.5 The Clinical Institute Withdrawal Assessment for Alcohol (CIWA-A) scale.

Heroin withdrawal

Heroin withdrawal is rarely life threatening and therefore can be managed with symptomatic relief only. Dehydration is the main complication and occurs if the patient has diarrhoea or vomiting. These symptoms should be treated with oral electrolyte solutions. Antiemetics and loperamide also help. Analgesia such as paracetamol or ibuprofen can be given for pain.

Case 23 Fever, muscle stiffness and tremor

Presentation

22-year-old David Elliott attends the out of hours GP surgery complaining of fever, muscle stiffness and a tremor in his hands. He had just started haloperidol at the instruction of his psychiatrist who had recently diagnosed David with psychosis.

Initial interpretation

Muscle stiffness and fever in someone taking an antipsychotic medication is suggestive of neuroleptic malignant syndrome (NMS). Other conditions such as serotonin syndrome or infections such as meningitis can present in a similar way. Immediate treatment and withdrawal of the antipsychotic is required in NMS to prevent cardiovascular collapse.

Further history and examination

David states that he has been taking twice the dose recommended by his psychiatrist as he thought it would help reduce the hallucinations he has been suffering from. Soon after starting the haloperidol David started to feel unwell. On examination he is tachycardic with a slightly raised blood pressure. He has significantly increased tone in his arms and legs and a shuffling gait. He has a tremor in both arms. His temperature is 39.4 despite use of paracetamol, which David took before attending the GP service.

Working diagnosis

The symptoms of fever and rigidity coupled with his recent use of antipsychotic medication indicate that David has neuroleptic malignant syndrome (NMS). Autonomic instability often occurs with NMS; however, NMS should be confirmed through further investigation.

Immediate intervention

As David shows signs of autonomic instability (with his heart rate and blood pressure being raised coupled with his high temperature) he is admitted urgently to hospital. Blood tests are done to rule out infection (**Table 15.7**) and assess levels of creatinine kinase, which is usually raised in NMS. A chest X-ray, head CT and lumbar puncture should be considered if there is any doubt regarding the diagnosis. The antipsychotic medication is stopped and David is given further doses of antipyrexial medication. He is rehydrated intravenously and benzodiazepines are given to aid muscle relaxation and reduce agitation. Bromocriptine is given if supportive measures alone do not reduce his symptoms.

David's investigation results		
Investigation	Result (normal)	Conclusion
Full blood count	WBC 14 x10⁹/L (3.5–11.0)	Leukocytosis is common in NMS
Urea and electrolytes	Urea 5 mmol/L (3–9)	
	Creatinine 1 mg/dL (0.6–1.3)	
C-reactive protein	16 mg/L (<6)	Common in NMS
Calcium	1.9 mmol/L (2.1–2.8)	Common in NMS
Creatine kinase	1029 U/L (24–174)	From rhabdomyolysis in NMS
Clotting	Prothrombin time 18 s (10–15)	Common in NMS
Liver function tests	ALT 10 U/L (5–21)	
	AST 11 U/L (6–40)	
	ALP 53 U/L (42–128)	
Thyroid	Free T3 5 pg/mL (3–7)	
Glucose	4.5 mmol/L (4.4–7.8)	
Arterial blood gas	Arterial pH 7.33 (7.34–7.45)	Metabolic acidosis is common in NMS
	Bicarbonate 15 mmol/L (18–23)	

Table 15.7 David's investigation results. ALP alkaline phosphatase; ALT alanine transaminase; AST aspartate transaminase; GGT gamma-glutamyl transferase; NMS, neuroleptic malignant syndrome; WBC, white blood count

Complications of psychiatric medication

Medications prescribed for mental illnesses can, rarely, cause NMS or serotonin syndrome. Both syndromes require immediate withdrawal of the medication and supportive treatment before considering an alternative medication. The symptoms of both syndromes are very similar (**Table 15.8**); however, serotonin syndrome has a lower mortality rate and tends to be milder than NMS. Other conditions and drugs can mimic the symptoms of NMS or serotonin syndrome; these should be excluded before making a diagnosis and include:

- Cocaine, amphetamine or MDMA use
- Malignant hyperpyrexia (can be caused by anaesthetic agents)

Symptoms of neuroleptic malignant syndrome and serotonin syndrome		
Symptom	Neuroleptic malignant syndrome	Serotonin syndrome
Neuromuscular dysfunctions, e.g. rigidity, hyperreflexia, tremor	Always present, usually marked rigidity	Present, usually with marked clonus
High temperature	Always present	Present
Autonomic instability, e.g. tachycardia, hyper or hypotension	Often significant and requiring hospitalisation	Minor and may go unnoticed
Altered mental state	Present, may be severe enough to cause a coma	Present, often in the form of agitation
Increased creatine kinase from rhabdomyolysis	Present to a significant degree	Occures to a minor degree
Abnormal blood results: coagulopathy, metabolic acidosis and deranged liver function tests	Occurs in severe cases	Occurs in severe cases
Kidney failure	Secondary to rhabdomyolysis	Rarely occurs
Cardiovascular collapse	10–20% of cases	Rare

Table 15.8 Symptoms of neuroleptic malignant syndrome and serotonin syndrome

- Catatonia
- Heat stroke
- Encephalitis or meningitis
- Poisoning or overdose.

Neuroleptic malignant syndrome

NMS is fatal in 10% of cases. It is caused by the actions of dopamine antagonists, i.e. the mechanism of action of most antipsychotics. Other drugs which can cause NMS include:

- Anticholinergic medication
- Metoclopramide
- Lithium

Management requires admission to an acute medical facility for monitoring and supportive treatment as needed. The drug which triggered NMS should be withdrawn. Supportive treatment involves:

- Reducing the hyperpyrexia through medication and cooling devices

- Muscle relaxants such as benzodiazepines
- Rehydration or dialysis for kidney dysfunction
- Heparin, platelets or coagulation factors for coagulopathies
- Intensive care for severe cases

Serotonin syndrome

Serotonin syndrome has many of the features of NMS but is usually milder in presentation. It occurs secondary to increases in serotonin and therefore can occur after taking antidepressants or other serotonergic drugs such as:

- Analgesics, e.g. tramadol
- Antiemetics, e.g. metoclopramide
- Buspirone
- Lithium
- Some antipsychotics

Supportive treatment and monitoring is similar to that of NMS for severe cases; however, most cases of serotonin syndrome are mild and can be managed in the community setting.

Chapter 16
Integrated care

Introduction................. 297
Case 24 Chronic psychosis
and weight gain 300
Management of mild and
moderate depression 302
Physical health problems in the
chronically mentally unwell 304

Depression in the chronically
physically unwell 305
Screening for postnatal
depression 307
Alcohol dependence 308
Community care of dementia.... 309

Starter questions

Answers to the following questions are on page 311.

1. What is the difference between primary and secondary care?
2. Why do patients with schizophrenia have a higher risk of cardiovascular disease?
3. Why do some alcohol-dependent patients undergo detoxification in hospital rather than in the community?

Introduction

In countries such as the UK, there has been a decline in the number of patients with mental illness whose care is delivered in hospitals. This reflects improvements in the treatment of psychiatric disorders, along with criticism of the failings of large inpatient psychiatric institutions. Currently, as in most other specialties, the majority of patients are assessed and managed in the community, receiving support from primary and secondary care services as required. The general structure of mental health services and rough divisions in the types of work they do are shown in **Figures 16.1** and **16.2**.

Primary care

In psychiatry more than in many other specialties, there is considerable overlap between health and social care. This is one of the reasons that the framework for integrated delivery of mental health care – the types of organisation and personnel – varies from country to country and in some aspects within a country. On the whole, this chapter sets out the general principles, but where specifics are unavoidable, it refers to English service structures.

Primary health care services are provided by general practitioners (GPs) or family physicians who are usually a patient's first point of contact with the health care and mental health care systems. GPs work alongside other professionals, such as practice nurses, midwives, health visitors and counsellors.

Mental illness accounts for a large proportion of GPs' workloads and up to 95% of mental illness is assessed and managed within primary care. GPs provide treatment options such as:

- self-help
- medication
- referral to a counsellor for short-term support based on talking therapy, to help cope with specific issues such as

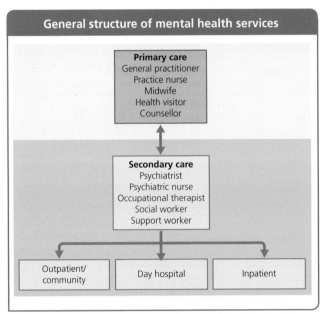

Figure 16.1 A generalised structure of mental health services.

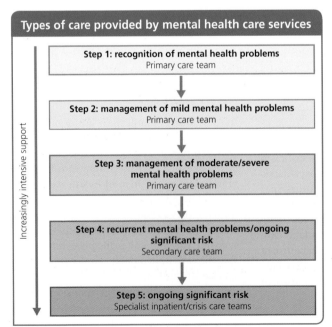

Figure 16.2 A generalised division of the types of care provided by primary and secondary mental health care services.

bereavement, relationship difficulties or mild depression

GPs and practice nurses are well placed to educate patients and their carers about mental illness and its management, and they monitor and manage physical health problems in patients who have mental illness.

Secondary care

In some cases, patients cannot be effectively or safely managed within primary care; GPs will therefore refer the patient to secondary care for additional support. Other reasons for referral include:

- uncertainty about diagnosis
- the presence of moderate to severe mental illness
- poor response to treatment

GPs use care pathways, such as those produced by the National Institute for Health and Care Excellence (NICE), to help them decide when to refer a patient to secondary care.

Secondary care teams

Secondary mental health care services include psychiatric hospitals and community-based care. These services are coordinated by community mental health teams (CMHTs)

formed of healthcare professionals from different specialties, including some or all of the following:

- psychiatrists
- community psychiatric nurses (CPNs)
- psychologists
- occupational therapists
- social workers
- support workers

CMHTs work within the community and often see patients in GP surgeries or in the patient's home. Psychiatrists working within CMHTs review patients at outpatient clinics.

A number of additional specialist teams provide secondary mental health care services to specific patient groups (**Table 16.1**). Usually, patients are referred via their GP.

Hospital admission

When a patient's behaviour and associated risks mean it is not possible to assess and manage them safely in the community, hospital admission to an inpatient psychiatric unit is required. The aim of admission is to enable assessment and/or treatment in a safe environment where risks can be managed. Patients are discharged back to the community as soon as it is safe to do so.

Specialist mental health teams in secondary care	
Team	Role
Child and adolescent mental health services	Assessment and management of children and young people with mental health or behavioural difficulties
	Work closely with patients' families and schools/colleges
Community drug and/or alcohol teams	Assessment and management of patients who consume excess alcohol or use illicit drugs
	Work closely with voluntary sector, e.g. Alcoholics Anonymous and Narcotics Anonymous
Community intellectual disability teams	Assessment and management of people with an intellectual disability and mental health or behavioural difficulties
	Work closely with families/carers, social care services, and generic physical health services
	Includes physiotherapists and speech and language therapists
Early intervention in psychosis teams	Assessment and management of patients with possible psychosis
	Offer education on psychosis to patients and their families
Assertive outreach teams	Similar to CMHTs, offering more flexible, frequent intense contact to high-risk patients with complex and enduring needs who are difficult to engage in other services, such as CMHTs
Intensive home treatment teams	Similar to CMHTs, providing short-term, intensive support to patients who might otherwise require hospital admission

Table 16.1 Specialist teams within the UK secondary mental health care service

If a patient is severely unwell they are admitted to a psychiatric intensive care unit (PICU). If an inpatient stay is prolonged (several years) the patient can 'step-down' into a rehabilitation unit to regain skills needed to live in the community, such as budgeting, cooking and managing relationships, before being discharged back to the community. Some recently discharged patients attend day hospitals for further support (e.g. psychological therapy, occupational therapy, education for carers); the patient goes home at the end of each day and at weekends. This approach is often used for elderly patients because they lose community life skills quicker than younger patients and re-acquire them more slowly.

Forensic inpatient units provide high-security settings for the assessment and management of people with mental illness who have committed, or are thought to be at high risk of committing, a serious criminal offence. There are also community forensic mental health services which care for patients after discharge from forensic inpatient units or prison-based forensic mental health services.

Case 24 Chronic psychosis and weight gain

Presentation

Frank Ogden is a 40-year-old, single, unemployed man with schizophrenia who lives alone in a ground floor flat. He sees his GP, Dr Cheema, concerned about the weight he has gained over the last few years.

Initial interpretation

Frank's current body mass index [BMI (weight in kg divided by weight in m²)] should be checked to assess how overweight he is. A medication history is needed because some antipsychotic medications cause weight gain. Other factors that contribute weight gain should be assessed such as Mr Ogden's eating habits, as well as any physical health consequences arising from his weight gain.

History

Frank says that he comfortably wore 32 inch (81 cm) waist trousers 2 years ago, but now struggles to fit into a 38 inch (97 cm) waist. He is unhappy about his size, but has found it difficult to reduce his weight. He describes feeling hungry most of the time and prefers to eat carbohydrate-rich snacks, such as crisps, between meals rather than fruit or vegetables.

He has not experienced any physical health problems as a consequence of his weight gain, with no joint pain or breathlessness on exertion. A systems review reveals no other symptoms.

He was started on his current antipsychotic medication around 2 and a half years ago. Prior to that, he was on a different antipsychotic medication and his weight was stable. He takes his medication regularly and he feels this helps reduce the number of voices he hears. He feels his mental state is currently good: he he continues to hear voices intermittently but these do not distress him. His mood is stable and he is sleeping well.

Interpretation of history

Frank has gained weight since starting his current antipsychotic medication. Being overweight is a risk factor for cardiovascular disease. Other risk factors for cardiovascular disease should be checked, such as family history, as well as Frank's smoking history and current lifestyle in terms of diet and exercise.

Further history

Frank recalls his father died from a heart attack at the age of 51. His mother is still alive and is being treated for breast cancer.

Case 24 *continued*

Schizophrenia: assessing cardiovascular risk

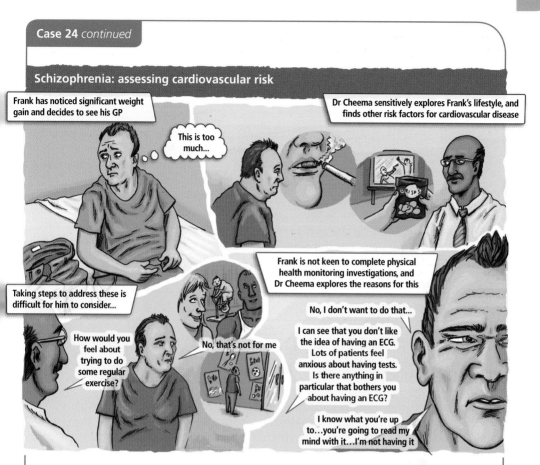

Frank has noticed significant weight gain and decides to see his GP

This is too much...

Dr Cheema sensitively explores Frank's lifestyle, and finds other risk factors for cardiovascular disease

Taking steps to address these is difficult for him to consider...

Frank is not keen to complete physical health monitoring investigations, and Dr Cheema explores the reasons for this

How would you feel about trying to do some regular exercise?

No, that's not for me

No, I don't want to do that...

I can see that you don't like the idea of having an ECG. Lots of patients feel anxious about having tests. Is there anything in particular that bothers you about having an ECG?

I know what you're up to...you're going to read my mind with it...I'm not having it

Frank smokes 25 cigarettes per day, increasing to 40 per day when he is 'stressed'. He denies using illicit drugs or alcohol. He does not have any structured daytime activities and spends most of his time in his flat watching DVDs or using his computer. He does not engage in regular exercise.

Physical examination

Frank's BMI is 28 kg/m². His fingers are tar-stained. His blood pressure and pulse are normal. The rest of his cardiovascular examination, and his respiratory, gastrointestinal and neurological examinations are all normal.

Interpretation of findings

Frank's physical examination reveals he is overweight. He has difficulties moderating his food intake, and these difficulties began following a change in his antipsychotic medication. His history reveals other risk factors for cardiovascular disease, including smoking, a sedentary lifestyle and a family history of cardiovascular disease in a first-degree male relative under 55 years old.

Investigations

Blood tests are arranged to evaluate Frank's cardiovascular risk factors, including a fasting blood glucose level to assess for the presence of diabetes and a blood lipid profile to assess for the presence of hypercholesterolaemia. The results of these tests are within normal ranges.

Case 17 *continued*

Diagnosis

Frank is overweight and this is increasing his risk of physical health problems, including cardiovascular disease. He is given advice and written information on healthy eating, and told he would benefit from exercising regularly, for at least 30 minutes per day, three days per week. Frank cannot afford any exercise equipment to use at home or to pay to go swimming or to the gym. He is offered a referral to free group exercise activities, but declines because he does not like being around other people as he does not trust them and fears they will be watching him.

Frank is advised of the risks of cigarette smoking and the support available to help him cut down is discussed. He says he is not going to stop smoking, as this helps him calm down, stops his voices when they are bad and that smoking is the only thing he has to look forward to each day.

Dr Cheema refers Frank to a consultant psychiatrist for a review of antipsychotic medication as this seems to be contributing to weight gain. Frank agrees to see Dr Cheema again next year for a further health check.

Management of mild and moderate depression

Most patients with mild to moderate depression are managed in primary care. A stepped approach is taken, in which primary care-based interventions are offered first and secondary care-based interventions are offered if these are ineffective or if symptoms worsen (**Figure 16.3**).

If a patient answers 'yes' to either of these questions, an assessment of their mental state and associated risks is completed by their GP. If this shows there are significant risks of self-harm, suicide, harm to others or neglect, a referral to secondary mental care services is required.

Step 1

The stepped approach requires GPs and practice nurses to identify those at risk of depression in the community by using screening questions whenever they suspect that a patient has a degree of depression (regardless of whether this was the reason for the consultation):

Screening questions to identify those at risk of depression include:

■ 'During the last month, have you often been bothered by feeling down, depressed or hopeless?'

■ 'During the last month, have you often been bothered by having little interest or pleasure in doing things?'

Step 2

People with mild to moderate depression and low associated risks are initially offered low-intensity psychosocial interventions from counsellors who work in general practice surgeries and other community-based locations. Interventions include:

■ structured group physical exercise programme
■ computerised cognitive behavioural therapy
■ individually guided self-help, for example, using prescribed books, based on cognitive behavioural therapy (CBT)

Follow-up appointments with a GP assess the patient's response to treatment and monitor the patient's risk.

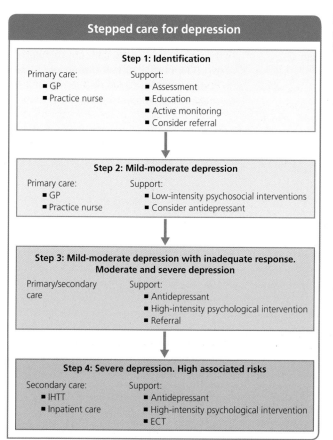

Figure 16.3 The stepped care approach to depression. IHTT, intensive home treatment team.

Stepped care for depression

Step 1: Identification

Primary care:
- GP
- Practice nurse

Support:
- Assessment
- Education
- Active monitoring
- Consider referral

Step 2: Mild-moderate depression

Primary care:
- GP
- Practice nurse

Support:
- Low-intensity psychosocial interventions
- Consider antidepressant

Step 3: Mild-moderate depression with inadequate response. Moderate and severe depression

Primary/secondary care

Support:
- Antidepressant
- High-intensity psychological intervention
- Referral

Step 4: Severe depression. High associated risks

Secondary care:
- IHTT
- Inpatient care

Support:
- Antidepressant
- High-intensity psychological intervention
- ECT

> **Computerised CBT is delivered by an interactive computer programme.** Patients can access their sessions at a time that suits them, rather than, for example, having to take time off work to attend sessions with a therapist. Many patients prefer the anonymity of undertaking CBT via computer rather than face-to-face with a therapist.

Step 3

Patients with mild to moderate depression who have declined or not benefitted from low-intensity interventions are offered higher-intensity psychological interventions, e.g. CBT. Alternatively, an antidepressant, e.g. an SSRI, is offered.

Those with moderate or severe depression are offered both medication and high-intensity psychological intervention; a referral to secondary care should also be considered.

Antidepressant medication

Patients prescribed antidepressant medication in primary care are reviewed by their GP after 2 weeks, and every 2–4 weeks thereafter to monitor mental state and suicidal ideation.

When prescribing antidepressants GPs talk to patients about:

- the reasons for prescribing and the importance of continuing treatment for a period of time after symptoms improve
- side effects
- discontinuation symptoms
- potential interactions with other drugs
- the possibility of increased suicidal thoughts in the early stages of treatment

Step 4

Those with severe depression, or whose associated risks cannot be safely managed within primary care, are referred to secondary care services for further support. This includes:

- medication, such as antidepressants
- high-intensity psychological interventions

- combined treatment, which may include ECT

In the most severe cases, patients are referred to an IHTT (**Table 16.1**) for intensive, short-term support or are admitted to hospital for further assessment and support.

Physical health problems in the chronically mentally unwell

People with chronic mental health difficulties are at increased risk of physical and sometimes life-shortening health problems. This reflects the higher prevalence of smoking, lack of exercise and poor diet. These problems are compounded in patients with schizophrenia or other disorders that similarly require long-term antipsychotic medication. A number of these drugs, particularly the atypical (second generation) antipsychotics, affect insulin function and glucose homeostasis and cause often substantial weight gain, further increasing the risk of diabetes and cardiovascular disease. All antipsychotic drugs are associated with increased risk of sedation, sexual dysfunction, postural hypotension, cardiac arrhythmia, and sudden cardiac death.

Other drugs used for mental disorders also have side effects for which all clinicians in primary and secondary healthcare should be vigilant. However, it is the antipsychotic medications for which an integrated approach to care is most needed and occurs most commonly.

Physical health investigations

Before antipsychotic medication is started, psychiatrists in secondary care liaise with GPs to investigate the patient's physical health, including an assessment of smoking habits, diet and level of physical activity and:

- body mass index
- blood pressure
- fasting blood glucose
- blood lipid profile

If the history, examination or investigations identify any cardiovascular risk factors, an ECG is undertaken to check for any undetected cardiac abnormalities which would rule out the use of particular antipsychotics.

Hydrocarbons in cigarette smoke interact with other drugs. Reduction/cessation of smoking affects metabolism of schizophrenia medications, particularly clozapine. With the latter, for example, serum clozapine rises, necessitating closer monitoring for side effects, e.g. hypersalivation, hypotension, sedation and seizures. If these occur, dose reduction to minimise side effects must be balance with avoiding a deterioration in mental state.

Smoking cessation

Patients with chronic mental illnesses who smoke should be offered help to stop. Medications to assist this can be considered, including bupropion (a noradrenaline and dopamine reuptake inhibitor that reduces cigarette cravings) and varenicline (a nicotinic acetylcholine receptor partial agonist that reduces the urge to smoke). However, they increase the risk of serious adverse psychiatric symptoms, including anxiety and suicidal ideation.

Monitoring medication

Once antipsychotic medication has been started, the psychiatrist and their team monitor the patient's physical health. After a year,

Annual health checks for patients with chronic psychosis		
Risk factor	Investigation	Action if abnormal
Obesity	Annual weight/body mass index	Advice on strategies to increase physical activity levels and improve diet
		Consider referral to weight management programme, physical activity programme or dietician
		Information on voluntary self-help groups
		Consider switching antipsychotic medication to one less likely to cause weight-gain
Hypertension	Annual blood pressure measurement	Lifestyle advice
		Consider antihypertensive medication
Diabetes	Annual fasting blood glucose and/or HbA1c	Lifestyle advice
		Consider medication to treat diabetes, e.g. metformin
		Consider switching antipsychotic medication
Hypercholesterolaemia	Annual blood lipid profile	Lifestyle advice
		Consider lipid-lowering medication
Smoking	History-taking: questions around smoking	Education on smoking risks
		Offer support for smoking cessation
		Consider nicotine replacement therapy with inhalators, gum, patches, lozenges or spray
		Consider medications for smoking cessation, such as bupropion or varenicline
Sedentary lifestyle	History-taking: questions around levels of physical activity	Advice on benefits of regular physical exercise
		Offer referral to physical activity programme
Poor diet	History-taking: questions around dietary intake	Advice on healthy eating
		Consider referral to dietician

Table 16.2 Annual physical health checks for people with chronic psychosis

the GP takes over this responsibility and provides annual health checks (**Table 16.2**), ensuring that results and actions taken are communicated to the secondary care team.

When patients on antipsychotic medication experience physical symptoms such as weight gain, hypertension, hypercholesterolaemia or blood glucose abnormalities, their GP and psychiatrist work together to consider if antipsychotic medication is contributing. In some cases, switching to a different antipsychotic is discussed, but this requires consideration of the potential benefits and the risks of a relapse in psychotic symptoms.

Depression in the chronically physically unwell

Chronic physical illness, such as cancer, increases the risk of developing a depressive disorder (see Chapter 11). Because comorbid depression can negatively impact on the prognosis of physical illness and the patient's ability to make decisions about their treatment it is important that depression is identified in chronically physically unwell patients so that appropriate treatment can be offered.

Screening

Within primary care, GP and practice nurses screen chronically physically unwell patients to identify those at risk of depression by asking a number of questions.

Screening questions to identify chronically, physically unwell patients at risk of depression include:

- 'During the last month, have you often been bothered by feeling down, depressed or hopeless?'

- 'During the last month, have you often been bothered by having little interest or pleasure in doing things?'

If a patient answers 'yes' to either question, a further three are asked:

- 'During the last month, have you often been bothered by...
  - 'Feelings of worthlessness?'
  - 'Poor concentration?
  - 'Thoughts of death?

Patients identified as being at risk of depression are assessed in more depth by their GP. Measures such as the Hospital Anxiety and Depression Scale (HADS), Beck Depression Inventory (BDI) or Patient Health Questionnaire (PHQ-9) are used to assess the severity of depressive or anxiety disorders.

Management

As with patients without co-morbid chronic physical illness, a stepped care approach is taken and most patients are managed within primary care. Management options within primary care for those with mild depression include:

- structured group physical activity
- group-based peer support programmes
- computerised CBT

Those with moderate depression are offered:

- group or individual CBT
- behavioural couples therapy in cases where the patient's relationship with their partner is contributing to the maintenance of their depression

Antidepressant medication

Antidepressant medication is offered to patients with severe depression or whose mild–moderate depression is complicating the care of their physical health problem. The potential impact of drug interactions and side effects are always taken into account before prescribing, for example SSRIs exacerbate hyponatraemia and have an antiplatelet effect. GPs and practice nurses monitor the response to treatment and associated risks, e.g. risk of harm to self or others.

Referral to secondary care

If a patient's response to psychological or pharmacological therapy is poor, or if there are significant risks, for example, of the patient causing harm to themselves or others, which cannot be safely managed in primary care, the patient is referred refer patients to secondary care, e.g. to a CMHT or IHTT, for further support.

Adjusting to a diagnosis of terminal illness causes feelings of despair or anger, but these emotional responses are different to clinical depression. Depression is not an inevitable consequence of terminal illness and can be treated effectively in patients with terminal illnesses.

Depression in a palliative care setting

Psychiatrists in palliative care settings work with other secondary care professionals, such as specialist palliative medicine doctors, as well as GPs, to ensure that psychosocial stressors, such as pain, which may negatively impact on a patient's mood and mental state, are adequately addressed.

Effective treatments for depression in patients with terminal illness include:

- psychological therapies, such as CBT
- intensive specialist nursing support
- social support
- antidepressant medication

Screening for postnatal depression

Diagnosing and managing postnatal depression takes place in primary care. In the UK, midwives and health visitors monitor the health of new mothers and are trained to detect indicators of postnatal depression.

During their first appointment with their midwife, pregnant women are asked questions to identify risk factors for postnatal depression:

- 'Do you have, or have you previously had, severe depression, bipolar affective disorder, schizophrenia or puerperal psychosis?'

- 'Have you previously received treatment from a psychiatrist or specialist mental health team?'

- 'Is there a family history of perinatal mental illness?'

Midwives, health visitors and GPs also ask all new mothers the following questions to identify those who require further assessment of their mental state:

- During the past month, have you often been bothered by feeling down, depressed or hopeless?'
- 'During the past month, have you often been bothered by having little interest or pleasure in doing things?'

If the answer to both questions is 'yes', ask the following question:

- 'Is this something you feel you need or want help with?'

Patients with postnatal depression often feel ashamed and afraid to disclose their thoughts and feelings. They worry that they will be separated from their child or that their child will taken away from them by social services.

Management

In the UK, GPs use the Edinburgh Postnatal Depression Scale to assess the severity of the patient's symptoms (see page 219). Postnatal (puerperal) depression is treated similarly to non-puerperal depression, although the decision to start medication, is influenced by whether the mother is breastfeeding or not (see page 219). A stepped care approach is taken and most patients are managed within primary care (**Figure 16.4**).

Referral to secondary care

Women with severe postnatal depression who cannot be effectively and safely managed in primary care require admission to a mother and baby psychiatric unit or to a general psychiatric ward if they live in a region that does not have a specialist unit and transfer is not possible. Examples of reasons for admission include suicidal or infanticidal ideation and development of post-partum (puerperal) psychosis.

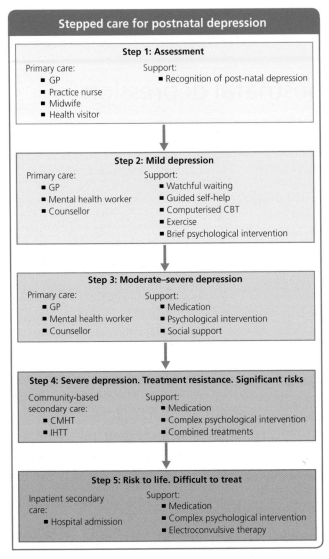

Figure 16.4 The stepped care approach to postnatal depression. CMHT, community mental health team; IHTT, intensive home treatment team

Alcohol dependence

GPs and practice nurses routinely ask patients about alcohol use and provide advice on the dangers of excessive drinking. They use screening questions to identify patients who are consuming excess alcohol; these patients are then offered a referral to a specialist secondary care alcohol team for support to address and reduce their alcohol intake (see page 195).

When enquiring about alcohol use in a primary care setting, be non-judgemental and remember:

- many patients are reluctant to discuss their drinking habits and may not provide accurate information
- patients may not wish to accept they have a problem

- maintaining rapport with patients is vital so that, over time, they can be encouraged to access support

Management

Patients referred to community alcohol teams are not always ready to cut down their alcohol intake to achieve abstinence. In these cases, community alcohol team nurses and psychologists offer motivational interviewing to explore the patient's ambivalence towards changing their alcohol-related behaviour (see page 196), with the aim of motivating the patient to address their alcohol intake.

Community alcohol teams provide CBT, couples therapy and family therapy. They support the patient's withdrawal from alcohol by detoxification, which may be community- or hospital-based. Patients who score 20 or more on the AUDIT questionnaire and/or who drink 15 or more units of alcohol per day are offered detoxification in the community. This involves:

- Daily supervision via home visits from the community alcohol team to support the patient's detoxification attempt and to monitor for complications, such as delirium tremens or a deterioration in their mental state
- Medications, such as chlordiazepoxide, to prevent symptoms of alcohol withdrawal (see page 298). Preferably, supportive family members ensure the patient takes their medication as prescribed
- Multivitamins to prevent Wernicke's encephalopathy (see page 193)

Some patients cannot complete detoxification in the community safely; the community alcohol team will offer admission to a specialist alcohol detoxification unit within a general psychiatric hospital for inpatient detoxification. Should the patient develop any significant physical health complications during their detoxification they are transferred to general medical hospitals for treatment of their physical health problems.

Inpatient alcohol detoxification is offered to patients with:

- poor social support, including homelessness
- an alcohol intake of 30 or more units per day
- a history of epilepsy or severe alcohol withdrawal symptoms
- significant physical health comorbidities (e.g. chronic liver disease)
- significant psychiatric comorbidities (e.g. psychosis, cognitive impairment)
- co-morbid misuse of illicit drugs

Discharge and follow-up

Following completion of detoxification from alcohol in hospital, patients are discharged back to the community. They are prescribed medication to help maintain abstinence (see page 196) and continue to receive support from the community alcohol team to help to maintain their abstinence and manage any periods of relapse.

Patients who develop cognitive impairment as a consequence of Korsakoff's syndrome are offered long-term care placement in supported independent or residential care where they receive ongoing support to maintain alcohol abstinence.

Community care of dementia

Two-thirds of people with dementia are cared for at home; most of the other third live in residential or specialist nursing care homes in the community. Almost all dementia care is delivered in the community, with input from the GP and from secondary care, including social care services and, when appropriate, a specialist memory or old age psychiatry service.

Identifying dementia

Many patients come to the attention of GPs after friends or family become aware of a memory problem. However, most elderly people who are no longer independent live in residential or nursing care homes within the community. The signs and symptoms of dementia can be missed in these settings; carers are therefore trained to recognise them and to liaise with general practitioners if further support is required.

Primary care GPs and practice nurses assess patients who have possible memory impairment (see page 76) and refer those with signs and symptoms of memory impairment to old age psychiatry memory assessment teams. These secondary care teams prescribe dementia-specific medication if required.

> **Be alert for possible dementia when performing health checks in patients at increased risk of dementia,** such as those with an intellectual disability, a neurological condition (e.g. Parkinson's disease) or cerebrovascular disease.

Care plans

Within secondary care, an integrated approach to the care of patients with dementia is taken, involving:

- healthcare services
- social care services
- voluntary organisations

Health and social care services work together to produce an individualised care plan which takes into account the patient's health care needs and their requirements for social support. Care plans are reviewed regularly to ensure each patient's needs are met given that as dementia progresses these can change over time.

Support for carers

As part of this integrated approach, the needs of family members or informal carers are assessed to ensure they are provided with support to cope with the demands of their role. A care plan is formulated for each principal carer in dicussion with the carer and includes:

- referral to voluntary organisations, such as the Alzheimer's Society, which provide support and information
- information on local groups of other carers, which offer peer-support
- education on dementia and how to care for and communicate with people with dementia

Carers are offered psychological interventions delivered by primary care counsellors if their role is causing them psychological distress or having a negative impact on their functioning.

Specialist and palliative care

If a patient develops behaviours associated with risks to the health and safety of themselves or of others, and these risks cannot be effectively and safely managed in the community, admission to a specialist inpatient unit is required. In England, for example, many elderly mental illness units are run as specialist divisions of care homes.

GPs and old age psychiatry services work together to monitor dementia and its associated risks and physical health problems over time. As patients enter the terminal stage of dementia, GP refer patients and their carers to specialist palliative care teams for additional support.

Answers to starter questions

1. Primary health care services are usually a patient's first point of contact with the healthcare system. In the UK, primary care providers are general practitioners working alongside practice nurses, midwives, health visitors and counsellors. Secondary health care services provide specialist expertise; patients generally access such services via a referral from their GP. Secondary care services may be community- or hospital-based.

2. The prevalence of smoking, lack of exercise and poor diet is higher in people with schizophrenia, and these are all risk factors for diabetes and cardiovascular disease. In addition, some antipsychotic medications used to treat schizophrenia impair insulin function, impacting on glucose homeostasis and causing significant weight gain, further increasing the risk of diabetes and cardiovascular disease.

3. Treatment to support patients withdrawing from alcohol can take place either in the community or in hospital. Patients undergoing detoxification in the community require a high level of social support and daily supervision to manage their medication, symptoms and risks of complications. For patients with poor social support, (e.g. those who are homeless), who drink 30 or more units per day, who have a history of epilepsy or severe alcohol withdrawal symptoms, significant physical or psychiatric comorbidity or comorbid misuse of illicit drugs it is not possible to manage the risks of alcohol withdrawal in the community and inpatient alcohol detoxification is required.

Chapter 17
Self-assessment

SBA questions. 313   SBA answers 325

SBA questions

Affective (mood) disorders

1. A 34-year-old woman visits her health visitor after the birth of her baby. She feels she is not bonding with her baby, does not enjoy being a mother and is not going out of the house except when she has to. She has difficulty sleeping, even when the baby is settled and has lost her appetite.
    What is the single most likely diagnosis?

    A Baby 'blues'
    B Bipolar disorder
    C No mental illness
    D Obsessive compulsive disorder
    E Postnatal depression

2. A 58-year-old man is brought to the emergency department after trying to hang himself in his garage. He has been feeling very low for some time and has not been enjoying his usual activities. Recently, he has started hearing people whispering, saying negative things to him. Occasionally, he has also seen dark shadows in his home which he feels symbolise demons. He feels the only way out is through suicide.
    What is the single most likely diagnosis?

    A Depression
    B Dementia
    C Post-traumatic stress disorder
    D Psychotic depression
    E Schizophrenia

3. A 24-year-old woman has a 4-month history of low mood, which has impacted on her ability to socialise and enjoy her usual hobbies. She used to cycle frequently, but no longer has the energy to do so. Her sleep is poor and she has lost a little weight because she doesn't have much of an appetite.
    What is the single most appropriate treatment?

    A Antipsychotic medication
    B Lithium
    C Psychoanalytical therapy
    D Selective serotonin reuptake inhibitors
    E Watchful waiting

4. A 67-year-old man is recovering from an anterior myocardial infarction (MI), but does not attend his appointments regularly or do the exercise prescribed. He feels hopeless and that there is no point trying. Since the MI he has not been out much because he has little energy. He is having trouble sleeping.
    What is the single most likely diagnosis?

    A Angina
    B Cerebrovascular accident
    C Depression
    D Heart failure
    E Post-traumatic stress disorder

5. A 45-year-old woman is detained in a psychiatric unit because she is refusing to eat. For some time she has had a low mood, anhedonia and little energy. Over the last month her symptoms have worsened, with poor sleep, reduced appetite and intense feelings of guilt that she was ruining her family's life. She has refused medication because she felt it would only prolong her and her family's suffering. She has refused all food for 10 days because she feels the only way to die is to starve herself.
    What is the single most appropriate treatment?

    A Antipsychotic medication
    B Cognitive behavioural therapy
    C Electroconvulsive therapy

D Lithium
E Selective serotonin reuptake inhibitors

6. A 22-year-old man has jumped off the roof of his bungalow. He has sustained minor injuries and during assessment talks about being able to fly and describes how it feels. He says he developed special powers a few weeks ago and is now learning to control them. He is very talkative and expressive. He has previously been diagnosed with depression after attempting suicide.
What is the single most likely diagnosis?

A Bipolar disorder
B Borderline personality disorder
C Narcissistic personality disorder
D Psychotic depression
E Schizophrenia

7. A 20-year-old woman has low mood, reduced energy, insomnia and poor appetite. She feels nothing is enjoyable anymore and would like help. Previously, she has had 2 episodes of mania which required short hospital admissions. She is keen to avoid anything that will cause another manic episode.
What is the single most appropriate treatment?

A Antipsychotic medication
B Carbamazepine
C Monoamine oxidase inhibitors
D Selective serotonin reuptake inhibitors
E Tricyclic antidepressant medication

8. A 34-year-old woman has felt increasingly 'hyper' over the last 4 weeks, rushing around her home tidying and organising. She feels very tired, but unable to stop and is not sleeping properly. She is often 'drenched' in sweat and feels very weak. She has recently lost weight despite eating more than usual.
What is the single most likely diagnosis?

A Attention deficit hyperactivity disorder
B Bipolar disorder
C Generalised anxiety disorder
D Hyperthyroidism
E Mania

Schizophrenia and psychotic illness

1. A 22-year-old man with no previous medical or psychiatric history is brought to the doctor by his worried sister. He does not think he is ill and says there is a conspiracy to have him assassinated because he is receiving messages from Elvis Presley about government corruption. He cannot stop Elvis Presley talking to him and is angry that no one else will admit to having these experiences too.
What is the single most appropriate next step?

A Arrange assessment under mental health legislation
B Arrange a urine drug screen
C Ask questions to explore his hallucinations and delusions in detail
D Obtain a collateral history from his sister
E Reassure him that these experiences are not real

2. A 20-year-old male student, who lives with his parents, has a 4-month history of increasingly bizarre behaviour. He is unconcerned, but his parents report that he has become increasingly withdrawn and is distracted in conversation, stating he can see the shadow of a man in the corner of the room. On mental state examination, he is unkempt, with flattened affect, thought withdrawal and visual hallucinations. He has no thoughts of harm to himself or others.
What is the single most appropriate next step?

A Arrange assessment under mental health legislation
B Complete physical examination and investigations
C Offer informal admission for further assessment of his mental state
D Prescribe a trial of atypical antipsychotic
E Refer to the early intervention in psychosis team

3. A 46-year-old man with no previous medical or psychiatric history is convinced his wife is being sexually unfaithful with a work colleague. He will not accept his wife's denial of this and has been searching her handbag regularly for the last 4 months. He recently found a discarded banana skin, which he is certain proves her infidelity although he cannot explain this further. He has followed her in his car, without her knowledge, on several occasions. He has no hallucinations and is euthymic on mental state examination. Physical examination and blood tests are normal.
What is the single most likely diagnosis?

A Acute and transient psychotic disorder
B Erotomania
C Othello syndrome
D Schizoaffective disorder
E Schizophrenia

4. A 28-year-old woman has a 10-day history of unusual behaviour. She has no past psychiatric or medical history. Her husband recently asked her for a divorce and moved out of their home. Her symptoms started with confusion and incoherent speech. Within 48 hours, she described hearing her husband's voice talking to her when she was alone at home. Her mood changes during each day from elation to being anxious and irritable. She does not drink alcohol and has never used illicit substances. Physical examination and investigations are normal.

What is the single most likely diagnosis?

A Acute and transient psychotic disorder
B Bipolar affective disorder
C Persistent delusional disorder
D Schizoaffective disorder
E Schizophrenia

5. A 33-year-old woman with schizophrenia is hearing voices commenting on her actions. She has previously stubbed cigarettes out on her arm when commanded to do so by these voices. She does not drink alcohol or take illegal substances. She is concordant with medication, but her symptoms continue despite taking olanzapine and now amisulpiride at optimum doses, each for 2 months.

What is the single most appropriate next step?

A Offer informal hospital admission for further assessment of her mental state
B Prescribe a trial of clozapine
C Prescribe a trial of depot antipsychotic medication
D Prescribe oral risperidone at optimum dose for 6 weeks
E Refer to psychology for CBT

6. A 19-year-old woman has a 6-month history of a change in her behaviour, becoming increasingly withdrawn, neglecting her personal hygiene and describing hearing her thoughts being spoken out loud. She has no previous psychiatric or medical history and lives with her mother and sister. There is no co-morbid substance misuse. Physical examination and investigations are normal. She has no thoughts of harm to herself or others.

What is the single most appropriate next step?

A Arrange urgent assessment under mental health legislation
B Offer informal hospital admission for further assessment of her mental state
C Refer to the early intervention team for urgent assessment
D Prescribe antipsychotic medication
E Watchful waiting in primary care

7. A 23-year-old man has a 6-month history of psychotic symptoms with no organic cause and following psychiatric assessment has been diagnosed with schizophrenia. He has

been engaging with cognitive behavioural therapy, lives with a supportive girlfriend and has decided he would like to try olanzapine, as discussed with him by the consultant psychiatrist. He has no past medical history, takes no other medications, but smokes 10 cigarettes per day with no intention to stop. On mental state examination, he has some insight, but no thoughts of harm to himself or others.

What is the single most appropriate next action?

A Check blood lipid levels
B Check breath carbon monoxide levels
C Prescribe a trial of olanzapine
D Prescribe a trial of nicotine replacement therapy (nicotine patches)
E Watchful waiting in primary care

Anxiety disorders

1. A 47-year-old woman has had persistent anxiety for 3 years with no particular trigger. She has abdominal pains, tachycardia, tachypnoea and feelings of restlessness and tension. She is becoming increasingly isolated and rarely leaves the house.

What is the single most likely diagnosis?

A Agoraphobia
B Claustrophobia
C Generalised anxiety disorder
D Obsessive compulsive disorder
E Post-traumatic stress disorder

2. A 24-year-old man has an intense fear of dying. He tries to reduce it by cleaning and washing his hands, which he does approximately 15 times a day. These habits provide temporary relief, but his fears soon return and he imagines how awful it would be if he contracted various diseases. An MSE suggests a diagnosis of obsessive compulsive disorder.

What single examination will provide evidence to support this diagnosis?

A Abdomen
B Cardiovascular system
C Eyes
D Feet
E Hands

3. A 32-year-old male soldier was diagnosed with PTSD after he was injured in a bomb that killed many of his colleagues. He has recently completed a course of CBT, but, despite engaging well with the therapy, he has not found it helpful for his symptoms.

What is the single most appropriate alternative treatment?

A Antidepressants

B Antipsychotics
C Counselling
D Dialectical behavioural therapy
E Dynamic psychotherapy

4. A 32-year-old woman frequently feels anxious, has palpitations and a tremor. Her anxiety is preventing her socialising and disturbing her sleep. It started 1 month ago with no known trigger and she has lost a significant amount of weight since then.
What is the single most appropriate next step?

A Reassure and advise to return if symptoms persist
B Refer to a dietician for help with weight loss
C Refer to a psychiatrist for further assessment
D Refer to a psychotherapist for cognitive behavioural therapy
E Take blood for testing

5. A 22-year-old male student has an episode of dizziness, hyperventilation and chest pains; and has had a few over the last few months. They mainly occur in tutorials, but recently also occurred when he attempted to give a presentation.
What is the single most appropriate treatment?

A Antidepressants
B Cognitive behavioural therapy
C Diazepam taken before social events
D Eye movement desensitisation and reprocessing
E No treatment

Suicide and self-harm

1. A 13-year-old girl often self harms with a razor, cutting her arms and legs. She has done this for 6 months, but now feels it is out of control as she cuts 4 or 5 times a day, including at school. She begs not to disclose her self-harm to her parents.
What is the single most appropriate next step?

A Acknowledge her distress and agree the information can be kept confidential
B Conduct a physical examination
C Discuss referral to her local child and adolescent mental health team
D Discuss why she is reluctant to allow her parents to know
E Tell her that, due to her age, her parents must be informed

2. A 56-year-old man has been struggling with depression despite the starting antidepressants, and his suicidal feelings are increasing.
He has thought of dying by taking an overdose and has been buying paracetamol for that reason, with quite a few packets at home. He feels life is worthless and that he is a burden on his relatives.
What is the single most appropriate course of action?

A Ask him to get rid of the paracetamol and increase his antidepressant medication
B Phone the emergency services
C Reassure him that many people feel this way and ask him to return in a week
D Refer to the local mental health team
E Telephone the crisis mental health team or on-call psychiatrist for an emergency assessment

3. A 40-year-old woman has taken an overdose of 30 paracetamol tablets with alcohol. She has been feeling low for some time, but took the paracetamol on the spur of the moment after being sacked. Her husband found her taking the paracetamol and brought her to the emergency department. She is compliant with treatment and agrees she needs help.
What is the single most appropriate treatment initially?

A Activated charcoal
B Alcohol advice
C N-acetylcysteine
D No treatment required
E Problem-solving therapy

Personality disorders

1. A 24-year-old woman has been self-harming since she was 15 years old and this has now escalated to very deep cuts on her arms, legs and stomach. The triggers for her self-harm are times when she feels 'left out', e.g. if a friend cancels a meeting or does not reply to a text message. She often feels suicidal and occasionally attempts suicide when cutting herself, which is why the cuts have become deeper. As this has not worked she is contemplating taking overdoses instead. She often feels 'empty', but is not low in mood as she enjoys herself when out with friends. She has not had a serious relationship, but has had several short-term relationships which are often intense and lead to frequent arguments.
What is the single most likely diagnosis?

A Anankastic personality disorder
B Antisocial personality disorder
C Bipolar disorder
D Borderline personality disorder
E Depression

2. A 32-year-old woman is assessed over a number of sessions due to repeated suicide attempts and a long history of short, intense relationships.
    What is the single most appropriate treatment?

    A Antidepressants
    B Antipsychotics
    C Dialectical behavioural therapy
    D Electroconvulsive therapy
    E Eye movement desensitisation and repro-cessing

3. A 22-year-old man is assessed at the request of the police, who arrested him for assaulting his girlfriend. He has been with his current girlfriend for only a couple of weeks and boasts of having had sexual relationships with over 100 women. He has never had a long-term relationship. He denies assaulting previous partners, but it is suspected he is lying. He has previously been arrested for assault on a stranger. He denies having close friends or feeling any need to have any. He does not have a career and has tried many different jobs. In his childhood, he was expelled from multiple schools for fighting.
    What is the single most likely diagnosis?

    A Antisocial personality disorder
    B Borderline personality disorder
    C Histrionic personality disorder
    D Morbid jealousy
    E Psychosis

4. A 27-year-old man has become convinced that he is being followed by the police and that they have surveillance equipment in his house recording his movements and thoughts. He is very distressed by this and is considering leaving the country to escape. He admits to hearing the police commenting on his actions in his home and occasionally when outside.
    What is the single most appropriate treatment?

    A Antipsychotics
    B Antidepressants
    C Cognitive behavioural therapy
    D Dynamic psychotherapy
    E Sedative antihistamines

Substance misuse and addictions

1. A 40-year-old unemployed man drinks 2 bottles of vodka each day. He craves alcohol and experiences shaking, nausea and anxiety when he has not had any. He recently left his job as a hospital porter as he preferred to spend his time drinking at home. On examination, he smells of alcohol and has gynaecomastia. His memory is not impaired.
    Which is the single most likely diagnosis?

    A Alcohol dependence
    B Acute alcohol withdrawal
    C Binge drinking
    D Delirium tremens
    E Wernicke's encephalopathy

2. A 43-year-old married man with a 2-year history of alcohol dependence has successfully completed a community-based alcohol detox with the support of his family, and continues to engage with the community alcohol team. He is concordant with the medication prescribed. He now has facial flushing, headache and nausea, which started suddenly after he had a shave.
    Which single medication is most likely to account for this?

    A Acamprosate
    B Chlordiazepoxide
    C Diazepam
    D Disulfiram
    E Naltrexone

3. A 59-year-old divorced man has no past medical or psychiatric history. He presents accompanied by his daughter, who is concerned about his mental state. He has just arrived home from a holiday in the Falklands and states that during this time the Queen of England died. He denies any hallucinations, thought disorder or mood disturbance, and has had no recent falls. On examination, he is ataxic with nystagmus. His daughter says she thinks he drinks too much alcohol. A CT of the brain shows no abnormalities.
    What is the single most likely diagnosis?

    A Acute subdural haematoma
    B Chronic subdural haematoma
    C Delirium tremens
    D Schizophrenia
    E Wernicke's encephalopathy

4. A 62-year-old woman has had a fall resulting in a wrist fracture that has been treated with a plaster cast. She is awaiting discharge home. She is otherwise well with no past psychiatric history. 2 days after admission she becomes agitated and has visual hallucinations. Her son says that she normally drinks 3 bottles of wine a day. She is hypertensive, sweaty and shaky on examination, but there are no other abnormalities and she does not smell of alcohol. Her urine dipstick and full blood count are normal.
    What is the single most likely diagnosis?

    A Acute alcohol intoxication
    B Delirium tremens
    C Panic disorder

D Schizophrenia
E Wernicke's encephalopathy

5. A 19-year-old female student attended a party 24 hours ago and has been troubled by paranoid ideas since. She is a smoker, but does not drink alcohol. She is frightened by the large spiders she can see crawling over the ceiling despite her friend's reassurance that there is nothing there. She feels that time has slowed down. On examination, she has reddened sclera and nystagmus.
What single substance is most likely to be accounting for her symptoms?

A Amphetamine
B Anabolic steroids
C Cannabis
D Cocaine
E Diamorphine

6. A 24-year-old man with schizophrenia uses amphetamines intermittently, with no intention to stop. He forgets to take his antipsychotic medication when under the influence of amphetamines. He has made superficial cigarette burns to his hand in response to auditory hallucinations in the past, but has had no recent thoughts of harm to himself or others. He has not attended any appointments with his community mental health team worker for the last 4 weeks.
What is the single most appropriate next step?

A Arrange assessment under mental health legislation
B Arrange hospital admission for amphetamine detoxification
C Offer motivational interviewing
D Referral to the assertive outreach team
E Watchful waiting by general practitioner

7. A 28-year-old, unemployed, single woman with heroin dependence has been working with the substance misuse team for 1 year. She now acknowledges that her heroin use is causing difficulties in her life. She believes she needs to change her heroin-related behaviour, but is unsure how to go about doing so and wants to talk about the options available. Which single stage of the Prochaska and Di Clemente's model best describes her current state?

A Action
B Contemplation
C Maintenance
D Pre-contemplation
E Preparation

Eating disorders

1. A 17-year-old girl's mother is concerned because her daughter she has lost a lot of weight recently. The daughter denies any illness or significant weight loss. She believes her mother is overreacting to her not eating with the family and her doing 'a bit' more exercise. She is image-conscious and does not like the look of her body. She refuses to be weighed, but appears extremely thin.
Which single symptom is uncommon in this condition?

A Amenorrhea
B Diarrhoea
C Lanugo hair
D Low blood pressure
E Palpitations

2. A 22-year-old man has a history of significant weight loss. He rarely eats a full meal and spends a lot of time at the gym trying to 'tone up'. Other people have noticed his weight loss, but he still feels fat. His diet has become more extreme, reducing his calorie intake to about 500 Kcal per day.
What would not be considered an appropriate treatment?

A Cognitive analytic therapy
B Dietary advice
C Exposure response prevention therapy
D Family therapy
E Interpersonal psychotherapy

3. A 16-year-old girl collapses at school and is brought to the emergency department. On examination she is pale, significantly underweight and has low blood pressure. She denies any problem with her weight and states she just fainted because she was exercising in the sun. The examining doctor feels an ECG is required.
What is the single most likely finding?

A Atrial fibrillation
B Bradycardia
C Tachycardia
D Tall, tented T waves
E Ventricular fibrillation

4. A 24-year-old woman attends her dentist because of toothache and bad breath. Her dentist finds 7 cavities and notices Russel's sign on her hands. The patient appears to be of normal or slightly above normal BMI. She denies any problems with eating, although she admits to sometimes binge eating when she is upset.

What is the single most likely diagnosis?

A   Anorexia nervosa
B   Binge eating disorder
C   Bulaemia nervosa
D   Eating disorder not otherwise specified
E   Obsessive compulsive disorder

5. A 27-year-old woman is admitted to the emergency department with muscle pain and weakness after fainting while out with friends. She admits that over the last 6 months she has been vomiting after eating up to three times per day. Recently she has also bought some laxitives and has been using these as well to help her purge after eating. Her ECG is abnormal with a wide PR interval and inverted T waves.
What is the single most likely cause of her ECG findings?

A   Dehydration
B   Hyperkalaemia
C   Hypoglycaemia
D   Hypokalaemia
E   Metabolic acidosis

Perinatal psychiatry

1. A 28-year-old woman with a 6-week-old baby born by forceps delivery has a routine postnatal appointment with the health visitor. She has no past psychiatric or medical history. She states she is fine and enjoys motherhood. On direct questioning, she states she feels exhausted all the time and has difficulty falling asleep when her baby is sleeping, or relaxing when her partner is looking after the baby. She also discloses that she feels she is not a good enough mother.
What is the single most appropriate next step?

A   Arrange assessment under mental health legislation
B   Arrange an urgent outpatient appointment with the community mental health team
C   Complete the Edinburgh Postnatal Depression Scale
D   Reassure her that she has the 'baby blues'
E   Watchful waiting with a further assessment of her mental state at the next health visitor appointment in 2 weeks' time

2. The husband of a 30-year-old woman who gave birth to her first child 10 days ago reports to the GP that she has been pacing around at night, with a changeable mood and frequent bouts of crying. She has no past psychiatric or medical history and does not drink alcohol or take illicit drugs. On MSE, she says the hospital midwives are watching her through hidden cameras because her baby is the son of God. She has thought about jumping from a local bridge with her baby to stop the midwives watching her. She does not think she is unwell and does not want to come into hospital.
What is the single most appropriate next step?

A   Arrange another GP appointment within the next 48 hours for further assessment of her mental state
B   Arrange an urgent outpatient appointment with the community mental health team for further assessment of her mental state
C   Arrange assessment under mental health legislation
D   Prescribe an antidepressant
E   Prescribe an antipsychotic

Physical and psychological co-morbidity

1. A 21-year-old female student is concerned because she had two episodes of loose stools, abdominal bloating and nausea during her final exams. Her symptoms have now resolved. She has no past medical or psychiatric history, and no relevant family history. Physical examination, including per rectum examination, reveals no abnormalities. On MSE, she is euthymic with no delusions, but is worried her symptoms are indicative of bowel cancer as she read about this on the internet.
Which is the single most appropriate next step?

A   Arrange colonoscopy
B   Explain that there are no abnormalities on examination and she is worrying for no reason
C   Prescribe a trial of antidepressant medication
D   Refer to a psychologist for mindfulness therapy
E   Watchful waiting

2. A 52-year-old man with no past medical or psychiatric history has a sudden onset of breathlessness associated with palpitations, occurring during an argument with his son. Physical examination is normal. A panic attack is suspected.
What is the single most appropriate next step?

A   Arrange further physical investigations
B   Discharge with GP follow up
C   Provide written information on self-management of panic attacks
D   Refer to on-call psychiatrist for psychiatric assessment
E   Refer to psychology for cognitive behavioural therapy

3. A 26-year-old woman has an abnormal gait and states her left leg feels weak. She previously worked as a waitress, but is currently on sick leave. She has no past medical or psychiatric history. She is cheerful and does not think there is a serious explanation. She is euthymic on MSE. Blood tests and a MRI of her spine show no abnormalities. Her husband says that her symptoms started shortly after he asked for a divorce her because he is in a relationship with another woman.
What is the single most likely diagnosis?

A Conversion disorder
B Depression
C Generalised anxiety disorder
D Lumbar spine disc prolapse
E Somatisation disorder

4. A 48-year-old medically-retired woman has low mood, fatigue and constipation. She recently completed a course of radiotherapy for non-metastatic breast cancer. Her cancer pain is well-controlled and she has no other new pain. She has a history of postnatal depression. Physical examination reveals no new abnormalities. Blood tests reveal megaloblastic anaemia and folate deficiency. On MSE, she says she feels guilty about the effect of her cancer and its treatment on her children, but has no thoughts of harm to herself or others and no suicidal ideation.
What is the single most appropriate next step?

A Commence antidepressant treatment
B Commence folic acid treatment
C Refer to community mental health team
D Refer to psychology for cognitive behavioural therapy
E Watchful waiting

5. A 79-year-old man who wears a hearing aid is on the orthopaedics ward for surgical repair of a fractured neck of femur. He lives independently, with no previous psychiatric history. His consultant feels he is at risk of developing delirium during admission and wants to monitor for signs of this.
What is the single most appropriate action?

A Arrange baseline CT brain scan
B Displaying a clock in the patient's room
C Display reminders of the date in the patient's room
D Perform regular Abbreviated Mental Test Score assessments
E Perform regular blood cultures and serology

6. A 33-year-old, single, female shop assistant has a 2-year history of primary insomnia. It takes up to 2 hours for her to fall asleep after getting into bed; she wakes feeling unrefreshed and feels tired during the day. She has no other psychiatric or medical history. She has implemented sleep hygiene measures with limited success. She has completed a 2-week course of zopiclone and is requesting a repeat prescription. She is euthymic with no features of psychosis.
What is the single most appropriate next step?

A Prescribe trial of methylphenidate
B Prescribe 2-week supply of lorazepam
C Prescribe 2-week supply of zopiclone
D Refer to a psychologist for cognitive behavioural therapy
E Watchful waiting

7. A 24-year-old man has had the desire to dress as a woman since he was 12 years old. He wishes to be female, and has been wearing women's clothing and make-up every day for the last 10 months. He does not experience sexual arousal when wearing women's clothes. He has a previous history of depression but is currently euthymic with no thoughts of harm to himself or others.
What is the single most likely diagnosis?

A Depression
B Gender identity disorder
C Othello syndrome
D Transvestic fetishism
E Schizophrenia

Dementia and old-age psychiatry

1. An 80-year-old man who lives alone has a 3-day history of unusual behaviour. He telephones his daughter in the middle of the night to ask where his wife is (she died 17 years ago) and his neighbours hear him shouting to himself in the early hours of the morning. He does not drink and has no past medical history. He is euthymic but disorientated in time and place.
What is the single most appropriate next step?

A Arrange assessment under mental health legislation
B Complete physical examination and investigations
C Complete the Geriatric Depression Scale
D Prescribe trial of antidepressant medication
E Prescribe trial of antipsychotic medication

2. A 20-year-old man asks to be tested for Huntington's disease, which his 48-year-old father has recently been diagnosed with. He is himself asymptomatic with a normal neurological examination and no abnormalities on mental state examination.

What is the single most appropriate next step?

A Arrange CT brain scan
B Arrange MRI brain scan
C Arrange urgent referral to the neurology outpatient clinic
D Refer for genetic counselling
E Refer for genetic testing

3. A 50-year-old man with Down's syndrome and mild intellectual disability lives alone, with carers visiting daily. He has a gradual worsening of his ability to prepare meals and has started to forget the names of his carers, becoming irritable when he gets them wrong. He is otherwise well with no past medical or psychiatric history. On MSE, he is euthymic and cognitive impairment is evident. On physical examination, he has features of Down's syndrome with no acute abnormalities. Blood tests, including thyroid function tests, are normal.
What is the single most likely diagnosis?

A Alzheimer's disease
B Delirium
C Depression
D Frontotemporal dementia
E Hypothyroidism

4. A 68-year-old widowed woman has memory loss which started 6 months ago. She finds it difficult to remember her everyday plans and is concerned she has dementia. She sleeps poorly and is constipated. She is fully orientated in time, place and person, but scores 25/30 on the MMSE, saying 'I don't know' for the questions she loses points for. Neurological examination and blood tests are normal.
What is the single most likely diagnosis?

A Alzheimer's disease
B Creutzfeldt–Jakob disease
C Depression
D Huntington's disease
E Intracranial tumour

5. A 53-year-old man, with no past medical history, has an 8-month history of gradually worsening behaviour changes, which he has little awareness of. His wife reports he has made sexually explicit comments to their friends and was caught stealing sweets from the local shop. He is less motivated to do things although his mood is unchanged. On physical examination, primitive reflexes are evident, but there are no other abnormalities.
What is the single most likely finding on brain imaging?

A Asymmetric atrophy of temporal and frontal lobes
B Diffuse atrophy
C Hyperdense collection of blood in subarachnoid space

D Multiple areas of infarction
E Space-occupying lesion in pituitary gland

6. A 71-year-old unmarried man complains that people are trying to harm him by sending radiation through the house walls. He has covered his walls in foil to protect himself. He is convinced he can hear the people using their radiation machine at night and can smell the radiation entering his house. He does not feel low in mood, has been eating well and reports no memory difficulties. On examination, he has mild hearing loss, but no other neurological abnormalities. He is guarded and suspicious, but is euthymic. CT head showed no abnormalities.
What is the single most likely diagnosis?

A Charles Bonnet syndrome
B Delirium
C Depression
D Intracranial tumour
E Late-onset schizophrenia

7. An 83-year-old woman with Alzheimer's disease lives in a residential home, where she has become gradually more irritable over the last 4 months with no clear cause. She has no acute physical health problems and her mental state is otherwise stable. She is receiving speech and language therapy and physiotherapy, but continues to become restless and irritable at times, shouting at staff to ask why they won't let her go home to see her mother. She is concordant with memantine.
What is the single most appropriate action?

A Prescribe an antipsychotic to be taken as required
B Prescribe an antipsychotic to be taken regularly
C Refer for acupuncture
D Refer for aromatherapy
E Reorientate her by reminding her that her mother is deceased

Child and adolescent psychiatry

1. A parent and their 7-year-old child present to the GP due to concerns about the child's behaviour. In school the child is very disruptive, often getting into fights and distracts other children from their work. He has very poor listening skills and has difficulty following the teachers instructions. At home he is difficult to manage, never sitting on his chair for meals and always running around.
What is the single most likely diagnosis?

A ADHD

B Autism spectrum disorder
C Bipolar disorder
D Conduct disorder
E No mental illness

2. A 5-year-old boy is referred to the child and adolescent unit due to concerns about his behaviour at school. He has made no friends and rarely engages in classroom activities. The teacher has noticed that he spends a lot of time lining up the toy dinosaurs, which he loves to play with. His father remembers that at preschool he never played with other children, only on his own, and has never been imaginative. At home he plays with his dinosaurs constantly and gets upset if his parents intervene in any way. As a baby his speech was delayed and even now it is behind the other children's despite input from a speech therapist.
What is the single most likely diagnosis?

A ADHD
B Autism spectrum disorder
C Depression
D Generalised anxiety disorder
E Oppositional defiant disorder

3. A 14-year-old girl is referred for assessment of her low mood. She has been feeling low for the last 5 months and recently has stopped socialising, instead spending most of her time in her room alone. She has lost some weight as she feels she feels 'too tired to eat' as her sleep is very poor. She is not sure what the trigger is but has struggled with bullying since moving to secondary school at age 11. She is diagnosed with depression.
What is the single most appropriate treatment?

A Antidepressant medication
B Antipsychotic medication
C CBT
D Dynamic psychotherapy
E Family therapy

4. A 14-year-old boy is referred to child and adolescent psychiatry as he is very disruptive in school, often getting into fights and refusing to obey school rules. He is often rude to teachers and has been expelled from his secondary school due to hitting a teacher. At home his parents state he is often violent towards them and towards the pet dog, sometimes kicking or hitting it. He has been brought home by the police for throwing rocks at people's windows and lighting fires in public areas. He is diagnosed with conduct disorder.
What is the single most appropriate initial treatment?

A Antipsychotics
B Antidepressants
C Dialectical behavioural therapy
D Parent training programme
E Play therapy

Psychiatry of intellectual disability

1. A 22-year-old man lives with his mother and struggles with tasks, including shaving, cooking, using the bus and managing his money. He has a part-time job at a recycling depot where he receives close support to sort the different types of paper. He has recently completed an IQ test.
What is the single most likely IQ score on his test result?

A <20
B 20–34
C 35–49
D 50–69
E >100

2. A 10-year-old boy with moderate intellectual disability has an elongated face, large prominent ears and strabismus. His maternal uncle has similar facial features and mild intellectual disability.
What is the single most likely diagnosis?

A Down's syndrome
B Foetal alcohol spectrum disorder
C Fragile X syndrome
D Neurofibromatosis
E Tuberous sclerosis

3. A 26-year-old woman with moderate intellectual disability attends the outpatient clinic with a carer from her residential home. Her carer says the woman won't understand your questions and tells you she thinks the patient is depressed as she has been withdrawn and crying frequently.
What is the single most appropriate next step?

A Continue collateral history-taking with the carer
B Prescribe a trial of antidepressant medication
C Provide the patient with easy-read English written information about depression
D Refer to speech and language therapy
E Speak to the patient to assess her ability to engage in the consultation

4. A 31-year-old man with Down's syndrome, mild intellectual disability and schizophrenia is concordant with antipsychotic medication and

is currently well in terms of his mental state. He requires annual blood tests, including a lipid profile and blood glucose, as part of routine monitoring for antipsychotic side effects. When he is told he needs a blood test, he becomes frightened and says he does not want one.

What is the single most appropriate next step?

A Arrange for the patient to be restrained by nursing staff whilst the blood test is performed
B Check the patient's understanding of what a blood test is
C Provide information about having a blood test in the form of pictures or symbols
D Prescribe pro re nata lorazepam prior to performing the blood test
E Tell the patient you have decided he does not need to have a blood test

5. A 34-year-old woman has severe intellectual disability and lives in residential care. She has an onset of new behaviours including slapping herself on the side of her face, screaming and attempting to slap her carers.

What is the single most appropriate next step?

A Arrange admission to an intellectual disability inpatient unit for further assessment
B Complete physical examination
C Prescribe a trial of antipsychotic medication
D Refer to occupational therapy for assessment of the suitability of her environment
E Refer to speech and language therapy for assessment of her communication needs

Psychiatric emergencies

1. A 32-year-old woman, who has a history of bipolar disorder, is admitted to hospital under mental health legislation after becoming manic. On the ward she is agitated and starts slamming doors, demanding to leave. The nursing staff try to talk to her to calm her down but this fails and she starts trying to push past the nursing staff to get into other patients' rooms.

What is the single most appropriate next course of action?

A Intramuscular lorazepam
B Intravenous lorazepam
C Lithium
D Oral lorazepam
E Zopiclone

2. A 28-year-old homeless man is admitted to the ward voluntarily after attempting suicide by attempted hanging while intoxicated. A couple of days after his admission he starts to experience hallucinations, hearing voices and seeing creatures in his room. He is agitated, not sleeping well and is disorientated. On examination he has a tremor and is tachycardic.

What is the single most likely diagnosis?

A Delirium tremens
B Depression
C Malingering
D Parkinson's disease
E Schizophrenia

3. A 26-year-old man attends the emergency department agitated, demanding to see a doctor. He states that he is a heroin user and is now desperate to stop. He has not used heroin today and is in withdrawal with diarrhoea, sweating, headache and joint pains. On examination he has dilated pupils and slight tachycardia.

What is the single most appropriate treatment?

A Codeine
B Ibuprofen
C Methadone
D Morphine
E No treatment advised

4. A 76-year-old elderly woman is taken to her GP by her husband as he is worried about how confused she is. Over the last 2 years she had become more forgetful, but this had been managed by her husband being vigilant and taking over some tasks such as cooking. Over the last week she has often been disorientated to time and place which is worse at night. She has been wondering outside twice which she had never done before. She is also often agitated and occasionally has hit her husband. He husband thinks she may be seeing things occasionally.

What is the single most likely diagnosis?

A Alzheimer's disease
B Delirium
C Lewy-body dementia
D Parkinson's disease
E Vascular dementia

5. An 18-year-old woman is brought to the emergency department after her family becomes concerned that she is not eating. The girl refuses to speak and hides her face, appearing distressed. Her mother states she has been acting oddly for a couple of weeks, refusing to go outside for fear someone will harm her and over the last few days has been refusing to eat any food due to the same fears. She stays in her room alone but is often heard talking to

herself about someone trying to kill her. What is the single most likely diagnosis?

A Acute psychosis
B Anorexia
C Bipolar disorder
D Borderline personality disorder
E Withdrawal from alcohol

Integrated care

1. A 28-year-old woman with mild depression is engaging well with cognitive behavioural therapy. She feels more motivated and has started exercising regularly. She has no past psychiatric history and takes no medications. On mental state examination, she is low in mood with flattened affect, has no thoughts of harm to herself or others and no suicidal ideation.
   What is the single most appropriate next step?

   A Arrange assessment under mental health legislation
   B Continue to monitor in primary care
   C Offer informal admission to inpatient unit
   D Refer to community mental health team
   E Refer to crisis team

2. A 42-year-old single, homeless man with alcohol dependence syndrome drinks 35 units of alcohol per day. He has engaged well with the community alcohol team and wishes to undergo detoxification. He previously had seizures when he tried to stop drinking independently. He has no other past psychiatric history. He occasionally smokes cannabis, but says he has not done for several months.
   What is the single most appropriate next step?

   A Arrange community detoxification
   B Arrange inpatient detoxification
   C Provide information on local voluntary self-help groups
   D Refer to social care services for assistance with finding housing
   E Refer to substance misuse team for support regarding cannabis use

3. The carers of an 81-year-old woman, who lives in a residential home because of mobility difficulties, have noticed that she has become gradually more forgetful, short-tempered and irritable over the last 10 months. She has no new physical health problems and no past psychiatric history. Her blood test results are normal. She scores 25 on MMSE, and her general practitioner feels she is likely to have dementia.
   What is the single most appropriate next step?

   A Arrange assessment under mental health legislation
   B Continue to monitor in primary care
   C Prescribe trial of anti-dementia medication in primary care
   D Refer to old age psychiatry specialist team
   E Refer to social care services for support to find alternative care placement

SBA answers

Affective (mood) disorders

1. E

Baby blues are common after birth, but the history suggests anhedonia which, along with difficulty sleeping and loss of appetite, suggest depression.

2. D

A low mood and anhedonia (loss of pleasure) preceeded the hallucinations. This means that the most likely diagnosis is depression rather than schizophrenia. There is no evidence of memory loss to suggest dementia or a traumatic event to suggest PTSD.

3. D

SSRI medication is the first choice for moderate depression. If she had mild depression watchful waiting with self-help stratergies could be considered. Antipsychotic medication and lithium is not indicated for depression unless it is treatment-resistant or occurs in the context of a bipolar disorder. Psychoanalytical therapy is not used first-line for depression.

4. C

Heart disease and depression are often seen in association with each other. His low mood, feelings of hopelessness coupled with his low energy and poor sleep are indicative of depression. A CVA can occasionally produce some similar symptoms however, there would also be neurological signs. Heart failure and angina can cause reduced energy but would not cause low mood or hopelessness. There is nothing to suggest he is suffering from PTSD.

5. C

ECT is effective in 80% of cases of severe depression. It is usually first-line in cases where the patient's life is in imminent danger. As the patient is refusing food and medication ECT would be appropriate.

6. B

The diagnosis is bipolar disorder because the patient has had an episode of depression and is now manic. During a manic episode people may have delusional beliefs, but would not be considered schizophrenic. There is no indication that he has chronic symptoms suggestive of a personality disorder.

7. A

Because this patient has bipolar disorder it would not be recommended that she take an antidepressant medication (SSRI, tricyclic or MAO) without a mood stabiliser being used first. Carbamazepine is not used first-line for bipolar disorder and is not recommended for women of child-bearing age.

8. D

Although the hyperactivity could be a sign of mania it does not cause the patient to feel 'tired' or 'weak'. This, along with the patient frequently being 'drenched' in sweat and losing weight, suggests hyperthyroidism rather than mania. There is no suggestion of anxiety and no indication that she has previously had depression.

Schizophrenia and psychotic illness

1. C

This patient appears to be experiencing delusions and hallucinations, which need to be explored in detail. It would be inappropriate to challenge his beliefs and experiences (E) as they are real and distressing to him. The other options (A, B, D) may be necessary but would be premature at this stage.

2. B

Although this patient has symptoms suggestive of a psychotic disorder, organic causes for his symptoms must be ruled out first. The other options (A, C, D, E) may be necessary after initial physical examination and investigation.

3. C

This patient has delusions that his partner is being sexually unfaithful: this is pathological jealousy (Othello syndrome). Erotomania (B) is a delusional disorder in which the affected person believes that someone else, often a stranger or famous person, is in love with them. The other options (A,D and E) may explain some but not all of his symptoms.

4. A

This patient has a 10-day history of acute onset of symptoms which have fluctuated over time in the presence of associated acute stress (marital breakdown). Her symptoms are suggestive of acute and transient psychotic disorder. The other options (B–E) may explain some but not all of her symptoms.

5. B

This patient has treatment-resistant schizophrenia, as her symptoms continue despite adequate trials of two different antipsychotics. Clozapine is the first-line medication for treatment-resistant schizophrenia. A depot antipsychotic (C) is not indicated as she is concordant with oral medication nor are further trials of other antipsychotic medication (D). E may be helpful but her psychotic symptoms must be treated first. As she is concordant with medication admission is not required at present.

6. C

This patient has symptoms suggestive of an evolving psychotic disorder, with no underlying organic cause. Urgent referral to the early intervention team will allow rapid assessment and management of her symptoms. A is not indicated in the absence of immediate risk, B may be necessary following initial assessment. Initiation of antipsychotic medication (D) should follow full specialist psychiatric assessment. Watchful waiting (E) is inappropriate as prognosis is poorer with longer duration of untreated psychosis.

7. A

Atypical antipsychotics are associated with dyslipidaemia, so blood lipid levels must be checked prior to starting antipsychotic medication and monitored throughout treatment. A trial of olanzapine (C) should not be commenced before this has been done. Other options (D, B) are not indicated as he does not wish to stop smoking. Watchful waiting in primary care (E) is inappropriate as the prognosis is worse with a longer duration of untreated psychosis.

Anxiety disorders

1. C

GAD is the most likely diagnosis as sufferers experience 'free floating' anxiety that has no specific triggers. They experience a variety of sysmptoms of anxiety which impacts on the quality of life. GAD is a long-term condition that is usually present over a number of years. Agrophobia and claustrophobia are specific phobias, which means they have a defined trigger.

2. E

An examination of the hands in this form of OCD is likely to show damage to the skin and nails from repetitive washing. In patients who present with repetitive washing examination of their hands is important to support their history and assess the physical damage the washing has caused. An examination of the other systems, although useful to exclude other conditions, is unlikely to provide evidence to support a diagnosis of OCD.

3. A

Antidepressants can help reduce the symptoms of PTSD and would be a suitable alternative treatment if the CBT had not been helpful or there were still residual symptoms. Another suitable alternative would be EMDR (Eye Movement Desensitisation and reprocessing). Antipsychotics are rarely used in PTSD.

4. E

Reassurance is not appropriate given her presentation and lack of a definitive diagnosis at this point. Referral to a psychiatrist or dietican is premature, as anxiety disorders should be made only after ensuring alternative diagnosis has been excluded. The most likely diagnosis is hyperthyroidism rather than an anxiety disorder in this situation. Although it is presenting with similarities to Panic disorder or GAD these conditions should not be diagnosed until other medical conditions that can cause anxiety have been excluded. In this case the blood tests which would be most useful are thyroid function tests. A full blood count, U and E, CRP and LFT's could also be useful in this situation.

5. B

Antidepressants are not the recommended first-line of treatment in social anxiety disorder as they are not as effective as CBT. CBT is the treatment of choice for social anxiety disorder as it targets the symptoms the person is having and links them to their thoughts and actions. Diazepam used to be prescribed frequently for anxiety, however, it is no longer recommended due to its addictive nature and poor ability to maintain its effect on reducing anxiety. EMDR is a treatment for PTSD not social anxiety disorder.

Suicide and self-harm

1. D

It is inappropriate to agree to keep significant levels of self-harm in a child under 18 years of age confidential from their parents or guardian unless there is reason to believe that doing so would place the child in significant danger. Although a physical examination is useful it is more important at this stage to understand the reason for the self harm. Referral to CAMHS may be appropriate but it is premature at this point. A discussion about why she is reluctant to allow her parents to know is the most appropriate next step in this case; it could be something as significant as sexual abuse from a parent. The reason why may significantly alter how you proceed and the services that are utilized to help the child. It is correct that for a 13-year-old child, disclosing self harm should have parental input and you should inform the parents. However, if the disclosure places the child in significant danger then this is no longer appropriate. If you had a strong suspicion that the child was being abused by a parent you should ensure advice is sought immediately from social services while the child remained in the surgery.

2. **E**

Reassurance is inappropriate at this time. His plans to attempt sucide should be taken seriously and appropriate help sought. It is not appropriate simply to remove his paracetamol and increase his antidepressants will only help in the longer term. Referring to the local mental health team, even urgently, would not be appropriate given that this man has already taken steps towards attempting suicide. Although this patient does require help urgently the presentation does not currently suggest an ambulance or the police needs to be called. The most appropriate action is to request an emergency assessment. This is often done through contacting the local crisis mental health team. An alternative if this is not available is to contact the on-call psychiatrist who will be able to advise how to proceed.

3. **A**

Acetylcystine may be required. However, as the patient has presented within 2 hours of taking the overdose activated charcoal would be a more appropriate initial treatment. Treatment from the mental health team or crisis team is possible give the presentation, but this would not be the initial treatment because the overdose needs to be treated first.

Personality disorders

1. **D**

Borderline personality disorder is the most likely explanation because she has a long history of emotional instability, sensitivity to rejection, difficult maintaining relationships, feeling 'empty', self harming and thoughts of suicide. There is no evidence in the history that she has any of the obsessive compulsive or perfectionist traits which is found in anakastic personality disorder. She does not display any antisocial behaviours which would make antisocial personality disorder unlikely.

2. **C**

Dialectical behavioural therapy has a good evidence base to support its use in those with borderline personality disorder. Antidepressants are only utilised if talking therapy does

not improve low mood or there is co-morbid depression. Antipsychotics are occasionally used in complex personality disorders, however they are not used first-line. ECT is not an appropriate treatment for borderline personality disorder. EMDR is not used to treat borderline personality disorder.

3. **A**

The history gives a picture of the patient being callous, having no close relationships, instead having multiple short relationships and engaging in criminal behaviour. He is grandiose and boastful with the psychiatrist. This suggests antisocial personality disorder. Borderline personality disorder tends to show an intense need to have relationships and be very sensitive to rejection, the opposite of which is seen in this case. Histrionic personality disorder presents less with a history of criminal behaviour and more with dramatic behaviours that are often attention seeking. Morbid jealousy is a delusional disorder in which the person (often male) believes their partner is cheating on them and goes to extreme lengths to uncover the cheating. There is nothing to suggest this in the history.

4. **A**

Patients who have schizotypal personality disorder are at risk of developing psychosis. In this case the patient is showing symptoms of psychosis, therefore an appropriate treatment would be antipsychotics.

Substance misuse and addictions

1. **A**

This patient has a strong desire to drink alcohol, withdrawal symptoms when his alcohol intake is reduced and has neglected his job due to the increasing salience of drinking alcohol in his life – all are features of alcohol dependence. There are no signs of alcohol withdrawal on examination so (B) is unlikely, and the pattern of drinking described is a consistent, stereotyped daily intake rather than binge drinking (C). He does not currently show signs of alcohol withdrawal delirium but should be advised not to suddenly stop drinking due to the risks of developing delirium tremens (D). Although he is likely to be at risk of thiamine deficiency due to his alcohol dependency, he does not currently show the features of Wernicke's encephalopathy (E).

2. **D**

This patient is experiencing unpleasant symptoms arising from the interaction of disulfiram with alcohol contained within his aftershave aerosol spray. Acamprosate (A) and naltrexone (E) are used in alcohol abstinence treatment, but do not interact with alcohol in this way. Chlordiazepoxide (B) and diazepam (C) are benzodiazepines used during alcohol detoxification.

3. E

This patient is confabulating to fill the gaps in his memory of past events, is ataxic and has nystagmus, indicative of ophthalmoplegia – all are features of Wernicke's encephalopathy, which is likely given his daughter's report that he drinks too much alcohol. Although he is at risk of subdural haematoma (A, B) this is unlikely given the lack of head injury noted during the history-taking and normal brain CT scan. He does not show features of delirium tremens (C) and (D) does not explain his symptoms.

4. B

Although she is sweaty and shaky, which may occur in panic disorder (C), and has visual hallucinations and agitation, which may occur in schizophrenia (D), this woman has a long history of excess alcohol intake and it is likely that her drinking has ceased since admission resulting in symptoms and signs suggestive of alcohol withdrawal delirium (delirium tremens) a medical emergency. She does not smell of alcohol making acute alcohol intoxication (A) unlikely. Her current symptoms and signs are not suggestive of Wernicke's encephalopathy (E).

5. C

This patient symptoms have been caused by cannabis use. The other options may explain some but not all of her symptoms and findings on examination.

6. D

This man has substance misuse and co-morbid schizophrenia, a history of harm to himself and has been difficult to engage in treatment, all of which increase his risk of suicide or harm to others, meaning watchful waiting (E) is not appropriate. However, he has no current thoughts of harm to himself or others, and mental health legislation assessment (B) is not currently warranted. Referral to the assertive outreach team would enable a focus on engaging him in his treatment and is the next most appropriate step. He may be able to work on reducing his amphetamine use in the future, which may include motivational interviewing (C) or hospital-based detoxification (A).

7. B

This woman has moved beyond the pre-contemplation stage (D) and now acknowledges that her substance misuse is a problem and is ready to consider ways of changing her behaviour – this is the contemplation stage. She has not yet decided on a course of action to take (E) nor taken action (A) to change her behaviour. She will require ongoing support to maintain (C) any changes made.

Eating disorders

1. B

Constipation is most commonly associated with anorexia nervosa, not diarrhoea. The other symptoms commonly occur in a patient with anorexia, particularly one with a short history during which significant weight loss has occurred, as this gives the body less time to adapt.

2. C

Various therapies can be used to treat anorexia nervosa. CBT, cognitive analytic therapy, interpersonal psychotherapy and family therapy have evidence supporting their use. Dietary advice is essential and usually given through a dietican. Exposure response prevention therapy is used to treat OCD and would be an unlikely choice for the treatment of anorexia.

4. B

Bradycardia is the most common finding in anorexia nervosa. Tall tented T waves occur in hyperkalaemia which is uncommon in anorexia as is atrial fibrillation and tachycardia. The patient would not concious if she had ventricular fibrillation.

5. C

Bulaemia is characterised by binging and purging. In this example the patient admits to binging and there is evidence that she is regularly vomiting to purge. Most patients with bulaemia have a normal BMI.

Perinatal psychiatry

1. C

This patient has symptoms suggestive of postnatal depression, although many patients with postnatal depression conceal their true feelings because they are ashamed of how they feel. The health visitor should have a high level of suspicion and should use the Edinburgh Postnatal Depression Scale to screen her for the possibility of postnatal depression. Her symptoms do not fit with baby blues. Watchful waiting would be inappropriate. The other options (B, A) may be needed some stage but are not necessary at this time.

2. C

This patient has symptoms suggestive of postnatal psychosis. This is a psychiatric emergency and admission to a mother and baby unit, under the mental health legislation if the patient is unwilling to be admitted informally, is required. It would not be appropriate to monitor her mental state in the community (A, B) given the risks of harm to herself and her baby. The other options (D, E) may be necessary, but are premature at this stage.

Physical and psychological co-morbidity

1. E

This patient experienced abdominal symptoms in the context of psychosocial stressors, and her symptoms have now resolved. Her history and normal physical examination suggest bowel cancer is unlikely, and there are no indications that colonoscopy (A) is required at this stage. Likewise, there is no clear evidence of a mood disorder and antidepressant treatment (C) is not indicated. Her physical symptoms may have a psychological cause, but this cannot be assumed and a dismissive attitude (B) would be unhelpful. Referral to psychology for mindfulness therapy (D) may be warranted in the future should she continue to experience distress and should it become clearer that there is a psychological basis to her symptoms, but would be premature at this time. The most appropriate step is watchful waiting (E).

2. A

Although this patient's symptoms may be suggestive of a panic attack, this should not be assumed and the next step must be further investigations to exclude a physical cause (A). The other options (B, C, D, E) presume a diagnosis of panic attacks is correct, and are not appropriate at this stage.

3. A

This patient has conversion disorder. She is unconcerned by her significant symptoms, which started in the context of an acute psychosocial stressor and which have no clear physical cause. Lumbar spine disc prolapse (C) is unlikely given her normal MRI. Depression (B) is unlikely given that she is euthymic. She does not show multiple, recurrent or frequently changing symptoms as expected in somatisation disorder (E) or features suggestive of generalised anxiety disorder (D).

4. B

Although this patient symptoms may indicate depression, she has folate-deficiency anaemia which must be corrected (B) before psychiatric disorder can be diagnosed. Should her symptoms continue despite correction of her folate deficiency, the possibility of depression should be further explored and this may require treatment with medication (A) or psychological treatments (D) by specialists (C). The risk of suicide is high in those with cancer and a proactive approach is needed – watchful waiting (E) is not appropriate.

5. D

This patient has a fractured neck of femur which puts him at risk of delirium. Regular monitoring of his cognitive functioning, for example, using Abbreviated Mental Test Score assessments (D), would assist prompt detection of delirium. Although delirium may be caused by infection, regular blood cultures and serology (E) are not recommended. Similarly, baseline CT scans (A) are not recommended. Displaying a clock (B) and reminders of the date (C) may help orientate the patient should he become delirious but are not indicated at this stage.

6. D

This patient has primary insomnia. Methylphenidate (A) is a stimulant used to treat primary hypersomnia or narcolepsy, and is not indicated. She has tried sleep hygiene measures and a 2-week course of zopiclone. The risks of dependence mean that zopiclone should not be prescribed for longer than 2 weeks, so a further prescription (B) is not appropriate, nor is a prescription of lorazepam (B). Cognitive behavioural therapy (E) is as effective as short-term use of hypnotics and is the most appropriate next step. Given the negative impact of ongoing poor sleep on mood, behaviour and functioning, watchful waiting (E) is not appropriate.

7. B

This patient's symptoms of a strong belief, starting pre-pubertally, that he wishes to be a woman, and his history of living as a woman for the last 10 months, fit with a diagnosis of gender identity disorder (B). He does not have transvestic fetishism (D) as there is no sexual arousal associated with wearing women's clothing. Although people with gender identity disorder are at risk of depression, there are currently no features of this (A), schizophrenia (E), or Othello syndrome (morbid jealousy) (C).

Dementia and old-age psychiatry

1. B

This patient has acute onset of confusion, visual hallucinations and disorientation. The most likely diagnosis is delirium and thorough physical examination and investigations are required. The other options may be indicated at a later stage, but it is vital to first exclude delirium.

2. D

The most appropriate step to address this patient's request for testing is to refer him for genetic counselling. Although genetic testing (E) is used to identify those at risk of Huntington's disease, it would be inappropriate to refer this man without first offering genetic counselling given the untreatable and progressive nature of the disease. CT (A) and MRI (B) scans are not useful early in the disease and are not indicated at this stage. Similarly, urgent referral to the neurology outpatient clinic (C) is not indicated at this stage.

3. A

This patient's history, along with the results of his physical examination and blood tests, are suggestive of Alzheimer's disease, which presents at a younger age in people with Down's syndrome. Delirium (B) is unlikely given the gradual onset of his symptoms. Hypothyroidism is unlikely given his normal blood test results (E). The other options (C, D) may explain some but not all of his symptoms.

4. C

This patient's subjective report of memory impairment is worse than objective findings on examination. She also has biological symptoms suggestive of depression, along with normal physical examination and blood test results. These findings make depression (pseudodementia) the most likely diagnosis.

5. A

This patient's personality and behaviour changes, along with the presence of primitive reflexes on examination, mean that frontotemporal dementia is the most likely diagnosis, which would be suggested by asymmetrical atrophy of temporal and frontal lobes on brain imaging. More diffuse atrophy (B) would be suggestive of Alzheimer's disease and multiple areas of infarction (D) would suggest vascular dementia. His symptoms and signs do not indicate subarachnoid haemorrhage, which would be suggested by hyperdensity in the subarachnoid space (C), nor do they indicate a pituitary tumour, which would be suggested by a space-occupying lesion in the pituitary gland (E).

6. E

This patient has partition delusions and hallucinations, is guarded and suspicious and has mild hearing loss with normal examination and investigation findings, making late onset schizophrenia the most likely diagnosis. Depression (C) is unlikely given there are no mood or memory changes and no biological symptoms of depression. Delirium (B) or an intra-cranial tumour (D) are unlikely given his normal physical examination and investigation results. Testing of his vision as part of neurological examination revealed no abnormalities, making Charles Bonnet syndrome (A) unlikely.

7. D

Aromatherapy is one intervention recommended for consideration in the management of co-morbid agitation in people with dementia. Although some research has suggested acupuncture (C) may be helpful, this is not a recommended intervention. Antipsychotic medication should not be used pro re nata (A) nor regularly (B) in people with Alzheimer's disease because of the increased risk of cerebrovascular events. Reminding the patient that her mother is deceased whilst she is acutely agitated may worsen her distress (E).

Child and adolescent psychiatry

1. A

The poor attention the child shows in the class by not listening, distracting others and finding it difficult to follow instructions, coupled with his hyperactivity indicated by his disruptive behavior and inability to sit through meals, suggests that this child has ADHD. In a patient with ASD you would expect to find more problems with social interaction, such as not making friends and having poor speech. In conduct disorder you would expect the history to contain more signs of antisocial behaviours such as cruelty to animals, destruction of property, lying or stealing.

2. B

Autism spectrum disorder is most likely given this presentation. He has delayed speech and difficulty with social interactions in multiple, different settings. He has little interest in engaging with other children or his parents, preferring instead to play with his dinosaurs. His play also appears to be abnormal as he only lines them up and does not engage in imaginative play. ADHD is unlikely because there is no evidence of hyperactivity and he is able to engage in sustain play with his dinosaur toys.

Depression or GAD is rare in young children and there is no indication that he is low in mood or particularly anxious.

3. C

In an adult, antidepressant medication or CBT is the first-line treatment for depression. However, in children CBT alone is the recommended first-line treatment. Antidepressants can be added in during therapy if the depression becomes more severe or to enhance the response to CBT if needed. In this patient there is nothing to indicate that family therapy would be beneficial. The trigger for the depression appears to be bullying therefore it may be more appropriate to liaise with the school.

4. D

Medication is not routinely prescribed for conduct disorder. It is considered if there are co-morbid conditions such as depression or psychosis. Occasionally, children with severe conduct disorder will have a low dose of antipsychotics but this would not be considered as the first-line of treatment. Parent training programmes have a good evidence base for improving outcomes in children with conduct disorder, often along with therapy such as CBT for the child. Dialectical behavioural therapy is the therapy used for borderline personality disorders. Play therapy is for younger children (usually 3–11) to explore emotional difficulties and would not be considered first-line for the treatment of conduct disorder.

Psychiatry of intellectual disability

1. C

This patient requires support with some self-care tasks and activities of daily living, and works in supported employment. This suggests moderate intellectual disability, which would be indicated by an IQ score of 35–49. Other IQ score ranges below 70 (A, B, D) suggest a different severity of intellectual disability. An IQ score >100 (E) is not in itself suggestive of intellectual disability.

2. C

This patient and his maternal uncle's physical characteristics and intellectual disability indicate fragile X syndrome, the most common inherited cause of intellectual disability. The other options (A, B, D, E) explain some but not all of his features.

3. E

A collateral history (A) will be important, but it would be inappropriate to assume the carer is correct in saying that the patient cannot engage in the consultation and you should first speak to the patient to assess their communication skills. Following your assessment, a referral to speech and language therapy (D) may be appropriate for advice on how best to communicate with her, which may include using easy read English written information (C). It is inappropriate to prescribe a trial of antidepressants (B) on the basis of the collateral history alone.

4. B

This patient has schizophrenia and annual blood tests are required. Given his initial refusal to comply, the most appropriate next step is to check his understanding of what a blood test is (B). He may then require pictorial or symbolised information to help him understand the procedure (C). This alone may reduce his distress and enable him to comply with the procedure without the need for further actions. The other options (A, D) may be required, but this decision would need to be made as a 'best interests' decision and premature at this point. It would be unacceptable to decide that the patient does not need the blood test at this stage (E).

5. B

This patient's behavioural change may be the only way she can indicate distress, for example, arising from pain; it is vital that physical health causes are excluded. Further multidisciplinary assessments (D, E) may be necessary but are premature at this stage. Similarly, admission to an inpatient unit (A) or a trial of antipsychotic medication (C) would be premature at this stage.

Psychiatric emergencies

1. D

When there is a significant risk of the patient harming themselves or others rapid tranquilisation should be considered. As talking to the patient has already been attempted the next step would be to offer oral lorazepam (an antipsychotic is sometimes used instead). Lithium and zopiclone are not medications used in rapid tranquilisation.

2. A

The symptoms of psychosis with disorientation, tremor and autonomic instability (evidenced by the tachycardia) make delirium tremens the most likely diagnosis even though there is not an explicit history of alcohol abuse. Some patients do not disclose alcohol abuse, even if asked directly.

3. **B**

Although opioid withdrawal is unpleasant it is rarely life-threatening. It therefore does not require emergency treatment with opioids. Methadone is only used as part of a planned, controlled programme of withdrawal and should not be prescribed in the emergency setting. Simple painkillers such as ibuprofen are appropriate along with loperamide and dioralyte.

4. **B**

Although there is a history of some forgetfulness, which could be a sign of dementia, the current presentation is an acute (only 1 week) onset of periodic disorientation, agitation (with aggression) and possibly some visual hallucinations. This would suggest delirium.

5. **A**

Many patients who present as psychotic will not be florid or open about their symptoms. She appears to have paranoid delusions indicative of her fears about going outside and eating. Her talking to herself suggests she is experiencing auditory hallucinations.

Integrated care

1. **B**

This patient is experiencing a first episode of mild depression and is engaging with psychological intervention with no evident risk of harm to herself or others. Continued management within primary care is appropriate, with regular monitoring of her mental state. The other options are all part of the stepped care model for management of depression, but are not indicated at this stage.

2. **B**

This patient should first be offered inpatient detoxification whilst he is motivated to attempt this. Community-based detoxification (A) would not be safe as he drinks more than 30 units of alcohol per day with a history of withdrawal seizures, poor social support and cannabis use. He may require all of the other interventions (C, D, E) subsequently but detoxification as an inpatient is the first priority.

3. **D**

Ongoing monitoring in primary care (B) is not appropriate given the possibility of dementia, and she should be referred to the old age psychiatry team. A trial of anti-dementia medication (C) may be prescribed but would be initiated by specialist old age psychiatrists. She may require alternative care placements in the future, but referral to social care services (E) is not indicated at this stage, nor is assessment under mental health legislation (A).

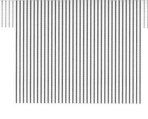

Index

Note: Page numbers in **bold** or *italic* refer to tables or figures, respectively.

A

Abbreviated Mental Test Score 231
Academic achievement, genes and 23
Acamprosate, for abstinence from alcohol 196
Acetylcholine **20**
 and cognitive impairment 248
Action potential 17–18, *18*
 depolarisation 17
 firing of action potential 17
 hyperpolarised cell 17
 refractory period 18
 repolarisation 18
Activated charcoal 163
Acute stress reaction 157–158
 dissociative stupor and 157
ADHD *see* Attention deficit hyperactivity disorder (ADHD)
Advance decisions 32
Advance directives 32, 283
Affective disorders 97–98
 aetiology *106*
 course and prognosis *115*
 depressive disorders 105–115
 epidemiology **116**
 investigations **100**
 mixed affective states 115
 persistent mood disorders 121
Agoraphobia 153–154
Alcohol dependence 186–196, *189, 192*
 CAGE screening questionnaire **188**, 194
 community alcohol teams 309
 consequences of excessive use 192, **192**
 couples therapy 196

discharge and follow-up 309
 epidemiology *192*
 inpatient alcohol detoxification 309
 investigations *194*
 management strategies *195*
 medications for abstinence from alcohol 195–196
 primary care 308–309
 Prochaska and DiClemente's transtheoretical model of change 195, *195*
 psychosocial interventions 196
 and thiamine deficiency 193
Alcoholics Anonymous (AA) 77, 196
Alcohol-related psychiatric disorders 201–202
Alcohol withdrawal 292, **292**, *293*
Alzheimer's disease 248–250
 see also Dementia
 brain imaging 249, *249*
 Down's syndrome and 248
 pathogenesis *248*
 reminiscence therapy 249
 risk factors 248
Amitriptyline 81
Amphetamine-related psychiatric disorders 202
Anabolic steroids **199**
Anaesthetics 199 *see also* Illicit drugs use
Anorexia nervosa 203–210
 aetiology **207**
 diagnostic approach **209**
 electrolyte imbalances 209
 epidemiology **207**
 management **210**
 physical symptoms and signs **208**, *208*

Antabuse, for abstinence from alcohol 196
Anticonvulsants 93–94
Antidepressants 7, 21, 80–81, 112–113, 306
 action mechanism 108
 bipolar disorder **120**
 discontinuation reactions 113–114
 emotional disorders 270
 monoamine oxidase inhibitors 84–85
 noradrenergic and specific serotonergic antidepressants 84
 panic disorder 150, 151
 patient concerns about **113**
 postnatal depression 219–220
 post-traumatic stress disorder 159
 selective serotonin reuptake inhibitors 83
 serotonin and noradrenaline reuptake inhibitors 83
 serotonin syndrome 81
 therapeutic effect 81
 tricyclic antidepressants 81–83
 withdrawal effects 81
Antiemetics 292
Antiepileptics, for bipolar disorder **120**
Antipsychotics *85*, 85–86
 acute psychosis 285
 agitation management 290
 atypical 88–90, **89**, 136
 bipolar disorder **120**
 conventional (typical) 86–88, 136
 depot antipsychotic medications 90

National Institute for Health and Care Excellence guidelines 85
neuroleptic malignant syndrome 87
persistent delusional disorders 139
postnatal period and **219**
prescription 85–86
schizophrenia 135–137, *137*
side effects 86, *86*, 136, *136*
use of *137*
weight gain 86, 300–302
withdrawal 86
Anxiety disorders 143, *144*
in older adults 256
women and 147
Anxiolytics 199 *see also* Illicit drugs use
benzodiazepines 90–91
β-Adrenergic antagonists 91–92
5-HT1$_A$ agonists 91
hypnotics and 90–91
postnatal period and **219**
Aripiprazole 88
ASD *see* Autism spectrum disorder (ASD)
Asperger's syndrome 263, *263 see also* Autism spectrum disorder (ASD)
Assertive outreach teams 7
Atenolol 92, 153
Atomoxetine 268
Attention deficit hyperactivity disorder (ADHD) 28, 260–262, 265, 267
aetiology 267–268
clinical features **268**
management *268*
Auditory hallucinations 60, 124–126, 132
Autism spectrum disorder (ASD) 262–265
child abuse/neglect and 264
clinical features **264**
diagnostic approach *264, 265*
increase in 262
mumps–measles–rubella (MMR) vaccine and 263
spectrum of autism *263*
Azapirones 91

B

Baby blues *see* Postnatal blues
Basal ganglia 16–17, *17*

Beck Depression Inventory (BDI) 306
Behaviour therapy **75**, 77
cognitive 78–79
dialectical 79–80
techniques and indications **78**
Benzodiazepines 80, 90
acute psychosis 285
acute stress reaction 158
adverse effects 91
agitation management 290
alcohol withdrawal 195, 292, **292**, *293*
bipolar disorder **120**
indications 91
mode of action 90, *90*
primary insomnia 237
withdrawal 90
Beta-blockers 91–92
phobias 153
Biopsychosocial model, for mental illness 51, **52**, *52*
Bipolar affective disorder 97, 105, 115–121 *see also* Affective disordersclassification **116**
clinical features **118**
course and prognosis **115**
diagnostic approach *119*
management **120**
Blood phobia 152
Borderline personality disorder 178–180, 182 *see also* Personality disorders
Brain 10
cerebral hemispheres 11–13, **12**
lateralisation of function 13
lobes of 10–11, *11*
Breathing-related sleep disorders **236** *see also* Sleep disorders
Bromocriptine 116
Bulimia nervosa 203, 210–212
binge eating behaviour 210, 211
diagnostic approach **209**
epidemiology **207**
management **212**
vomiting, repeated 211
Buprenorphine 200
Bupropion 304
Buspirone 91

C

Caffeine consumption, and anxiety 148

CAGE screening questionnaire, for alcohol misuse *188*
Cancer, and depressive disorder 232, 305
Cannabis 197, **199** *see also* Illicit drugs use
Cannabis-related psychiatric disorders 202
Capacity assessment 281–283, *282*, **283**
Carbamazepine 93
CBT *see* Cognitive behavioural therapy (CBT)
Central nervous system (CNS) 8, *10, 11*
Charles Bonnet syndrome 256
Childhood trauma, and depression 107, *107*
Chlordiazepoxide 90
Chlorpromazine 85, 87
Chronic mental health, and physical health problems 304–305, **305**
Circadian rhythm sleep disorders **236** *see also* Sleep disorders
Citalopram 83
CJD *see* Creutzfeld-Jakob disease (CJD)
Clinical Institute Withdrawal Assessment for Alcohol scale (CIWA-A) score 291, 292, *293*
Clomipramine 81
Clozapine 88–90
Cocaine 197 *see also* Illicit drugs use
Cognition-enhancing drugs 94
Cognitive behavioural therapy (CBT) 26, **75**, 78–79
alcohol dependence 196
depression 108, 112
emotional disorders 270
generalised anxiety disorder 148
illicit drug use 201
obsessive compulsive disorder 155, *157*
panic disorder 151
phobias 152, 154
primary insomnia 238
stages of *79*
trauma-focused 159
Community mental health teams (CMHTs) 299
Community Treatment Order 31
Conduct disorder 265–267
Confidentiality 32
Connors questionnaire 268

Conversion disorders 228–229
  'la belle indifference' 229
  types **229**
Corpus callosum 13
Cotard's syndrome 101
Counselling **75**, 76
Creutzfeld-Jakob disease (CJD)
  253
  iatrogenic 253–254
  new-variant 254
Crisis intervention services 7
Cultural beliefs, influence of 4
Curare 19
Cyclothymic personality disorder
  117, 121, **121**
Cytogenetics 23

D

Declaration of Madrid 28
Delirium 35, 229–231, 287
  causes **230**
Delirium tremens 195, 290, 292
Delusions 61–62
  and associated conditions **63**
  depression 101, 110
  persistent delusional disorders
    138–139
  primary **64**
  schizophrenia 128, 132
  secondary **64**
Dementia 244–248 see also
  Alzheimer's disease
  causes **247**
  clinical features **247**
  community care of 309–310
  frontotemporal 252–253
  integrated care plans 310
  with Lewy bodies 251,
    251–252
  memory impairment in,
    causes of **247**
  specialist and palliative care
    310
  vascular 250–251
Depression 21, 97, 98–102,
  105–115 see also Affective
  disorders
  aetiology 106, 107
  cancer patients and 232, 305
  in chronically physically unwell
    305–306
  classification **105**
  clinical features **109**, 110
  cognitive distortions in 108,
    108
  course and prognosis **115**
  electroconvulsive therapy 114
  epidemiology **105**
  genetic susceptibility to 107

global variation in prevalence
  of 37
life events and 107
in older adults **255**, 255–256
in palliative care setting
  306–307
pharmacological treatment
  112–114, **113**
psychological treatment
  111–112
relapse prevention 114
social phobia 153
social treatment 112
stepped care approach to
  111, 112, 302–304, 303
Desensitisation of neurone 21
Developmental disorders 262,
  263 see also Autism spectrum
  disorder (ASD)
Dialectical behavioural therapy
  75, 79–80, 175, 183
Diazepam 90
Disulfiram, for abstinence from
  alcohol 196
Donepezil 94, 249
Dopamine (DA) **20**
Dothiepin 81
Downregulation 20, 21
Down's syndrome
  genetic testing 277
  intellectual disability and 276,
    277
Drug-induced psychiatric
  disorders 201
  alcohol and 201–202
  amphetamine and 202
  cannabis and 202
  clinical effects 201
  key features 201
Drugs and psychoactive
  substances see Illicit drugs use
Duloxetine 83
Dyscalculia **263**
Dyslexia **263**
Dyspraxia **263**
Dysthymia 121, **121**

E

Early intervention services 7
ECT see Electroconvulsive
  therapy (ECT)
Edinburgh Postnatal Depression
  Scale (EPDS) 215, 219, 307
Elderly, mental illness in 255
  anxiety disorders 256
  depression **255**, 255–256
  late-onset schizophrenia
    256–257
Elective mutism **269**

Electroconvulsive therapy (ECT)
  94–95
  adverse effects 95
  bipolar disorder **120**
  contraindications 95
  depression 114
  postnatal depression 220
  postnatal psychosis 220
Emotional disorders 269–270
  specific to childhood **269**
  types of attachment and 269,
    270
Encopresis **269**
Enteric nervous system 9
Enuresis **269**
Epworth Sleepiness Scale 236
Erectile dysfuction see Sexual
  dysfunction
Escitalopram 83
Ethical and legal issues, in
  psychiatry 28–29
  advance directives 32
  common law 29–30
  confidentiality 32
  deprivation of liberty
    safeguards 29
  involuntary treatment and
    28–29
  mental capacity 29
  mental health legislation **30**,
    30–31, **31**
  voluntary treatment and 28
Eye movement desensitisation
  and reprocessing therapy 159

F

Familial Alzheimer's disease 248
  see also Alzheimer's disease
Family therapy 75
  alcohol dependence 196
Fight or flight response 10
Fluoxetine 83, 113, **212**, 270
Fluvoxamine 83
Formulation of case 70
  aetiology 71
  case summary 70
  differential diagnosis 70–71
  management 71
  prognosis 71
  risk 71
Fragile X syndrome, and
  intellectual disability 276, **277**
Frontal leucotomy 13
Frontotemporal dementias
  252–253
  clinical features **252**
  palmar grasp reflex 253
  palmomental reflex 253
  snout reflex 253

G

GABA (γ-amino butyric acid) **20**
GAD *see* Generalised anxiety
   disorder (GAD)
Galantamine 94, 249
Gender dysphoria 242
Gender identity disorders
   241–242
   depression in 242
Generalised anxiety disorder
   (GAD) 144–149
   aetiology **147**
   clinical features **149**
   comorbidities **149**
   investigations **149**
   pathogenesis *148*
Genetics, and psychiatric
   disorders 21, 23–24, **24**
   cytogenetics 23
   epidemiological studies 23,
      23, *24*
   molecular genetic studies 23
   pharmacogenetics 23–24
Genogram *49*
Geriatric Depression Scale 255
Glutamate **20**
Glycine **20**
Group psychotherapy **75**, 77

H

Hachinski Ischaemic Score 250
Hallucinations 60–61
   and associated conditions **62**
   depression 110
   schizophrenia 128, 132
Hallucinogens 199 *see also* Illicit
   drugs use
Haloperidol 87, 116
Hamilton Anxiety and Depression
   scale 74
Health checks, annual 305, **305**
Hepatitis B vaccination, for illicit
   drug users 200
Heroin 20, 189–191, 197, 200
   see also Illicit drugs use
Heroin withdrawal 293
History taking 44
   biopsychosocial model and
      three Ps 51, **52**, *52*, **53**
   collateral history 51
   communication skills 44, **46**
   family psychiatric history 48,
      49
   forensic history 50
   history of presenting
      complaint 47

past medical history 48
past psychiatric history 47
patient's premorbid
   personality 50–51
personal history 48
safety considerations **45**
significant relationships and
   events 48–49
skills for 44–47, **45, 46**
social history 49, **50**
substance misuse 49–50
Home treatment teams 7
Hospital Anxiety and Depression
   Scale (HADS) 306
Huntington's chorea *see*
   Huntington's disease
Huntington's disease 254
   genetic testing 254
Hypochondriacal disorder 228
Hypomania 116 *see also* Bipolar
   affective disorder
Hypothalamic axes 15, *15*
Hypothalamic–pituitary–adrenal
   axis 15
Hypothalamus 14–15, *15*

I

Illicit drugs use 197–201, *197*
   clinical features **199**
   investigations *200*
   management *195*
   Misuse of Drugs Act 1971,
      UK 197
   psychosocial interventions 201
   reward pathway and 198
   types of drug 197
Illness behaviour **27**
Illusions 60
Imipramine 81
Inhalants **199**
Intellectual disability 271–278
   causes **276**
   classification **275**
   core features 275
   diagnostic approach *277*, *278*
   genetic syndromes associated
      with 276, **277**
   mental illness and (*see* Mental
      illness, in people with
      intellectual disability)
Interpersonal therapy **75**, 76
Investigations 70, 72
   blood tests 72, **73**
   infection screening 72
   radiological imaging and
      electrocardiography 72, **74**
   rating scales 72, 74

Involuntary outpatient treatment
   31
Isocarboxazid 84

K

Korsakoff's syndrome 15, 193,
   309

L

Lamotrigine 94
Late-onset schizophrenia
   256–257
Learning difficulty 271
Learning disability 271
Legal issues *see* Ethical and legal
   issues, in psychiatry
Lesch–Nyhan syndrome 167
Levodopa 201, 252
Lewy bodies, in dementia with
   Lewy bodies 251, *251*
Life events **27**
Limbic system *13*, 13–14, *14*
Lithium 92
   adverse effects 92–93
   bipolar disorder **120**
   contraindications 92
   indications 92
   interactions 93
   mode of action 92
   monitoring 93
   postnatal period and **219**
   toxicity 93
   withdrawal 92
Lobotomy 13
Lofepramine 82
Lofexidine 200
Loperamide 292
Lorazepam 90, 290
Lurasidone 88
Luxury disorder *see* Depression

M

Management 74 *see also*
   specific treatment
      pharmacological 80–94
      physical treatments 94–95
      psychological 75–80
Mania 97, 115, 116 *see also*
   Bipolar affective disorder
Manic episodes 102–104,
   116 *see also* Bipolar affective
   disorder
Memantine 94, 249
Mental capacity 29
Mental Health Act 2007 of England
   and Wales **30**, 30–31, **31**

Mental health care
  asylum era 5–6, **6**
  chemical revolution 6–7, *7*
  community care 7
  evolution of *5*, 5–7
  global variation in access to
    38–39
  moral therapy 6
  neuroscience, development
    in 7
  primary care, collaboration
    with 7
  provision of **38**
  psychoanalysis 6
Mental health disorders 1 *see*
  also Psychiatric disorders
  allocation of resources to **39**
  Gap Action Programme 39
  global initiatives 39
  global variation in 36–38,
    37, *37*
  impact of 39
  prevalence of 36
  prevention of 2
  stigma with **3**, 3–4
Mental health services 297, *298*
  primary care 297–299
  secondary care **299**, 299–300
  types of care by *298*
Mental illness, in people with
  intellectual disability 278–280
  psychological therapies 280
Mental state examination (MSE)
  43, 53–54
  abnormal movements,
    spontaneous **56**
  appearance and behaviour
    54–56, *55*, **56**, 65–66
  attitude 56
  carrying out of 65–69
  caution and 54
  cognition 62, 64, **65**, 68
  descriptive psychopathology
    54
  empathy and 54
  expression 55–56
  insight 64–65, 68, *69*
  mood and affect 58–60,
    60, 67
  normal 54
  perceptions 60–61, *61*, **62**,
    67–68
  psychomotor function 56,
    56, 57
  speech *57*, 57–58, **59**, 66
  suicidal ideation 60, 67
  summary 65, **66**
  thoughts 61–62, **63**, 64, 68

Methadone 200, 292
3,4-methylenedioxy-
  methamphetamine (MDMA)
  197
Methylphenidate 268
Migrant populations,
  considerations in assessment
  of 4–5
Migration **27**
Mini-mental state examination
  (MMSE) 62
  Folstein's 62, **65**
Mirtazapine 84, 159
Moclobemide 84
Molecular genetics 23
Monoamine oxidase inhibitors
  (MAOIs) 84–85
Mood disorders *see* Affective
  disorders
'Mother's little helper' 149
MSE *see* Mental state
  examination (MSE)

N

Naltrexone, for abstinence from
  alcohol 196
Narcolepsy 236 *see* also Sleep
  disorders
Nervous breakdown 157
Nervous system 8
  autonomic nervous system
    9, 10
  central nervous system 8,
    10, 11
  divisions of *10, 11*
  glial cells 8, **9**
  neurones 8, *9*
  peripheral nervous system
    8–9, *10*
  somatic system 9
Neuroanatomical changes, in
  psychiatric disorders 21, **22**
Neuroleptic malignant syndrome
  (NMS) 87, 293–295, **295**
Neuroplasticity 21
Neurotransmitters 8, **19**, 19–21,
  20
  and psychological symptoms
    22
  receptors 19, *21*
Nightmares and night terrors
  236 *see* also Sleep disorders
Nihilistic delusions 220
Nitrazepam 90
NMS *see* Neuroleptic malignant
  syndrome (NMS)
Noradrenaline (NA) **20**
Noradrenergic and specific

serotonergic antidepressants
  (NaSSA) 84

O

Obsessive compulsive disorder
  (OCD) 154–157
  breaking cycle of *157*
  clinical features **156**, 156
  management 157
  streptococcal infection in
    children and 155
  sustaining *156*
  types of **156**
  Yale–Brown Obsessive
    Compulsive Scale 155
Olanzapine 88, 290
Older adults, mental illness in
  see Elderly, mental illness in
Opiates **199** *see also* Illicit drugs
  use
Oppositional defiant disorder
  265 *see also* Conduct disorder
Organic personality change
  233–234
  go/no go test 234
  letter fluency test 234
  motor test 234
Othello syndrome 139
Overdose 162–164, 167

P

Pabrinex 196
Paliperidone 88
Panic attacks 150
Panic disorder 150–151
  ischaemic heart disease and
    150
Paraphilias 241, **241**
Parasympathetic nervous system
  9
Parkinson's disease 17
Paroxetine 83, 113, 159
Pathological jealousy 139
Patient Health Questionnaire
  (PHQ-9) 74, 306
Persistent delusional disorders
  138–139
Persistent mood disorders 121,
  121
Persistent somatoform pain
  disorder 228
Personality disorders 177,
  180–184
  borderline 178–180, 182
  clinical features **183**
  conditions comorbid with
    183

diagnostic approach **183**
epidemiology *181*
psychopathy checklist **184**
types and subtypes *179*
Phaeochromocytoma 146
Pharmacogenetics 23–24
Pharmacological therapy 80
    antidepressants 80–85
    antipsychotics 85–90
    anxiolytics and hypnotics
        90–92
    cognition-enhancing drugs
        94
    concordance 80
    mood stabilisers 92–94
Phenelzine 84
Phobias 151
    agoraphobia 153–154, *154*
    social phobia 152–153
    specific **151**, 151–152
Physical examination 69–70
Pica **269**
Pick's disease 11, 252, 253
Polysomnography 237
Postnatal blues 217–218
    contributory factors **218**
Postnatal depression 214–216,
    217, 218–220, **218**
    stepped care for *308*
    and suicidal ideation 219
Postnatal psychosis 220
Post-traumatic stress disorder
    (PTSD) 158–159
Pregabalin 148
Primary health care services
    297–299
Primary insomnia 236 *see also*
    Sleep disorders
Prion diseases 253 *see also*
    Creutzfeld–Jakob disease (CJD)
Propranolol 92
Psychiatric disorders 1, 43 *see
    also* Mental health disorders
    classification of 33–35
    Diagnostic and Statistical
        Manual of Mental Disorders
        (DSM) 34, **35**
    diagnostic hierarchy of 35, *35*
    International Classification of
        Disease (ICD) 34, **34**
    neuroanatomical changes in
        21, **22**
    organic disease *vs.* functional
        disease 33
    syndromes 33–34
Psychiatric disorders, with
    physical illness 231–233
Psychiatric emergencies 281

acute psychosis **284**,
    284–285
agitation/violent behaviour
    289–290, 290f
alcohol withdrawal 290–293,
    291, **292**, *292, 293*
assessment of capacity to
    refuse treatment 281–283,
    282, **283**
dementia and acute confusion
    286, 286–287
suicidal behaviour 287–289
Psychiatric intensive care unit
    (PICU) 300
Psychiatric medication,
    complications of 293–295, **295**
    see also Neuroleptic malignant
    syndrome (NMS); Serotonin
    syndrome
Psychiatry 1, 2, 43
    culture and 4–5
    genetics and 21, 23–24
    history 5–7 (*see also* Mental
        health care, evolution of)
    neurology and 7, 8
    stigma and **3**, 3–4
    students and 3
Psychodynamic psychotherapy
    75, 76, 76–77
Psychological treatments **75**,
    75–76
    behaviour therapy 77–80
    counselling 76
    group psychotherapy 77
    interpersonal therapy 76
    psychodynamic psychotherapy
        76, 76–77
    therapeutic communities 77
Psychology 24
    areas of study in *25*
    behavioural 26
    biological 25
    cognitive 26
    mechanisms in **25**
Psychopath 180
Psychosis 213
Psychotropic medications 7, 80
    see also specific drug
PTSD *see* Post-traumatic stress
    disorder (PTSD)

Q

Quetiapine 88

R

Reactive attachment disorder
    269

Rehabilitation teams 7
Risperidone 88, 265
Ritalin *see* Methylphenidate
Rivastigmine 94, 249, 252
Russell's sign 211

S

Schizoaffective disorders
    139–140
    depressive 140
    manic 140
Schizophrenia 123, 127–138
    acute syndrome 128
    aetiology **130**
    antipsychotic medications
        135–137, *136, 137*
    'at-risk mental state,' phase
        128
    chronic syndrome 128
    classification 129, **129**
    diagnostic approach 134
    dopamine theory 131, **131**
    Early Intervention in Psychosis
        Services, UK 134
    epidemiology *129*
    global variation in prevalence
        of 37
    investigations **135**
    lack of insight 132
    late-onset 256–257
    negative symptoms 132, **133**
    neuroimaging techniques
        131
    prognosis **138**
    psychological treatment 137
    risk assessment 135, **135**
    social treatments 137–138
    treatment-resistant 137
Secondary mental health care
    services **299**, 299–300
Selective serotonin reuptake
    inhibitors (SSRIs) 83
    generalised anxiety disorder
        148
    obsessive compulsive disorder
        155
    phobias 153, 154
    postnatal period and **219**
    post-traumatic stress disorder
        159
    risk of suicidal thoughts 175
Self-harm 161, 164–171
    aetiology **168**
    clinical features *170*
    common sites *170*
    as coping strategy 168, *169*
    'deliberate self-harm' 166
    epidemiology **167**

management *171*
in mental illnesses **167**
pathogenesis *169*
safer alternative methods
of *171*
and suicide attempt *170*, 172
types *167*
Separation anxiety **269**
Serotonin (5-HT) **20**
Serotonin and noradrenaline
(norepinephrine) reuptake
inhibitors (SNRIs) 83
Serotonin syndrome 81, 114,
294, 295, **295**
Sertraline 83
Sexual dysfunction 238–240
management *240*
psychological/physical
co-morbidity with 240
sexual response cycle and
239, **239**, *239*
Sexual preference, disorders of
241, **241**
Sibling rivalry disorder **269**
Sick role **27**
Sildenafil 240
Sleep disorders 235–238
primary 235, **236**
psychological treatments
238, *238*
secondary 235, **235**
sleep cycle stages and 235,
235
Sleepwalking 236 *see also* Sleep
disorders
Smoking cessation 304
Social anxiety disorder *see* Social
phobia
Social mobility **27**
Social phobia 152–153
Social role **27**
Social support
alcohol dependence 196
illicit drug use 201
Sociology 26, **27**
Sodium valproate 93
Somatisation disorder 226–228
aetiology *227*
clinical features **227**
Somatoform disorders 226

hypochondriacal disorder
228
persistent somatoform pain
disorder 228
somatisation disorder
226–228
Speech and language therapy
253
SSRIs *see* Selective serotonin
reuptake inhibitors (SSRIs)
Stigma **27**
Stimulants **199** *see also* Illicit
drugs use
Stress *see* also Acute stress
reaction
hypothalamic–pituitary–
adrenal axis, role of 15
mental health disorders and
15
psychological response to **16**
short- and long-term
responses *16*
Substance misuse and addictions
185
alcohol dependence 186–
189, 192–196
drug-induced psychiatric
disorders 201–202
drugs and psychoactive
substances 197–201
Suicide 161, 172–175, 287–289
aetiology **173**
biological interventions 175
community care 174
crisis care 174–175
diagnostic approach **174**
global variation in prevalence
of 38
psychological interventions
175
social interventions 175
types *172*
Sulpiride 87
Supportive psychotherapy *see*
Counselling
Sympathetic nervous system 9

T

TCAs *see* Tricyclic
antidepressants (TCAs)

Temazepam 90
Tetris (computer game) 159
Thalamus 14, **14**
Therapeutic communities **75**, 77
Thioridazine 87
Tic disorders **269**
Tofranil 80
Tranylcypromine 84
Trazodone 82
Tricyclic antidepressants (TCAs)
81–83, 113
adverse effects 82
contraindications 82
indications 82
interactions 82–83
mode of action 82, *82*
postnatal period and **219**
Trifluoperazine 87

U

Unipolar depressive illness 105
Upregulation of receptors 21
Urine drug testing 198, *200*

V

Varenicline 304
Vascular dementia 250–251
Alzheimer's disease and 250
brain imaging 250, *251*
Venlafaxine 83, 113
Viagra *see* Sildenafil

W

Wernicke's encephalopathy 193
Weschler Intelligence Scale for
Children 276
Withdrawal (substance) 292
alcohol 292, **292**, *293*
heroin 293
symptoms of substance
withdrawal 292
World Health Organization
(WHO)
Gap Action Programme 39
health, definition of 2

Z

Zolpidem 91, 237
Zopiclone 91, 237